T0135114

Springer Series on Epidemiology and Public Health

Series Editors

Wolfgang Ahrens, BIPS, Leibniz Institute, Bremen, Germany

Iris Pigeot, Bremen, Germany

The series has two main aims. First, it publishes textbooks and monographs addressing recent advances in specific research areas. Second, it provides comprehensive overviews of the methods and results of key epidemiological studies marking cornerstones of epidemiological practice, which are otherwise scattered across numerous narrow-focused publications. Thus the series offers in-depth knowledge on a variety of topics, in particular, on epidemiological concepts and methods, statistical tools, applications, epidemiological practice and public health. It also covers innovative areas such as molecular and genetic epidemiology, statistical principles in epidemiology, modern study designs, data management, quality assurance and other recent methodological developments. Written by the key experts and leaders in corresponding fields, the books in the series offer both broad overviews and insights into specific areas and topics. The series serves as an in-depth reference source that can be used complementarily to the "The Handbook of Epidemiology," which provides a starting point of orientation for interested readers (2nd edition published in 2014 http://www. springer.com/public+health/book/978-0-387-09835-7). The series is intended for researchers and professionals involved in health research, health reporting, health promotion, health system administration and related aspects. It is also of interest for public health specialists and researchers, epidemiologists, physicians, biostatisticians, health educators, and students worldwide.

More information about this series at http://www.springer.com/series/7251

Miriam Sturkenboom · Tania Schink

Editors

Databases
for Pharmacoepidemiological
Research

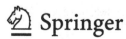 Springer

Editors
Miriam Sturkenboom
Erasmus MC
Rotterdam, The Netherlands

Julius Center for Health Sciences
and Primary Care, Global Health
University Medical Center Utrecht
Utrecht, The Netherlands

Tania Schink
Department of Clinical Epidemiology
Leibniz Institute for Prevention Research
and Epidemiology—BIPS
Bremen, Germany

ISSN 1869-7933 ISSN 1869-7941 (electronic)
Springer Series on Epidemiology and Public Health
ISBN 978-3-030-51457-0 ISBN 978-3-030-51455-6 (eBook)
https://doi.org/10.1007/978-3-030-51455-6

© Springer Nature Switzerland AG 2021
This work is subject to copyright. All rights are reserved by the Publisher, whether the whole or part of the material is concerned, specifically the rights of translation, reprinting, reuse of illustrations, recitation, broadcasting, reproduction on microfilms or in any other physical way, and transmission or information storage and retrieval, electronic adaptation, computer software, or by similar or dissimilar methodology now known or hereafter developed.
The use of general descriptive names, registered names, trademarks, service marks, etc. in this publication does not imply, even in the absence of a specific statement, that such names are exempt from the relevant protective laws and regulations and therefore free for general use.
The publisher, the authors and the editors are safe to assume that the advice and information in this book are believed to be true and accurate at the date of publication. Neither the publisher nor the authors or the editors give a warranty, expressed or implied, with respect to the material contained herein or for any errors or omissions that may have been made. The publisher remains neutral with regard to jurisdictional claims in published maps and institutional affiliations.

This Springer imprint is published by the registered company Springer Nature Switzerland AG
The registered company address is: Gewerbestrasse 11, 6330 Cham, Switzerland

Preface

The use of secondary data resources for pharmacoepidemiological research has gained increasing interest in the past decade. These databases allow the analysis of drug and vaccine utilization after approval in the daily routine of care as well as the investigation of their comparative effectiveness and safety. They are especially useful for the identification of rare risks and rare drug exposures over long periods of time, thus sustainably enlarging the basis for drug safety research.

This book is dedicated to Prof. Edeltraut Garbe, who was a distinguished Professor of Clinical Epidemiology at the University of Bremen and Head of the Department of Clinical Epidemiology at the Leibniz Institute for Prevention Research and Epidemiology—BIPS. Throughout her career, but especially during her time at BIPS, Professor Garbe has conducted numerous pharmacoepidemiological studies in large healthcare databases examining the association of drugs and disease outcomes. Professor Garbe was—together with Professor Iris Pigeot—instrumental in the development and maintenance of the German Pharmacoepidemiological Research Database (GePaRD).

Chapter "Role of Real World Data in Pharmacoepidemiology Research: From Single Database Towards Global Collaboration" gives an introduction to the role of secondary data in pharmacoepidemiological research and important developments in the last years. Chapter "Worldwide Availability of Pharmacoepidemiological Databases" provides a comprehensive overview of general classification characteristics of databases together with their strengths and limitations. In the following chapters, the databases are described separately in more detail according to a clear standardized structure. These database descriptions have each been written by the professionals who work with or maintain these databases. By describing practical experiences, the authors give the readers a more in-depth understanding of the strengths and limitations of the respective databases with regard to pharmacoepidemiological research.

Bremen, Germany   Dr. Tania Schink
Rotterdam/Utrecht, The Netherlands   Prof. Dr. Miriam Sturkenboom

Contents

Databases for Pharmacoepidemiological Research

Databases in Europe

Databases for Pharmacoepidemiological Research

Role of Real World Data in Pharmacoepidemiology Research: From Single Database Towards Global Collaboration

Miriam Sturkenboom

Abstract Since the thalidomide disaster in the 1960s, post-marketing surveillance has progressed rapidly: Spontaneous reporting systems were developed on national and international scale and in parallel methods for active surveillance such as in hospital case control surveillance systems were developed. Healthcare data sources such as electronic medical records, insurance claims, and disease registries have been used in the past four decades to identify, refine, and evaluate potential safety signals of marketed medical products.

1 Introduction

Since the thalidomide disaster in the 1960s, post-marketing surveillance has progressed rapidly: Spontaneous reporting systems were developed on national and international scale and in parallel methods for active surveillance such as in hospital case control surveillance systems were developed. Healthcare data sources such as electronic medical records, insurance claims, and disease registries have been used in the past four decades to identify, refine, and evaluate potential safety signals of marketed medical products. In the USA, use of single databases for pharmacoepidemiological research began in 1979 when Hershel Jick's group evaluated the association between post-menopausal oestrogens and endometrial cancer using the Group Health Cooperative (GHC) of Puget Sound database. Since then, the use of already available electronic patient healthcare data for research has exponentially increased, mostly driven by the computerization of healthcare supply, the occurrence of drug safety issues and the recognition of the value of these data for benefit-risk monitoring of drugs and devices. Recently, the increased interest in data science and real-world evidence has put even more focus on the secondary use of this data. Regulatory agencies across the world are actively seeking ways to include real world evidence

M. Sturkenboom (✉)
University Medical Center Utrecht, 3508 GA Utrecht, The Netherlands
e-mail: m.sturkenboom@erasmusmc.nl

© Springer Nature Switzerland AG 2021
M. Sturkenboom and T. Schink (eds.), *Databases for Pharmacoepidemiological Research*, Springer Series on Epidemiology and Public Health,
https://doi.org/10.1007/978-3-030-51455-6_1

in regulatory decision making. The condition for this to happen is to have good information on the quality and characteristics of the data sources.

This introductory chapter to the book on descriptions and characteristics of different healthcare data sources around the world summarizes the main trends in use of this real-world data in the last 15 years and illustrates how we moved from single database to multi-database research.

2 Paradigm Shift in the Use of Healthcare Data to Assess Drug Effects

A key incident in raising concerns about the status of active surveillance of drug safety in the USA appeared with the 2004 withdrawal of rofecoxib (Vioxx) by Merck because of an apparent increased risk of serious cardiovascular events. The withdrawal came amid questions about the Food and Drug Administration's (FDA) handling of a possible association between selective serotonin-reuptake inhibitors and suicidal ideation in adolescents. Further concerns were raised about the agency's handling of staff disagreements about these and other drugs. In this context, the FDA sought a review from the Institute of Medicine (IOM) (McClellan 2007). The IOM's September 2006 report included a broad range of recommendations and the realization that the USA relied too much on the spontaneous reporting system but did follow new drugs actively in a systematic way (Institute of Medicine. Committee on the Assessment of the US Drug Safety System 2007). An important contribution of Richard Platt that started a paradigm shift in pharmacoepidemiology was: 'With a (now feasible) data network including information on 100 million patients, a statistically significant "signal" of serious cardiovascular risk could have been detected after less than 3 months of experience with rofecoxib' (Institute of Medicine. Committee on the Assessment of the US Drug Safety System 2007). This notion was the basis for the Sentinel system that the FDA announced in May 2008. The Sentinel system is a distributed data network (rather than a centralized database) that allows participating health plans and other organizations to create data files in a standard format and to maintain possession of those files, while sharing and allowing for pooling. This way of working had already been implemented by the same group in the Vaccine Safety Datalink and was an example for the start of many networks of databases implemented after it had been realized that it is better to work together than in isolation (Brown et al. 2010).

Traditionally, pharmacoepidemiological studies were conducted independently in one data source according to different protocols and definitions and later brought together through a meta-analysis of the published effect estimates. Good examples are the studies on NSAIDs and cardiovascular effects (McGettigan and Henry 2011; Varas-Lorenzo et al. 2013). Although meta-analyses of different and independent studies on isolated data sources allow for pooling of results, it is possible to be much more efficient. The heterogeneity in design, definitions of outcomes and exposures, and conduct of the studies may limit our ability to combine the studies and interpret results. Also, when studies are done in single data sources estimates can only be obtained from the most frequently used drugs in each of the single databases. Although meta-analyses of the results from individual database studies have been the state of the art for a long time we have come to realize that we can make a quantum leap forward. This can be achieved by the conduct of multi-data source studies which work with the same protocol, the same definitions, and the same analytical program (Trifiro et al. 2014).

The motivation behind the multi-data source studies within the USA, Canada, and Europe or even globally is the earlier detection and validation, and hence earlier management, of potential safety issues (Coloma et al. 2012; de Bie et al. 2015). Overall, multi-data source studies increase statistical sample size and heterogeneity of exposure for post-marketing drug and vaccine safety surveillance. Examples of the advantages of international multi-data source studies in Europe were provided in the VAESCO project whilst monitoring the risk of Guillain-Barré syndrome (GBS) and narcolepsy associated with the pandemic influenza vaccine and the Safety of NSAIDs project (SOS) in the referral procedure for diclofenac (Arlett et al. 2014; VAESCO Consortium 2012; Dieleman et al. 2011; Romio et al. 2014; Wijnans et al. 2013). Moreover, new drugs (or infrequently used drugs for rare diseases) that slowly penetrate the market will require a greater amount of patient data to obtain a significant user population within a reasonable time frame.

The recognition of the need to work together has resulted in the creation of several distributed data source networks, some have been established by the U.S. and Canadian governments (e.g., Sentinel and CNODES) in a sustainable fashion, others (in Europe) have been project-based with limited funding and duration. Based on the accrued experience voluntary communities/alliances or charities have been initiated to make the efforts sustainable (e.g., Sigma Consortium, Vaccine Collaboration for Europe).

3 North America

The Sentinel Initiative was established in 2008 after the FDA Amendments Act mandated the creation of a new post-marketing surveillance system utilizing electronic health records (EHRs) to prospectively monitor the safety of marketed medical products. Two pilot projects were initiated. First, the Mini-Sentinel which would enable the FDA to examine privately held electronic healthcare data representing over 100 million individuals (Behrman et al. 2011; Platt et al. 2012, 2009; Robb et al. 2012). The second pilot project was the Post-Licensure Rapid Immunization Safety Measurement (PRISM) programme (Nguyen et al. 2012). Both pilots were successfully transitioned into the SENTINEL program in 2016 (U.S. Food and Drug Administration 2020). The Sentinel Initiative has grown into the largest multisite distributed database dedicated to medical product safety in the world. It is constantly growing and improving to meet FDA needs. In September 2019, the FDA announced the expansion of Sentinel into three distinct coordinating centers: Sentinel Operations Center, Innovation Center, and Community Building and Outreach Center to increase its impact even further. As of 2019, Sentinel had 17 data partners, which transform their data into the Sentinel Common Data Model. Together they have access to health data on 70 million persons that are actively accruing data.

In Canada, the Drug Safety and Effectiveness Network (DSEN) was established in 2011 by the government to augment available evidence on drug safety and effectiveness by leveraging existing resources from 'real-world' settings such as the National Prescription Drug Utilization System (Canadian Institutes for Health Information 2018). The DSEN established a collaborating center, the Canadian Network for Observational Drug Effect Studies (CNODES), which is a distributed network of investigators and linked databases in British Columbia, Alberta, Saskatchewan, Manitoba, Ontario, Quebec, and Nova Scotia, plus the Clinical Practice Research Database in the United Kingdom and Marketscan database in the USA (Suissa et al. 2012). CNODES is funded by the Canadian Institutes of Health Research (CIHR, Grant #DSE—146021). Initially, sites conducted analyses separately, according to common protocol, but currently pilots are ongoing to use the Sentinel Common Data model.

4 Europe

The European Medicines Agency (EMA) has recognized the need to promote pharmacoepidemiological research after the issues around rofecoxib, cerivastatin, and rosiglitazone in Europe and created the European Network of Centres for Pharmacoepidemiology and Pharmacovigilance (ENCePP) in 2006. This initiative is coordinated by EMA and aims to build capacity for and increase trust in post-authorization studies to further support medicine decision making. ENCePP centers collaborate in a non-funded voluntary way to set standards, guidance, and methods (Blake et al. 2012). In addition, EMA has requested the European Commission to fund specific drug safety studies in which multiple healthcare databases are combined such as: (i) nonsteroidal anti-inflammatory drug-related gastrointestinal and cardiovascular risks (SOS) (CORDIS 2019f); (ii) the arrhythmogenic risk of drugs (ARITMO) (CORDIS 2019b); (iii) the cardio/cerebrovascular and pancreatic safety of blood glucose-lowering agents (SAFEGUARD) (CORDIS 2015); (iv) the risk of congenital anomalies related to new anti-epileptic agents, insulin analogues, anti-asthmatic drugs and antidepressants (EUROmediCAT) (CORDIS 2019d); (v) the long-term adverse effects of methylphenidate in attention deficit and hyperactivity disorder (ADDUCE) (CORDIS 2019c); (vi) the safety of biological agents in patients with juvenile idiopathic arthritis (PHARMACHILD) (CORDIS 2019e); (vii) the safety of epoetins (EPOCAN) (CORDIS 2016); and (viii) the risk of cancer associated with insulin analogues (CARING) (CORDIS 2017). EMA itself also tenders for different drug safety studies.

The European Centre for Disease Prevention and Control (ECDC) funded two vaccine-related projects that involve collaborative database approaches: The Influenza-Monitoring Vaccine Effectiveness (I-MOVE) consortium coordinated by EpiConcept (Valenciano and Ciancio 2012) and the Vaccine Adverse Event Surveillance and Communication project (VAESCO) coordinated by the Brighton Collaboration Foundation on the safety of vaccines (European Centre for Disease Prevention and Control 2011). VAESCO has ended and I-MOVE is continuing as a voluntary network.

The Innovative Medicines Initiative, which aims to establish public private partnerships, has funded several projects that are key to this development of networks for pharmacoepidemiological research, examples are: PROTECT, EMIF, ADVANCE, and ConcePTION. The Pharmacoepidemiological Research on Outcomes of Therapeutics by a European Consortium (PROTECT) project finished in 2014 (Innovative Medicines Initiative 2017). Its goal was to strengthen the monitoring of the benefit-risk of medicines in Europe. Several methodologies were created and tested, but unfortunately the project could not be sustained. The European Medical Informatics Framework (EMIF) project (2013–2018) was to build an integrated, efficient framework for consistent re-use and exploitation of currently available patient-level data to support novel research. The EMIF-Platform intended to provide a means for researchers to 'browse' available data in Europe—a full 'medical information browser' that allows for rapid exploration and exploitation of the wealth of information that at present remains largely 'hidden' in numerous isolated and scattered healthcare environments across Europe (EMIF 2019). Several tools were created such as a data catalogue and a task management system for distributed studies. Also, the Jerboa Java-based data transformation software, that had been developed in prior projects as a prototype, was reprogrammed. Unfortunately, apart from the tools, the network was not sustained after the project funding ended. Instead, a novel project was initiated in 2018 with a similar goal as EMIF. It is called the European Health Data and Evidence Network (EHDEN) (Innovative Medicines Initiative 2020b). The goal of EHDEN is to build a federated data network of allowing access to the data of 100 million EU citizens standardized to the OMOP common data model.

The ADVANCE—Accelerated Development of VAccine beNefit-risk Collaboration in Europe project was running between 2013 and 2019 (CORDIS 2019a). It aimed to help health professionals, regulatory agencies, public health institutions, vaccine manufacturers, and the general public make more informed decisions on benefits and risks of marketed vaccines. The project created a framework and several tools (e.g., Codemapper to harmonize codes, a Vaccine Ontology, a dashboard for monitoring benefits and risks, a Blueprint) to rapidly deliver reliable data on vaccine benefits and risks. ADVANCE was a unique collaboration between key players in the sector, including the ECDC, EMA, national public health and regulatory bodies, vaccine manufacturers, small and medium entrepreneurs (SMEs), and academic institutions in 19 European countries (CORDIS 2019a). All partners decided that the project should be sustained after the funding ended, and the Vaccine monitoring Collaboration for Europe (VAC4EU) was established as a non-for profit international association (VAC4EU 2020). VAC4EU will use the tools that were developed in ADVANCE and use common protocols, a common data model, and common analytics across all data sources. As of January 2020, 19 organizations joined, providing access to health data on more than 100 million persons. Another IMI-funded project that relies on a distributed data network for generation of real-world evidence on the effects of drugs is ConcePTION, which started in 2019. The ultimate goal of ConcePTION is to create a trusted biomedical ecosystem capable of providing evidence-based information on the safety of medications during pregnancy and breastfeeding in an efficient, systematic, and ethically responsible way. It creates a data source catalogue and data quality indicators and uses a common data model, common R analytics, and transparency in workflows (Innovative Medicines Initiative 2020a).

The Nordic countries have established the NOrPEN network, a collaboration between 11 academic pharmacoepidemiology centers that work with population-based registries. The Nordic countries have a long tradition of registry-based epidemiological research. Many population-based health registries were established in the 1960s, with use of unique personal identifiers facilitating linkage between registries. The databases together cover 25 million inhabitants (Denmark: 5.5 million; Finland: 5.3 million; Iceland: 0.3 million; Norway: 4.8 million; and Sweden: 9.2 million) (Furu et al. 2010).

5 Global Networks/Initiatives

By recognizing that global diversity may be beneficial to study the effects of drugs several globally oriented networks and projects have been tested/established. The focus may be on methods development (OMOP, OHDSI) and capacity building in special groups/areas of interest (GVSI), or on addressing specific research questions (ASPEN, SOMNIA). The main projects are as follows.

The Observational Medical Outcomes Partnership (OMOP) was a US public-private partnership between the FDA, academia, data owners, and the pharmaceutical industry and was administered by the Foundation for the National Institutes of Health (Stang et al. 2010). It was initiated to identify the needs of an active drug safety surveillance system and to develop the necessary methodologies to enhance secondary use of observational data for maximizing the benefit and minimizing the risk of pharmaceutical agents. The project has had an important impact on the field of pharmacoepidemiology. A general common data model was developed and it was demonstrated with an engineering approach that the same epidemiological methods can yield totally different results in different databases while different methods can yield totally different results in the same database (Foundation for the National Institutes of Health 2019). The many publications and lessons learned can be obtained from the website. While the OMOP data and research lab transitioned to IMEDS at the Reagan Udall Foundation, the investigators initiated the OHDSI community (Observational Health Data Sciences and Informatics). OHDSI is a multi-stakeholder, inter-disciplinary collaboration striving to bring out the value of observational health data through large-scale analytics. The research community enables active engagement across multiple disciplines (e.g., clinical medicine, biostatistics, computer science, epidemiology, life sciences) and spans multiple stakeholder groups (e.g., researchers, patients, providers, payers, product manufacturers, regulators) (Observational Health Data Sciences and Informatics 2020).

5.1 Capacity Building

The Global Vaccine Safety Initiative (GVSI) was launched under the auspices of the World Health Organization in March 2012. It is based on the Global Vaccine Safety Blueprint, the safety strategy of the Global Vaccine Action Plan (GVAP). The GVSI vision is to establish effective vaccine pharmacovigilance systems in all countries by 2020. Focus is specifically on lower and middle income countries which will see most of the new vaccines first and should have adequate safety surveillance systems. As part of the active surveillance activities a multi country pilot study was conducted to test the systems in 15 countries around the world (World Health Organization 2015).

6   How Do People Work Together?

Currently, several projects and networks are developing or have developed their own methods, guidance, and codes of how these collaborations should be done across multiple databases. The standard of using data from different data sources for active safety surveillance is currently the use of a distributed data approach in which data holders maintain control over their protected data and its uses. A common protocol is written and data holders transform their data of interest into a common data model that enforces uniform data element naming conventions, definitions, and data storage formats. The common data format allows data checking, transformation, and analysis via identical computer programs (e.g., SAS, R, JAVA) shared by all data holders. Existing distributed networks typically distribute these computer programs via task management systems, data access providers execute the programs and return the output via secure mechanisms to a coordinating center for aggregation and, possibly, additional analysis (Brown et al. 2010).

This is the typical workflow but there are some key differences in implementation across the networks. Notably, some networks request the data access providers to transfer all or parts of their data into a general common data model (CDM), whereas others request only study-specific data to be transformed to the CDM or request local data owners to aggregate the data.

Adopting a common or reference data model lays the groundwork for achieving syntactic and semantic interoperability so that comparable analyses can be performed across research study sites. A CDM makes it possible to centralize the development of queries and testing of methodologies. Several CDMs exist; the most famous are the Sentinel and OMOP CDM. For the OMOP CDM, the original data is mapped to a common terminology and phenotypes are created, independent of study questions. On the contrary, in Sentinel algorithms, the creation of variables is done per study.

Data transformation scripts are usually developed centrally in SAS, R or JAVA based language (e.g., Jerboa) and aggregated data that can be shared are produced (Trifiro et al. 2014). Final analysis is also organized differently across the networks: In Sentinel and DSEN, aggregated counts and estimates will be provided by the sites and pooled in meta-analytic ways. In several European and some global projects (ADVANCE, Conception, EMIF), aggregated patient-level data can be shared to a protected remote research environment facilitating pooling of data on the individual level and combined analyses (Trifiro et al. 2014).

Networks of data access providers have tremendous utility for addressing drug safety issues while benefiting from a common and transparent evidence generation approach that is now proven to be acceptable to many data access providers. A distributed approach keeps the data with the people who know the data best and who can best consult on proper use of the data and investigate findings or anomalies. Obstacles to effective implementation of both centralized and distributed approaches include differences in computing environments and information systems, the need for data standardization and checking, organization-by-organization variation in contracting policies and procedures, concerns related to the ethics of human subjects' research and data privacy, and cross-institution variation in the rules and guidelines related to privacy and proprietary issues (Brown et al. 2010).

7   Conclusion

The future is bright for the use of electronic healthcare data to generate evidence on medications. There is increasing recognition of the value of real-world evidence and the use in clinical and regulatory decision making. Pharmacoepidemiologists have a 40-year history of using this type of data. As a result of the drug safety scandals 15 years ago, distributed data network initiatives have appeared, each of them recognizing the uniqueness of the data sources that comprise them and the need to have local expertise on the data, but also the recognition that we should work together.

This book, a tribute to professor Edeltraut Garbe, is written from this point of view, a compilation of unique data sources that come together to celebrate the unique contributions that Edeltraut Garbe has made to pharmacoepidemiology, both in terms of establishing GePaRD as well as the critical attitude towards making sense out of the healthcare data to serve public health and improve patient safety. She was a pioneer in these networks and a teacher to all of us in how to close the loop between pharmacology, epidemiology, and electronic data and to translate this into valuable knowledge.

References

Arlett P, Sarac SB, Thomson A et al (2014) The European Medicines Agency's use of prioritised independent research for best evidence in regulatory action on diclofenac. Pharmacoepidemiol Drug Saf 23(4):431–434. https://doi.org/10.1002/pds.3594

Behrman RE, Benner JS, Brown JS et al (2011) Developing the sentinel system—a national resource for evidence development. N Engl J Med 364(6):498–499. https://doi.org/10.1056/NEJ Mp1014427

Blake KV, Devries CS, Arlett P et al (2012) Increasing scientific standards, independence and transparency in post-authorisation studies: the role of the European Network of Centres for Pharmacoepidemiology and Pharmacovigilance. Pharmacoepidemiol Drug Saf 21(7):690–696. https://doi.org/10.1002/pds.3281

Brown JS, Holmes JH, Shah K et al (2010) Distributed health data networks: a practical and preferred approach to multi-institutional evaluations of comparative effectiveness, safety, and quality of care. Med Care 48(6 Suppl):S45–S51. https://doi.org/10.1097/MLR.0b013e3181d9 919f

Canadian Institutes for Health Information (2018) Drug safety and effectiveness network. https://cihr-irsc.gc.ca/e/40269.html. Accessed 6 Feb 2020

Coloma PM, Trifiro G, Schuemie MJ et al (2012) Electronic healthcare databases for active drug safety surveillance: is there enough leverage? Pharmacoepidemiol Drug Saf 21(6):611–621. https://doi.org/10.1002/pds.3197

CORDIS (2015) Safety evaluation of adverse reactions in diabetes (Safeguard). https://cordis.eur opa.eu/project/id/282521. Accessed 6 Feb 2020

CORDIS (2016) Gaining sage on the Epoetins' saga: assessing long term risks and advancing towards better Epoetin driven treatment modalities (EPOCAN). https://cordis.europa.eu/project/ id/282551. Accessed 6 Feb 2020

CORDIS (2017) CAncer Risk and INsulin analoGues. https://cordis.europa.eu/project/id/282 526/de. Accessed 6 Feb 2020

CORDIS (2019a) Accelerated development of vaccine benefit-risk collaboration in Europe (ADVANCE). https://cordis.europa.eu/project/id/115557. Accessed 6 Feb 2020

CORDIS (2019b) Arrhythmogenic potential of drugs (ARITMO). https://cordis.europa.eu/project/ id/241679. Accessed 6 Feb 2020

CORDIS (2019c) Attention deficit hyperactivity disorder drugs use chronic effects (ADDUCE). https://cordis.europa.eu/project/id/260576. Accessed 6 Feb 2020

CORDIS (2019d) EUROmediCAT: safety of medication use in pregnancy in relation to risk of congenital malformations. https://cordis.europa.eu/project/id/260598. Accessed 6 Feb 2020

CORDIS (2019e) Long-term PHARMacovigilance for adverse effects in childhood arthritis focussing on immune modulatory drugs (PHARMACHILD). https://cordis.europa.eu/project/ id/260353. Accessed 6 Feb 2020

CORDIS (2019f) Safety of non-steroidal anti-inflammatory drugs (SOS). https://cordis.europa.eu/ project/id/223495. Accessed 6 Feb 2020

de Bie S, Coloma PM, Ferrajolo C et al (2015) The role of electronic healthcare record databases in paediatric drug safety surveillance: a retrospective cohort study. Br J Clin Pharmacol 80(2):304–314. https://doi.org/10.1111/bcp.12610

Dieleman J, Romio S, Johansen K et al (2011) Guillain-Barre syndrome and adjuvanted pandemic influenza A (H1N1) 2009 vaccine: multinational case-control study in Europe. BMJ 343:d3908. https://doi.org/10.1136/bmj.d3908

EMIF (2019) European medical information framework (EMIF). https://www.emif.eu/. Accessed 6 Feb 2020

European Centre for Disease Prevention and Control (2011) VAESCO investigation into narcolepsy. https://www.ecdc.europa.eu/en/news-events/ecdc-vaesco-investigation-narcolepsy. Accessed 6 Feb 2020

Foundation for the National Institutes of Health (2019) Observational medical outcomes partnership (OMOP). https://fnih.org/what-we-do/major-completed-programs/omop. Accessed 6 Feb 2020

Furu K, Wettermark B, Andersen M et al (2010) The Nordic countries as a cohort for pharmacoepidemiological research. Basic Clin Pharmacol Toxicol 106(2):86–94. https://doi.org/10.1111/j.1742-7843.2009.00494.x

Innovative Medicines Initiative (2017) Pharmacoepidemiological research on outcomes of therapeutics by a European ConsorTium (PROTECT). https://www.imi-protect.eu/. Accessed 6 Feb 2020

Innovative Medicines Initiative (2020a) ConcePTION. https://www.imi.europa.eu/projects-results/project-factsheets/conception. Accessed 6 Feb 2020

Innovative Medicines Initiative (2020b) European health data and evidence network (EHDEN). https://www.imi.europa.eu/projects-results/project-factsheets/ehden. Accessed 6 Feb 2020

Institute of medicine. Committee on the assessment of the US drug safety system (2007) The future of drug safety: promoting and protecting the health of the public. National Academies Press, Washington, D.C.

McClellan M (2007) Drug safety reform at the FDA—pendulum swing or systematic improvement? N Engl J Med 356(17):1700–1702. https://doi.org/10.1056/NEJMp078057

McGettigan P, Henry D (2011) Cardiovascular risk with non-steroidal anti-inflammatory drugs: systematic review of population-based controlled observational studies. PLoS Med 8(9):e1001098. https://doi.org/10.1371/journal.pmed.1001098

Nguyen M, Ball R, Midthun K et al (2012) The Food and Drug Administration's Post-Licensure Rapid Immunization Safety Monitoring program: strengthening the federal vaccine safety enterprise. Pharmacoepidemiol Drug Saf 21(Suppl 1):291–297. https://doi.org/10.1002/pds.2323

Observational Health Data Sciences and Informatics (2020) Welcome to OHDSI! https://www.ohdsi.org/. Accessed 6 Feb 2020

Platt R, Wilson M, Chan KA et al (2009) The new sentinel network—improving the evidence of medical-product safety. N Engl J Med 361(7):645–647. https://doi.org/10.1056/NEJMp0905338

Platt R, Carnahan RM, Brown JS et al (2012) The U.S. Food and Drug Administration's Mini-Sentinel program: status and direction. Pharmacoepidemiol Drug Saf 21(Suppl 1):1–8. https://doi.org/10.1002/pds.2343

Robb MA, Racoosin JA, Worrall C et al (2012) Active surveillance of postmarket medical product safety in the Federal Partners' Collaboration. Med Care 50(11):948–953. https://doi.org/10.1097/MLR.0b013e31826c874d

Romio S, Weibel D, Dieleman JP et al (2014) Guillain-Barre syndrome and adjuvanted pandemic influenza A (H1N1) 2009 vaccines: a multinational self-controlled case series in Europe. PLoS ONE 9(1):e82222. https://doi.org/10.1371/journal.pone.0082222

Stang PE, Ryan PB, Racoosin JA et al (2010) Advancing the science for active surveillance: rationale and design for the Observational Medical Outcomes Partnership. Ann Intern Med 153(9):600–606. https://doi.org/10.7326/0003-4819-153-9-201011020-00010

Suissa S, Henry D, Caetano P et al (2012) CNODES: the Canadian network for observational drug effect studies. Open Med 6(4):e134–e140

Trifiro G, Coloma PM, Rijnbeek PR et al (2014) Combining multiple healthcare databases for postmarketing drug and vaccine safety surveillance: why and how? J Intern Med 275(6):551–561. https://doi.org/10.1111/joim.12159

U.S. Food and Drug Administration (2020) FDA's Sentinel Initiative. https://www.fda.gov/safety/fdas-sentinel-initiative. Accessed 6 Feb 2020

VAC4EU (2020) VAccine monitoring Collaboration for Europe. https://vac4eu.org/. Accessed 6 Feb 2020

VAESCO Consortium (2012) Narcolepsy in association with pandemic influenza vaccination—a multi-country European epidemiological investigation. https://www.ecdc.europa.eu/en/publications-data/narcolepsy-association-pandemic-influenza-vaccination-multi-country-european

Valenciano M, Ciancio B (2012) I-MOVE: a European network to measure the effectiveness of influenza vaccines. Euro Surveill 17(39). https://doi.org/10.2807/ese.17.39.20281-en

Varas-Lorenzo C, Riera-Guardia N, Calingaert B et al (2013) Myocardial infarction and individual nonsteroidal anti-inflammatory drugs meta-analysis of observational studies. Pharmacoepidemiol Drug Saf 22(6):559–570. https://doi.org/10.1002/pds.3437

Wijnans L, Lecomte C, de Vries C et al (2013) The incidence of narcolepsy in Europe: before, during, and after the influenza A(H1N1)pdm09 pandemic and vaccination campaigns. Vaccine 31(8):1246–1254. https://doi.org/10.1016/j.vaccine.2012.12.015

World Health Organization (2015) The global vaccine safety initiative activities portfolio. https://www.who.int/vaccine_safety/news/highlight_3/en/. Accessed 6 Feb 2020

Worldwide Availability of Pharmacoepidemiological Databases

Iris Pigeot, Maike Tahden, Dimitrios Zampatis, Douglas J. Watson, Ulla Forssen, and Bianca Kollhorst

Abstract Randomized clinical trials are conducted to prove the efficacy of a new drug or more generally of a new pharmaceutical product. However, phase III-studies are usually not able to provide a full picture of the benefit-risk-profile of a new drug for several reasons which increases the likelihood that adverse drug reactions will occur after marketing approval that were not observed during phase III of clinical development. The knowledge gap regarding the benefit-risk-profile of a newly approved drug may be closed by pharmacoepidemiological studies based on large electronic healthcare databases after marketing approval. Databases increasingly represent an important worldwide data resource for pharmacoepidemiological research, but their information content, the covered timespan and the population size may heavily differ. In this chapter, we will provide an overview of existing databases worldwide that seem to be appropriate to conduct pharmacoepidemiological research. For this purpose, we will first briefly characterize and compare the major features of main types of databases and highlight their advantages and limitations in comparison to epidemiological field studies. We will then describe our search strategy to identify adequate

I. Pigeot (✉) · M. Tahden · B. Kollhorst
Biometry and Data Management, Leibniz Institute for Prevention Research and Epidemiology—BIPS, Achterstrasse 30, 28359 Bremen, Germany
e-mail: pigeot@leibniz-bips.de

M. Tahden
e-mail: maike.tahden@uni-oldenburg.de

B. Kollhorst
e-mail: kollhorst@leibniz-bips.de

D. Zampatis
Global Patient Safety, Merck Healthcare KGaA, Frankfurter Str. 250, 64293 Darmstadt, Germany
e-mail: dimitrios.zampatis@merckgroup.com

D. J. Watson
PharmaEpi Consulting, LLC, 9 Gull Point Rd, Hilton Head Island, SC 29928, USA
e-mail: pharmaepiconsulting@gmail.com

U. Forssen
Clinical Epidemiology, CSL Behring, 1020 First Avenue, 19406-0901 King of Prussia, PA, USA
e-mail: ullfor@gmail.com

© Springer Nature Switzerland AG 2021
M. Sturkenboom and T. Schink (eds.), *Databases for Pharmacoepidemiological Research*, Springer Series on Epidemiology and Public Health,
https://doi.org/10.1007/978-3-030-51455-6_2

databases for pharmacoepidemiological studies which are then presented in summary tables. We conclude with some remarks on necessary prerequisites for the successful use of existing databases.

1 Introduction

In phase III of drug development, randomized clinical trials (RCTs) are conducted to prove the efficacy of a new drug or more generally of a new pharmaceutical product. However, phase III-studies are usually not able to provide a full picture of the benefit-risk-profile of a new drug for several reasons (Garbe and Suissa 2014): the number of patients included in such RCTs is too small to detect and to quantify rare and serious adverse drug effects; the patient group is highly selected and excludes patients with a considerable number of comorbidities, children and elderly patients; the duration of such studies is too short to reveal long-term risks; the clinical setting is highly controlled and does not reflect daily practice where often various drugs are combined; recommendations regarding dietary behavior are ignored; and so-called "off-label use" is common. These limitations increase the likelihood that some adverse drug reactions (ADRs) will occur after marketing approval that were not observed during phase III of clinical development.

The knowledge gap regarding the benefit-risk-profile of a newly approved drug may be closed by adverse event reporting systems containing spontaneous reports of adverse events and pharmacoepidemiological studies after marketing approval. Signal generation and drug safety studies facilitate a prospective monitoring of drug safety if they are based on large electronic healthcare databases. Such databases are well established in North America, but also in many European countries (Garbe and Suissa 2014; Strom 2012; Suissa and Garbe 2007). Most recently, they have also been established in various Asian countries (AsPEN Collaborators et al. 2013; Kimura et al. 2011).

Databases increasingly represent an important worldwide data resource for pharmacoepidemiological research, but their information content, the covered timespan and the population size may heavily differ from database to database (see also the various databases described in this book). Thus, the appropriateness of a specific database to answer a certain research question has to be critically evaluated in each single situation.

In this chapter, we will provide an overview of existing databases worldwide that seem to be appropriate to conduct pharmacoepidemiological research. This overview is not intended to be complete but should give an idea of the variety of available databases. We will first briefly characterize and compare the major features of main types of databases and highlight their advantages and limitations in comparison to epidemiological field studies (see also Garbe and Pigeot 2015). We will then describe our search strategy to identify adequate databases for pharmacoepidemiological studies. The databases that we identified and rated as relevant are summarized in several tables stratified by type of database, continent and country (see Tables 2,

3, 4, 5, 6, 7 and 8). We conclude with some remarks on necessary prerequisites for the successful use of existing databases.

2 Types of Databases

Electronic healthcare databases may be roughly categorized into two types: (1) medical record databases that mainly contain excerpts of electronic patient records typically provided by general practitioners (GPs) and (2) administrative databases that are based on health insurance claims data or on state-funded health systems (Strom 2012). Although the information contained in both types is comparable there are some major differences. In the ideal case, both types should at least provide information on age, sex, inpatient and/or outpatient diagnoses, prescription date, drugs prescribed, date of hospital admission, types of surgery, date of discharge, and reason for discharge. However, as can be seen in Tables 2, 3, 4, 5 and 6 this is not always the case. Compared to administrative databases, medical record databases have the advantage of also containing data on lifestyle factors such as smoking, alcohol or body mass index, prescribed daily dose for medications, and laboratory findings. Other important clinical data such as inpatient diagnoses or information on secondary care might be added by the physician to the patient record, but are not always complete.

The advantages of healthcare databases become obvious when compared to epidemiological field studies where primary data collection is needed to receive the necessary information. To collect such data may be time and cost intensive whereas studies based on healthcare databases are cost-efficient and can be conducted within a reasonable time frame. Epidemiological field studies also typically face the problem that certain vulnerable groups, such as the elderly, multi-morbid patients or patients with lower socio-economic status are difficult to reach leading to the inclusion of a selected group of subjects in the study. In addition, studies based on healthcare databases usually do not require an informed consent for each study which mitigates against potential selection bias. Moreover, information on prescribed drugs provided by healthcare databases is considered as more reliable than corresponding statements by patients in field studies (Kelly et al. 1990) which is of special importance in the elderly (Tamblyn et al. 1995).

The major advantage of healthcare databases, however, results from their large numbers of patients and the potential for long follow-up time for outcomes with minimal subjects lost to follow-up. The population size of such databases is usually large enough to investigate uncommon or rare ADRs. An example in this respect is the occurrence of febrile convulsions as a rare adverse reaction to vaccines (Schink et al. 2014). Moreover, maintenance of such databases over long time periods with minimal loss of patients over time allows the investigation of ADRs with long latency times, such as various cancers. Whereas exposure and outcome data collected from physicians and patients in some field studies may suffer from recall bias, especially if long-term memory is required, healthcare database studies are free from this limitation. Automated healthcare databases also provide the opportunity to study drug effects that would be unethical to investigate in a clinical study such as off-label use of drugs in children (Dörks et al. 2013).

Despite these clear benefits of healthcare databases for pharmacoepidemiological research there are some limitations. Missing information and the fact that the data have not been initially collected for research purposes might impair their validity, which is especially true for administrative databases (Strom 2012). Missing information may result from time periods before the establishment of a database or from data typically not recorded for administrative purposes. Most administrative databases do not contain any information on non-prescription (over-the-counter) drugs, on the prescribed daily dose, on drug use during a stay in hospital, lifestyle factors, socio-economic status, or on laboratory values. Some missing information may be added by linkage to primary data or to other registries such as, e.g., cancer registries. However, such linkage requires a very stringent data protection concept and is only possible for a limited number of databases since a unique personal identifier common to the databases being linked is needed (Herk-Sukel et al. 2012). A good practice example in this respect is provided by the Scandinavian databases (Furu et al. 2010).

3 Search Strategy

Searching for electronic healthcare databases worldwide that are suitable for pharmacoepidemiological research, especially drug safety and drug utilization research was a quite challenging task since the assessment of the usefulness of a specific database required some basic understanding of the health system in each country. Also, in our search strategy we did not limit ourselves to the term database. Other terms used in this context were for instance data repository (e.g., Population Research Data Repository, Manitoba, Canada), virtual data warehouse (e.g., Health Care Systems Research Network (HCSRN) Virtual Data Warehouse, US), record linkage system (e.g., PHARMO, Netherlands) or register (e.g., National Patient Register, Denmark). In the following, the term "database" is used as synonym for a set of linked files or a single file that can be linked to others where each of the files contains demographic data and specific information regarding healthcare encounters, e.g., on diagnoses and procedures associated with hospitalizations or physician visits and drug exposure. The possibility to link such data files by a personal identifier is an important prerequisite for pharmacoepidemiological research. Hence, a file for instance with drug dispensation data only becomes a useful "database" for drug safety research if it can be linked to another file with information on outpatient and/or inpatient diagnoses. This had to be considered when we assessed the various electronic databases.

Various steps were taken to identify large computerized databases, so-called automated databases, containing healthcare data as sources for pharmacoepidemiological research. Our search focused only on databases that contain information irrespective of the disease status of a person. This means that, for instance, registries including only patients with specific diseases such as cancer or diabetes were not taken into account.

In a first step, the Website Bridge to Data (www.bridgetodata.org) was used to explore available databases. This site is a unique non-profit online reference describing population healthcare databases for use in epidemiology and health outcomes research. It provides useful and detailed information on pharmacoepidemiological and other population data sources for use in epidemiology, health services research, and healthcare economics and as models for designing healthcare systems and data resources worldwide.

Second, an internet-based search in PubMed and Google using pre-defined keywords in order to identify any further databases in published articles and in the references of articles was conducted (see Table 1).

Table 1 List of keywords for conducting free text search

Adjectives to the terms Data/database	Data/database
Large	Data
Automated	Data?
Computerised[a]	Database?
Clinical	Datenbank?
Medical record?[b]	Information
Medical	Collect?
Secondary	Resource?
Healthcare	Source?
HEALTH care	Data? AND collect?
Health insurants	Data? AND resource?
Registry (data?)	Data? AND source?
?Register?	
Claims	
Hospital	
Outpatient	
Prescription	
(Medical) treatment	
Record system	
Pharmacoepi?	
Pharmacovigilance	

[a]Dollar sign is used to represent one character within a keyword, e.g., computerised represents computerized and computerised
[b]Question mark is used as a truncation symbol to ensure that we get as many relevant hits as possible

Third, scientists or pharmacoepidemiologists from industry with experience in research with healthcare databases were contacted in order to identify databases not found by the above search strategy.

In a fourth step, the websites of the databases and research articles found in the previous steps were consulted to obtain information on the features of the identified databases. Several database administrators were contacted by email and asked to fill out a questionnaire prepared by the authors to obtain missing information. The questionnaire was developed to gather information on the main features of these databases and to assess their quality as well as their usefulness with respect to pharmacoepidemiological research. The questions were classified according to the following six categories: (1) description of the database, (2) source population, (3) type of data, (4) variables, (5) inpatient setting, and (6) outpatient setting. Besides the general description, the first category covers questions regarding the total number of subjects and the period of data collection. With the help of the second category, information about the source population, such as age and sex, was collected. Furthermore, information on the type of data collected (e.g., claims data or medical records) and whether or not the data are at an individual patient level were collected by the third category. The availability of demographic data was also requested in the fourth category. Categories five and six contained information as to whether either or both in- and outpatient drug and diagnoses data were available.

In the final step, all databases were evaluated with regard to their relevance or usefulness to conduct pharmacoepidemiological studies of pharmaceutical products. Each database was categorized independently by two researchers as relevant or not relevant. Disagreements were discussed and in case of no consensus a third researcher was consulted. The relevance or usefulness of each database was assessed based on the availability of (1) data at individual patient level, (2) information on age and sex, (3) in- and/or outpatient treatment data, (4) in- and/or outpatient diagnoses, and (5) on the ability to track patients over time. Databases rated as relevant were those meeting criteria (1), (2), (5), and (3) or (4) and/or databases that could be linked to other data sources to add the missing information. Databases assessed as not relevant were those missing most or all of the criteria without an option of linkage to other databases.

After categorization, the list of relevant databases was checked for plausibility and comprehensiveness. Further relevant databases were searched for by manual search.

4 Results

In total, we identified 75 relevant databases, displayed in Tables 2, 3, 4, 5, 6, 7 and 8. References with relevant information on these databases are provided below these tables and are not added to the overall reference list at the end of this chapter.

4.1 Asia

We identified four administrative databases in Asia, one each in Taiwan and Korea and two in Japan (Table 2). The National Health Insurance Research Database in Taiwan, the National Insurance Claims Database in Japan and the Health Insurance Review and Assessment Service (HIRA) databases in Korea cover approximately the whole population and hold data on in- and outpatient diagnoses, and medication. Moreover, it is possible to link additional information to the databases.

4.2 Australia

In Australia, nine administrative databases were rated as relevant, six of which result from data linkage initiatives in eight states/territories in Australia that provide access to administrative hospital data (Table 3). Furthermore, we found two databases (MBS and PBS claims) administered by the government statutory authority Medicare Australia that can be linked to each other and one administered by the Department of Veterans' Affairs. The databases of the data linkage initiatives can be linked to other population-based datasets such as birth or death registries, survey data, and also to the two Medicare databases. Moreover, the Population Health Research Network has been established: a linkage project to build data linkage units in all Australian states/territories and facilitate cross-jurisdictional data integration (Doiron et al. 2013). All administrative databases have in common that they do not provide information on outpatient diagnoses. One medical record database was identified (Table 4).

4.3 Europe

Nordic Countries (Denmark, Finland, Norway, Sweden, and Iceland)
Each of the five Nordic countries has a nationwide prescription registry that provides information on dispensed outpatient medications (Furu et al. 2010). In each country, the use of a unique personal identifier included in all national registries allows linkage of the prescription registries to other data sources such as birth, death, cancer registries, and especially registries that contain information on hospital encounters including diagnoses. In Demark and Sweden, databases lack information on outpatient diagnoses (Table 5). Moreover, we identified two regional administrative databases, namely OPED and AUHD, in Denmark.

United Kingdom (UK)
We identified seven medical record databases, three of which cover all regions of the UK, three cover Scotland only, and one covers the whole of Wales (Table 6). All seven databases contain information on outpatient diagnoses and medications, and

Table 2 Administrative Databases Asia

Country, Region	Name (acronym)	Data volume	Period of data collection	Frequency of update	Individual patient level data [Yes/No]	Longitudinal data [Yes/No]	Data on sex and age [Yes/No]	Diagnoses [In/Out]	Medications [In/Out]	Linkage with other data sources possible [Yes/No][a]
Taiwan	National Health Insurance Research Database (National Health Insurance Research Database 2019; Cheng et al. 2011; Kimura et al. 2011)	99% of Taiwan residents (~24 Mio.)	Since 1995	Annually	Yes	Yes	Yes	In/Out	In/Out	Yes
Japan	Japan Medical Data Center (JMDC) Claims Database (Fujimoto et al. 2015; Tanaka et al. 2015; Kimura et al. 2010; JMDC 2020)	~5.6 Mio. insurants	Since 2005	Monthly	Yes	Yes	Yes	In/Out	In/Out	Yes

(continued)

Table 2 (continued)

Country, Region	Name (acronym)	Data volume	Period of data collection	Frequency of update	Individual patient level data [Yes/No]	Longitudinal data [Yes/No]	Data on sex and age [Yes/No]	Diagnoses [In/Out]	Medications [In/Out]	Linkage with other data sources possible [Yes/No][a]
	National Insurance Claims Database (NDB) (Okamoto 2014; Kimura et al. 2011)	~127 Mio. residents	Since 2009	Monthly/Annually	Yes	Yes	Yes	In/Out	In/Out	No
Korea	Health Insurance Review & Assessment Service (HIRA) Database (Seong et al. 2011; Kim et al. 2014; Kimura et al. 2011)	~52 Mio. residents	Since 2000	Annually	Yes	Yes	Yes	In/Out	In/Out	Yes

[a]Data sources include mortality, birth, and cancer registries or occupational data, etc.

Table 3 Administrative Databases Australia

Region	Name (acronym)	Data volume	Period of data collection	Frequency of update	Individual patient level data [Yes/No]	Longitudinal data [Yes/No]	Data on sex and age [Yes/No]	Diagnoses [In/Out]	Medications [In/Out]	Linkage with other data sources possible [Yes/No][a]
National	Australian Department of Veterans' Affairs (DVA) Administrative Claims Database (Ramsay et al. 2013; Lu 2009)	220,000 veterans	Since 2001		Yes	Yes	Yes	In/Out	Out	Yes
National	Medicare Benefits Schedule (MBS) Claims (Lu 2009)	25 Mio. residents	Since 1984		Yes	Yes	Yes	Out		Yes
National	Pharmaceutical Benefits Scheme (PBS) Dispensing Database (Lu 2009)	25 Mio. residents	Since 2002	Regularly, every few months	Yes	Yes	Yes		In/Out (partially)	Yes
Australian Capital Territory + New South Wales	Centre for Health Record Linkage (CHeReL) (Centre for Health Record Linkage 2019)	15 Mio. residents	Since 2001	Quarterly	Yes	Yes	Yes	In		Yes

(continued)

Table 3 (continued)

Region	Name (acronym)	Data volume	Period of data collection	Frequency of update	Individual patient level data [Yes/No]	Longitudinal data [Yes/No]	Data on sex and age [Yes/No]	Diagnoses [In/Out]	Medications [In/Out]	Linkage with other data sources possible [Yes/No][a]
Northern Territory + South Australia	SA-NT Datalink (SA-NT Datalink 2019)	~1.9 Mio. residents	Since 2000		Yes	Yes	Yes	In/Out	In	Yes
Queensland	Data Linkage Queensland (Queensland Government Queensland Health 2019)	~5 Mio. residents	Since 2000	Monthly	Yes	Yes	Yes	In		Yes
Tasmania	Tasmanian Data Linkage Unit(University of Tasmania 2020)	~500,000 residents	Since 2000		Yes	Yes	Yes	In		Yes

(continued)

Table 3 (continued)

Region	Name (acronym)	Data volume	Period of data collection	Frequency of update	Individual patient level data [Yes/No]	Longitudinal data [Yes/No]	Data on sex and age [Yes/No]	Diagnoses [In/Out]	Medications [In/Out]	Linkage with other data sources possible [Yes/No][a]
Victoria	Victorian Data Linkages (VDL) (Victoria State Government 2019)	~2.6 Mio. residents	Since 1993		Yes	Yes	Yes	In		Yes
Western Australia	Western Australian Data Linkage System (WADLS) (Holman et al. 2008; Data Linkage Western Australia 2019)	~3.7 Mio. residents	Since 1970	Monthly	Yes	Yes	Yes	In		Yes

[a]Data sources include mortality, birth, and cancer registries or occupational data, etc.

Table 4 Medical Record Databases Australia

Region	Name (acronym)	Data volume	Period of data collection	Frequency of update	Individual patient level data [Yes/No]	Longi-tudinal data [Yes/No]	Data on sex and age [Yes/No]	Diagnoses [In/Out]	Medications [In/Out]	Dosing regimen [Yes/No]	Linkage with other data sources possible [Yes/No][a]
National	General Practice Research Network (GPRN) (Kerr et al. 2003; Saltman et al. 2005; Sayer et al. 2003; Trinh et al. 2017)	~4 Mio. patients	Since 1999	Weekly	Yes	Yes	Age/Sex	Out	Out	Yes	

[a]Data sources include mortality, birth, and cancer registries or occupational data, etc.

Table 5 Administrative Databases Europe

Country, Region	Name (acronym)	Data volume	Period of data collection	Frequency of update	Individual patient level data [Yes/No]	Longitudinal data [Yes/No]	Data on sex and age [Yes/No]	Diagnoses [In/Out]	Medications [In/Out]	Linkage with other data sources possible [Yes/No][a]
Denmark	National Patient Register (Thygesen et al. 2011; Lynge et al. 2011; Schmidt et al. 2019)	~5.8 Mio. residents	Since 1977	Weekly	Yes	Yes	Yes	In/Out (only emergency room visits)	No	Yes
	National Prescription Registry (Thygesen et al. 2011; Kildemoes et al. 2011; Schmidt et al. 2019)	~5.8 Mio. residents	Since 1995	Weekly	Yes	Yes	Yes		Out	Yes
Southern Denmark	Odense University Pharmacoepidemiological Database (OPED) (Furu et al. 2010; Hallas et al. 2017)	~2 Mio. residents	Since 1990	Monthly	Yes	Yes	Yes		Out	Yes
North Denmark, Central Denmark	Aarhus University Hospital Database (AUHD) (Sorensen et al 2009; Ehrenstein et al. 2010; Valkhoff et al. 2014; Furu et al. 2010)	~2 Mio. residents	Since 1989	Monthly	Yes	Yes	Yes	In	Out	Yes

(continued)

Table 5 (continued)

Country, Region	Name (acronym)	Data volume	Period of data collection	Frequency of update	Individual patient level data [Yes/No]	Longitudinal data [Yes/No]	Data on sex and age [Yes/No]	Diagnoses [In/Out]	Medications [In/Out]	Linkage with other data sources possible [Yes/No][a]
Estonia	Estonian Health Insurance Fund (EHIF) Database (Jurisson et al. 2015)	~1.3 Mio. residents	Since 2004	Daily	Yes	Yes	Yes	In/Out	Out	Yes
France	Système National des Données de Santé (SNDS) (Health Data Hub 2020)	~68 Mio. residents	Since 2003	Bi-annually	Yes	Yes	Yes	In/Out (only chronic diseases)	Out	Yes
Finland	Care Register for Health Care incl. the Finnish National Discharge Register (Finnish Institute for Health and Welfare 2020)	~5.5 Mio. residents	Since 1967	Annually	Yes	Yes	Yes	In/Out		Yes
	Finnish Register of Primary Health Care Visits (Finnish Institute for Health and Welfare 2020)	~5.5 Mio. residents	Since 2011	Annually	Yes	Yes	Yes	Out	Out	Yes
	Finnish Prescription Registry (Furu et al. 2010)	~5.5 Mio. residents	Since 1994	Monthly	Yes	Yes	Yes		Out	Yes

(continued)

Table 5 (continued)

Country, Region	Name (acronym)	Data volume	Period of data collection	Frequency of update	Individual patient level data [Yes/No]	Longitudinal data [Yes/No]	Data on sex and age [Yes/No]	Diagnoses [In/Out]	Medications [In/Out]	Linkage with other data sources possible [Yes/No][a]
Germany	German Pharmacoepidemiological Research Database (GePaRD) (Pigeot and Ahrens 2008)	~25 Mio. residents	Since 2004	Annually	Yes	Yes	Yes	In/Out	Out	Yes
	Institute for Applied Health Research Berlin (InGef) Database (formerly German Health Risk Institute (HRI) Database) (Andersohn and Walker 2016)	~9 Mio. residents	Last six years	Bi-annually	Yes	Yes	Yes	In/Out	Out	No
Germany, Hesse	Versichertenstichprobe AOK Hessen/KV Hessen (Ihle et al. 2005; Abbas et al. 2012)	~360,000 residents	1998–2017		Yes	Yes	Yes	In/Out	Out	Yes
Iceland	Icelandic Hospital Discharge Registry (Gudbjornsson et al. 2010)	~0.3 Mio. residents	Since 1999		Yes	Yes	Yes	In		Yes

(continued)

Table 5 (continued)

Country, Region	Name (acronym)	Data volume	Period of data collection	Frequency of update	Individual patient level data [Yes/No]	Longitudinal data [Yes/No]	Data on sex and age [Yes/No]	Diagnoses [In/Out]	Medications [In/Out]	Linkage with other data sources possible [Yes/No][a]
	Icelandic Medicines Registry (Furu et al. 2010; Gudbjornsson et al. 2010)	~0.3 Mio. residents	Since 2002	Daily	Yes	Yes	Yes		Out	Yes
	Icelandic Registry of Contact with Primary Health Care	~0.3 Mio. residents	Since 2004		Yes	Yes	Yes	Out		Yes
Ireland	Irish Health Service Executive-Primary Care Reimbursement Service (HSE-PCRS) pharmacy database (Sinnott et al. 2017)	~1.6 Mio residents (~33% of the Irish population)	Since 1998	Monthly	Yes	Yes	Yes		Out	Yes
Italy, Veneto, Liguria, Tuscany, Marche, Lazio, Abruzzo, Campania	ARNO Observatory (Marchesini et al. 2014; Maggioni et al. 2016)	~11 Mio. residents	Since 1987	Annually	Yes	Yes	Yes	In	Out	Yes

(continued)

Table 5 (continued)

Country, Region	Name (acronym)	Data volume	Period of data collection	Frequency of update	Individual patient level data [Yes/No]	Longitudinal data [Yes/No]	Data on sex and age [Yes/No]	Diagnoses [In/Out]	Medications [In/Out]	Linkage with other data sources possible [Yes/No][a]
Italy, Lombardy	Regional Database Lombardy (SISR) (Avillach et al. 2013)	~10 Mio. residents	Since 1997	Annually	Yes	Yes	Yes	In	In/Out	Yes
Italy, Emilia Romagna	Emilia Romagna Regional Database (ERD) (Oteri et al. 2010; Oteri et al. 2016)	~6 Mio residents	1997–2013	Monthly	Yes	Yes	Yes	In	Out	Yes
Italy, Tuscany	ARS Tuscany Regional Database (Valkhoff et al. 2014; Avillach et al. 2013)	~3.6 Mio. residents	Since 2003	Quarterly	Yes	Yes	Yes	In	In (only probabilistically linked to patient)/Out	Yes
Italy, Como, Cremona, Lecco, Lodi, Mantova, Milano 2, Pavia, Varese	Osservatorio Interaziendale per la Farmacoepidemiologia e la Farmacoeconomia (OSSIFF) Database (Valkhoff et al. 2013; Masclee et al. 2018)	~3.8 Mio. residents	Since 2000		Yes	Yes	Yes	In	Out	Yes

(continued)

Table 5 (continued)

Country, Region	Name (acronym)	Data volume	Period of data collection	Frequency of update	Individual patient level data [Yes/No]	Longitudinal data [Yes/No]	Data on sex and age [Yes/No]	Diagnoses [In/Out]	Medications [In/Out]	Linkage with other data sources possible [Yes/No][a]
Netherlands	Achmea Health Database (formerly AGIS Health Database) (Smeets et al. 2011; Nielen et al. 2018)	~5 Mio. residents	Since 1997	Annually	Yes	Yes	Yes	In	Out	Yes
Norway	Norwegian Patient Register (Hoiberg et al. 2014; Bakken et al. 2020)	~5.3 Mio. residents	Since 2008	Annually	Yes	Yes	Yes	In/Out	Out	Yes
	Norwegian Registry for Primary Health Care (Bakken et al. 2020)	~5.3 Mio. residents	Since 2017		Yes	Yes	Yes	Out		Yes
	Norwegian Prescription Database (Furu et al. 2010)	~5.3 Mio. residents	Since 2004	Monthly	Yes	Yes	Yes		Out	Yes
Sweden	Swedish National Patient Registry (Socialstyrelsen 2020)	~10.1 Mio. residents	Since 1987	Monthly	Yes	Yes	Yes	In/Out		Yes
	Swedish Prescribed Drug Register (Furu et al. 2010)	~10.1 Mio. residents	Since 2005	Monthly	Yes	Yes	Yes		Out	Yes
UK	Hospital Episode Statistics (HES) Database (NHS digital 2020)	>200 Mio. records	Since 1990	Annually	Yes	Yes	Yes	In		Yes

[a]Data sources include, e.g., mortality, birth, and cancer registries; occupational and survey data

some of them also provide information on the prescribed dose. The MEMO and ISD databases also contain data on hospitalizations. Moreover, besides medical records, the SAIL database in Wales includes administrative data on inpatient diagnoses. One administrative database was identified in the UK (HES) that contains data on inpatient diagnoses and allows linkage to other databases in the UK (Table 5).

Netherlands
We identified one administrative database, Achmea Health Base, which includes data on inpatient diagnoses and outpatient medications only. To overcome the lack of, e.g., outpatient diagnoses, it is possible to link this database to other data sources such as medical record databases or cancer registries. Moreover, three medical record databases could be found, one of which, the PHARMO record linkage system, provides data on in- and outpatient diagnoses, and medications as well as other data sources such as administrative data and cancer registries (Table 6).

Italy
We found five regional administrative databases which have in common that they all lack data on outpatient diagnoses (Table 5). Only in the region of Lombardy information on inpatient medications is available. Furthermore, three medical record databases were found, one of which includes exclusively data on children treated by pediatric general practitioners and family pediatricians (Table 6). Two contain data on in- and outpatient diagnoses and outpatient medications. Moreover, the Caserta record linkage database contains linked data from medical records (GP prescription database) and administrative databases including inpatient diagnoses and outpatient medications.

4.4 Other European Countries (Estonia, France, Germany, Ireland, Spain)

For the remainder of Europe, we rated eight databases as relevant located in five countries, namely three administrative databases in Germany, one each in France, Estonia, and Ireland, and two medical record databases in Spain (Tables 5 and 6).

4.5 North America

Canada
We identified several administrative databases that are provincially managed by nine of the ten Canadian provinces; almost all cover approximately the whole population in the provinces (Table 7). Moreover, four of the databases in British Columbia, Manitoba, Nova Scotia, and Ontario are managed by linkage initiatives that provide access to linked datasets (Doiron et al. 2013). In other provinces such as Quebec,

Table 6 Medical Record Databases Europe

Country, Region	Name (acronym)	Data volume	Period of data collection	Frequency of update	Individual patient level data [Yes/No]	Longitudinal data [Yes/No]	Data on sex and age [Yes/No]	Diagnoses [In/Out]	Medications [In/Out]	Dosing regimen [Yes/No]	Linkage with other data sources possible [Yes/No][a]
Netherlands	Julius General Practitioners Network (JGPN) (formerly Utrecht Health Project and the Utrecht General Practitioners Network) (Kasteleyn et al. 2014; Venmans et al. 2009; Smeets et al. 2018)	~370,000 patients	Since 1996	Quarterly	Yes	Yes	Yes	Out	Out		Yes
	PHARmacoMOrbidity linkage system (PHARMO data base network) (PHARMO Institute 2020)	~9 Mio. residents	Since 1989	Annually	Yes	Yes	Yes	In/Out	In/Out	Yes	Yes
	Interdisciplinary Processing of Clinical Information (IPCI) (IPCI 2020; Horton et al. 2020)	~2.4 Mio. residents	Since 1994	Annually	Yes	Yes	Yes	In (partial discharge diagnosis)/Out (only indication for prescription)	Out	Yes	Yes

(continued)

Table 6 (continued)

Country, Region	Name (acronym)	Data volume	Period of data collection	Frequency of update	Individual patient level data [Yes/No]	Longitudinal data [Yes/No]	Data on sex and age [Yes/No]	Diagnoses [In/Out]	Medications [In/Out]	Dosing regimen [Yes/No]	Linkage with other data sources possible [Yes/No][a]
Italy, Southern Italy	Caserta record linkage database (formerly Arianna Database)(Oteri et al. 2010)	~1.1 Mio. residents	Since 2000	Bi-annually	Yes	Yes	Yes	In/Out (only indication for prescription)	Out	Yes	Yes
Italy	Health Search/Longitudinal Patient Database (HSD) (Valkhoff et al. 2014)	~2 Mio. residents	Since 1998	Bi-annually	Yes	Yes	Yes	In/Out	Out	Yes	No
	PEDIANET (Avillach et al. 2013)	~265,000 children	Since 2000	Daily	Yes	Yes	Yes	In/Out	Out	Yes	Yes
Spain	BIFAP (Base de Datos para la Investigación Farmacoepidemiologica en Atención Primaria) Database (Ruigómez et al. 2014; Hernandez-Rodriguez et al. 2020)	~12 Mio. residents	Since 2001	Annually	Yes	Yes	Yes	In (partial)/Out	Out	Yes	No

(continued)

Table 6 (continued)

Country, Region	Name (acronym)	Data volume	Period of data collection	Frequency of update	Individual patient level data [Yes/No]	Longitudinal data [Yes/No]	Data on sex and age [Yes/No]	Diagnoses [In/Out]	Medications [In/Out]	Dosing regimen [Yes/No]	Linkage with other data sources possible [Yes/No][a]
Spain, Catalonia	Sistema d'Informació per al Desenvolupament de l'Investigació en Atenció Primària (SIDIAP) Database (Pérez-Sáez et al. 2015; SIDIAP 2020)	~7 Mio. residents	Since 2006	Annually	Yes	Yes	Yes	Out	Out	No	Yes
UK	The Health Improvement Network (THIN) (The Health Improvement Network 2020)	~12 Mio. residents	Since 1994	Three times per year	Yes	Yes	Yes	Out	Out	Yes	Yes
	Clinical Practice Research Datalink (CPRD) (CPRD 2020)	~45 Mio. residents	Since 1987	Monthly	Yes	Yes	Yes	Out	Out	Yes	Yes
	QRESEARCH (QRESEARCH 2020)	~35 Mio. residents	Since 1989	Regularly	Yes	Yes	Yes	Out	Out	Yes	Yes
UK, Scotland	The Primary Care Clinical Informatics Unit (PCCIU) Database (University of Aberdeen 2020)	~1.7 Mio. residents	Since 2000	Bi-annually	Yes	Yes	Yes	Out	Out	No	No

(continued)

Table 6 (continued)

Country, Region	Name (acronym)	Data volume	Period of data collection	Frequency of update	Individual patient level data [Yes/No]	Longitudinal data [Yes/No]	Data on sex and age [Yes/No]	Diagnoses [In/Out]	Medications [In/Out]	Dosing regimen [Yes/No]	Linkage with other data sources possible [Yes/No][a]
	Health Informatics Centre (HIC) linked Databases, formerly Tayside Medicines Monitoring Unit (MEMO) Databases (Evans and MacDonald 1999)	~800,000 residents	Since 1989		Yes	Yes	Yes	In	Out	Yes	Yes
	Information Services Division (ISD) Data Warehouse (ISD Scotland 2020)	~5.4 Mio. residents	Since 1975	Annually	Yes	Yes	Yes	In	Out	No	Yes
UK, Wales	Secure Anonymised Information Linkage (SAIL) Databank (Lyons et al. 2009; John et al. 2016; SAIL Databank 2020)	~3 Mio. residents	Since 1987		Yes	Yes	Yes	In/Out	Out	Yes	Yes

Table 7 Administrative Databases Canada

Province	Name (acronym)	Data volume	Period of data collection	Frequency of update	Individual patient level data [Yes/No]	Longitudinal data [Yes/No]	Data on sex and age [Yes/No]	Diagnoses [In/Out]	Medications [In/Out]	Linkage with other data sources possible [Yes/No][a]
Alberta	Alberta Administrative Health Datasets (Suissa et al. 2012; Government of Alberta Department of Health and Wellness 2017)	~4.4 Mio. residents	Since 1993	Annually	Yes	Yes	Yes	In/Out	Out	Yes
British Columbia	Population Data BC (PopData) (Suissa et al. 2012; Population Data BC 2020)	~4.7 Mio. residents	Since 1985	Annually	Yes	Yes	Yes	In/Out	Out	Yes
Manitoba	Population Research Data Repository (MCHP) (Roos et al. 2008; Suissa et al. 2012; Manitoba Centre for Health Policy 2020)	~1.3 Mio. residents	Since 1976	Annually	Yes	Yes	Yes	In/Out	Out	Yes

(continued)

Table 7 (continued)

Province	Name (acronym)	Data volume	Period of data collection	Frequency of update	Individual patient level data [Yes/No]	Longitudinal data [Yes/No]	Data on sex and age [Yes/No]	Diagnoses [In/Out]	Medications [In/Out]	Linkage with other data sources possible [Yes/No][a]
Newfoundland and Labrador	Newfoundland and Labrador Centre for Health Information (Hurd et al. 2018; Newfoundland and Labrador Centre for Health Information 2020)	~520,000 residents	From 1995/96–2012/13		Yes	Yes	Yes	In/Out	Out	Yes
New Brunswick	New Brunswick Institute for Research, Data and Training (University of New Brunswick 2020)	~770,000 residents	Since 1997		Yes	Yes	Yes	In	Out	Yes
Nova Scotia	Health Data Nova Scotia (HDNS), formerly Population Health Research Unit (PHRU) (Dalhousie University 2020)	~970,000 residents	Since 1989	Quarterly	Yes	Yes	Yes	In/Out	Out	Yes

(continued)

Table 7 (continued)

Province	Name (acronym)	Data volume	Period of data collection	Frequency of update	Individual patient level data [Yes/No]	Longitudinal data [Yes/No]	Data on sex and age [Yes/No]	Diagnoses [In/Out]	Medications [In/Out]	Linkage with other data sources possible [Yes/No][a]
Ontario	Institute for Clinical Evaluative Sciences (ICES) Data Repository (Suissa et al. 2012; Institute for Clinical Evaluative Sciences 2020)	~14.5 Mio. residents	Since 1991	Annually	Yes	Yes	Yes	In/Out	Out	Yes
Québec	Régie de l'Assurance Maladie du Québec (RAMQ) databases (Kawasumi et al. 2011; Tamblyn et al. 1995; Suissa et al. 2012; Douros et al. 2019)	~3.5 Mio. residents	Since 1983	Monthly	Yes	Yes	Yes	Out	Out	Yes

(continued)

Table 7 (continued)

Province	Name (acronym)	Data volume	Period of data collection	Frequency of update	Individual patient level data [Yes/No]	Longitudinal data [Yes/No]	Data on sex and age [Yes/No]	Diagnoses [In/Out]	Medications [In/Out]	Linkage with other data sources possible [Yes/No][a]
	Maintenance et exploitation des données pour l'étude de la clientele hospitalière (MED-ÉCHO) database (Douros et al. 2019)	~8.2 Mio. residents	Since 1987	Annually	Yes	Yes	No	In		Yes
Saskatchewan	Saskatchewan Health Services Databases (Suissa et al. 2012; Culpepper et al. 2019; Government of Saskatchewan 2020)	~1.1 Mio. residents	Since 1970	Quarterly	Yes	Yes	Yes	In/Out	Out	Yes

[a]Data sources include, e.g., mortality, birth, and cancer registries; occupational and survey data

two health databases are available for research purposes containing information on hospitalization, outpatient diagnoses, and medications that can be linked by a unique patient identifier. All databases have in common that they do not have information on inpatient medications, but that they can be linked to other population datasets such as birth, death, and cancer registries and survey data.

United States
We found three administrative databases based on the following health care programs of the US government: Medicare, Medicaid and the Department of Veterans Affairs (VA) Health Care System (Table 8). All three databases have in common that only specific populations are covered: residents equal or older 65 (Medicare), low income elderly persons or pregnant women (Medicaid), chronically disabled persons (Medicaid), and US armed services veterans (VA) (Hennessy et al. 2012). All three databases provide information on in- and outpatient diagnoses and outpatient medications. Only the VA database additionally holds information on inpatient medications. All three databases can be linked to other data sources such as mortality or cancer registries. Moreover, we identified two networks/initiatives of data obtained from Health Care Systems Research Network (HCSRN) Virtual Data Warehouse and the Kaiser Permanente (KP) Center for Effectiveness and Safety Research that comprise 15 regional health plans in the HMO Research Network and eight KP regions with partially overlapping data. Both have in common that they hold claims data on in- and outpatient diagnoses and outpatient medications, but also medical record data on laboratory test results, smoking status, and body mass index (Andrade et al. 2012). Moreover, we identified three databases based on commercial insurances that contain information on out- and inpatient diagnoses and procedures as well as outpatient pharmacy claims.

5 Conclusion

We were able to identify a large number of databases throughout the world, but their content, size, duration and geographic coverage at the local and national level differed remarkably. This variation is partly due to differences in legal requirements among countries, which may not only hinder the collection of specific information and the longitudinal maintenance of social and medical data but may also hinder linkage of a pharmacoepidemiological database with other data sources, especially with primary data. Primary data are an especially important add-on to many pharmacoepidemiological studies both to validate the information available in the database and to provide data missing from the database. Thus, a researcher is strongly advised to contact the administrator of a database beforehand to make sure that the information available in the respective database suits the needs of a specific project and to learn about advantages and limitations of this specific type of database. In addition, a researcher should clarify all necessary legal and/or administrative steps to get access to the data. Last, it is recommended to check if it is possible to link the records in

Table 8 Administrative Databases USA

State	Name (acronym)	Data volume	Period of data collection	Frequency of update	Individual patient level data [Yes/No]	Longitudinal data [Yes/No]	Data on sex and age [Yes/No]	Diagnoses [In/Out]	Medications [Yes/No]	Linkage with other data sources possible [Yes/No][a]
National	Medicare Database (Center for Medicare and Medicaid Services (CMS) 2019; Strom 2012)	~60 Mio. residents (96% of all US citizens aged 65 and older)	1999–2018	Annually	Yes	Yes	Yes	In/Out	Out	Yes
National	Medicaid Database (Strom 2012; Center for Medicare and Medicaid Services (CMS) 2019)	~65 Mio. residents	1999–2016	Annually	Yes	Yes	Yes	In/Out	Out	Yes

(continued)

Table 8 (continued)

State	Name (acronym)	Data volume	Period of data collection	Frequency of update	Individual patient level data [Yes/No]	Longitudinal data [Yes/No]	Data on sex and age [Yes/No]	Diagnoses [In/Out]	Medications [Yes/No]	Linkage with other data sources possible [Yes/No][a]
National	Veterans Affairs Database (US Department of Veterans Affairs 2019; Strom 2012)	~14.5 Mio. veterans	Since 1997		Yes	Yes	Yes	In/Out	In/Out	Yes
Colorado, Georgia, Hawaii, Maryland and Virginia, Northern California, Oregon, Ohio, Southern California	Kaiser Permanente (KP) Center for Effectiveness and Safety Research (Strom 2012)	~13 Mio. residents			Yes	Yes	Yes	In/Out	Out	Yes

(continued)

Table 8 (continued)

State	Name (acronym)	Data volume	Period of data collection	Frequency of update	Individual patient level data [Yes/No]	Longitudinal data [Yes/No]	Data on sex and age [Yes/No]	Diagnoses [In/Out]	Medications [Yes/No]	Linkage with other data sources possible [Yes/No][a]
	Health Care Systems Research Network (HCSRN) Virtual Data Warehouse (VDW), former HMO Research Network Virtual Data Warehouse (Strom 2012; Health Care Systems Research Network 2019)	~16 Mio. residents	Since 1994		Yes	Yes	Yes	In/Out	Out	Yes

(continued)

Table 8 (continued)

State	Name (acronym)	Data volume	Period of data collection	Frequency of update	Individual patient level data [Yes/No]	Longitudinal data [Yes/No]	Data on sex and age [Yes/No]	Diagnoses [In/Out]	Medications [Yes/No]	Linkage with other data sources possible [Yes/No][a]
State	HealthCore Integrated Research Database (HIRD[SM]) (Petersen et al. 2010; AbuDagga et al. 2014; Singhal et al. 2019)	~45 Mio. residents	Since 2001	Monthly	Yes	Yes	Yes	In/Out	Out	
	OptumInsight Research (OIR) Database (Goodin et al. 2014; OPTUM 2013)	~111 Mio. residents	Since 1993		Yes	Yes	Yes	In/Out	Out	Yes
National	Truven Health Analytics MarketScan® Research Databases (Kulaylat et al. 2019)	~230 Mio. residents	Since 1995	Annually	Yes	Yes	Yes	In/Out	Out	Yes

[a]Data sources include, e.g., mortality, birth, and cancer registries; occupational and survey data

a database with primary health care records or other databases with data related to health care.

Based on our experience it is additionally strongly recommended to have a basic understanding of the health system of the specific country where the data have been collected to avoid misinterpretation and misuse of the data. If databases of various countries have to be pooled, e.g., to achieve the required sample size for the investigation of very rare outcomes or exposures (as, e.g., in the EU-funded project "Safety Evaluation of Adverse Reactions in Diabetes–SAFEGUARD") this information is especially necessary in order to be able to harmonize the variables included in the respective study.

For many databases only roughly described here, necessary and more detailed information is provided in the following chapters of this book.

Acknowledgements This chapter is based on work partly funded by CSL Behring.

References

Abbas S, Ihle P, Koster I et al (2012) Estimation of disease incidence in claims data dependent on the length of follow-up: a methodological approach. Health Serv Res 47(2):746–755

AbuDagga A, Stephenson JJ, Fu A-C et al (2014) Characteristics affecting oral anticoagulant therapy choice among patients with non-valvular atrial fibrillation: a retrospective claims analysis. BMC Health Serv Res 14:310

Andersohn F, Walker J (2016) Characteristics and external validity of the german health risk institute (HRI) database. Pharmacoepidemiol Drug Saf 25 (1):106–109. https://doi.org/10.1002/pds.3895

Andrade SE, Raebel MA, Boudreau D et al (2012) Health maintenance organizations/health plans. In: Strom BL, Kimmel SE, Hennessy S (eds) Pharmacoepidemiology. Wiley-Blackwell, Chichester, pp 163–188

AsPEN Collaborators, Andersen M, Bergman U et al (2013) The Asian pharmacoepidemiology network (AsPEN): promoting multi-national collaboration for pharmacoepidemiologic research in Asia. Pharmacoepidemiol Drug Saf 22(7):700–704

Avillach P, Coloma PM, Gini R et al (2013) Harmonization process for the identification of medical events in eight European healthcare databases: the experience from the EU-ADR project. J Am Med Inform Assn 20(1):184–192

Bakken IJ, Ariansen AMS, Knudsen GP et al (2020) The norwegian patient registry and the norwegian registry for primary health care: Research potential of two nationwide health-care registries. Scand J Public Health 48 (1):49–55. https://doi.org/10.1177/1403494819859737

Cheng CL, Kao YH, Lin SJ et al (2011) Validation of the national health insurance research database with ischemic stroke cases in Taiwan. Pharmacoepidemiol Drug Saf 20(3):236–242

Centre for Health Record Linkage (2019) What we do. http://www.cherel.org.au/. Accessed 18 Dec 2019

Center for Medicare and Medicaid Services (CMS) (2019) Research Data Assistance Centre. http://www.resdac.org/cms-data. Accessed 18 Dec 2019

CPRD (2020) Clinical practice research datalink. https://www.cprd.com Accessed 3 Jan 2020

Culpepper WJ, Marrie RA, Langer-Gould A et al (2019) Validation of an algorithm for identifying MS cases in administrative health claims datasets. Neurology 92 (10):e1016-e1028. https://doi.org/10.1212/wnl.0000000000007043

Data Linkage Western Australia (2019) Enabling Health & Medical Research in Western Australia. http://www.datalinkage-wa.org.au/. Accessed 18 Dec 2019

Dalhousie University (2020) Health data nova scotia. https://medicine.dal.ca/departments/depart ment-sites/community-health/research/hdns.html. Accessed 6 Jan 2020

Doiron D, Raina P, Fortier I et al (2013) Linking Canadian population health data: maximizing the potential of cohort and administrative data. Can J Public Health 104(3):e258–e261

Dörks M, Langner I, Dittmann U et al (2013) Antidepressant drug use and off-label prescribing in children and adolescents in Germany: results from a large population-based cohort study. Eur Child Adoles Psy 22(8):511–518

Douros A, Renoux C, Yin H et al (2019) Concomitant Use of Direct Oral Anticoagulants with Antiplatelet Agents and the Risk of Major Bleeding in Patients with Nonvalvular Atrial Fibrillation. Am J Med 132 (2):191–199.e112. https://doi.org/10.1016/j.amjmed.2018.10.008

Ehrenstein V, Antonsen S, Pedersen L (2010) Existing data sources for clinical epidemiology: Aarhus University Prescription Database. Clin Epidemiol 2:273–279

Evans JM, MacDonald TM (1999) Record-linkage for pharmacovigilance in Scotland. Brit J Clin Pharmaco 47(1):105–110

Finnish Institute for Health and Welfare (2020) Register descriptions. https://www.thl.fi/en/web/ thlfi-en/statistics/information-on-statistics/register-descriptions. Accessed 3 Jan 2020

Furu K, Wettermark B, Andersen M et al (2010) The Nordic countries as a cohort for pharmacoepi-demiological research. Basic Clin Pharmacol Toxicol 106(2):86–94. https://doi.org/10.1111/j. 1742-7843.2009.00494.x

Fujimoto M, Higuchi T, Hosomi K et al (2015) Association between statin use and cancer: Data mining of a spontaneous reporting database and a claims Database. Int J Med Sci 12 (3):223–233

Garbe E, Pigeot I (2015) Benefits of large healthcare databases for drug risk research. Bundesge-sundheitsblatt Gesundheitsforschung Gesundheitsschutz 58(8):829–837. https://doi.org/10.1007/ s00103-015-2185-7

Garbe E, Suissa S (2014) Pharmacoepidemiology. In: Ahrens W, Pigeot I (eds) Handbook of epidemiology. Springer, Berlin, pp 1875–1925

Government of Alberta Department of Health and Wellness (2017) Overview of administra-tive health datasets. https://open.alberta.ca/dataset/657ed26d-eb2c-4432-b9cb-0ca2158f165d/ resource/38f47433-b33d-4d1e-b959-df312e9d9855/download/research-health-datasets.pdf. Accessed 27 Jan 2020

Government of Saskatchewan (2020) Saskatchewan Health. Health Data and Analytics. https:// www.ehealthsask.ca/health-data/analytics/. Accessed 28 Jan 2020

Goodin DS, Corwin M, Kaufman D et al (2014) Causes of death among commercially insured multiple sclerosis patients in the United States. PLoS One 9 (8):e105207

Gudbjornsson B, Thorsteinsson S, Sigvaldason H et al (2010) Rofecoxib, but not celecoxib, increases the risk of thromboembolic cardiovascular events in young adults—a nationwide registry-based study. Eur J Clin Pharmacol 66 (6):619–625

Hallas J, Hellfritzsch M, Rix M et al (2017) Odense Pharmacoepidemiological Database: A Review of Use and Content. Basic Clin Pharmacol Toxicol 120 (5):419–425. https://doi.org/10.1111/ bcpt.12764

Health Data Hub (2020) https://www.health-data-hub.fr/?lang=en. Accessed 3 Jan 2020

Health Care Systems Research Network (2019) VDW Data Model. http://www.hcsrn.org/en/Res ources/VDW/. Accessed 18 Dec 2019

Hennessy S, Freeman CP, Cunningham F (2012) US Government Claims Databases. In: Strom BL, Kimmel SE, Hennessy S (eds) Pharmacoepidemiology. Wiley-Blackwell, Chichester, pp 209–223

Hernandez-Rodriguez MA, Sempere-Verdu E, Vicens-Caldentey C et al (2020) Evolution of polypharmacy in a spanish population (2005-2015): A database study. Pharmacoepidemiol Drug Saf. https://doi.org/10.1002/pds.4956

Herk-Sukel MP, Lemmens VE, Poll-Franse LV et al (2012) Record linkage for pharmacoepidemi-ological studies in cancer patients. Pharmacoepidemiol Drug Saf 21(1):94–103

Holman CD, Bass AJ, Rosman DL et al (2008) A decade of data linkage in Western Australia: strategic design, applications and benefits of the WA data linkage system. Aust Health Rev 32(4):766–777

Hoiberg MP, Gram J, Hermann P et al (2014) The incidence of hip fractures in Norway -accuracy of the national Norwegian patient registry. BMC Musculoskelet Disord 15:372

Horton DB, Bhullar H, Carty L et al (2020) Electronic Health Record Databases. In: Strom BL, Kimmel SE, Hennessy S (eds) Pharmacoepidemiology. Wiley, pp 241–289. https://doi.org/10.1002/9781119413431.ch13

Hurd J, Pike A, Knight J et al (2018) Health and health service use of very elderly Newfoundlanders. Can Fam Physician 64(10):e453–e461

Institute for Clinical Evaluative Sciences (2020) The ICES data repository. https://www.ices.on.ca/Data-and-Privacy/ICES-data/. Accessed 27 Jan 2020

Ihle P, Koster I, Herholz H et al (2005) Sample survey of persons insured in statutory health insurance institutions in Hessen - Concept and realisation of person-related data base. Gesundheitswesen 67:638–645

IPCI (2020) Interdisciplinary processing of clinical information. http://www.ipci.nl/Framework/Framework.php. Accessed 3 Jan 2020

ISD Scotland (2020) National data catalogue. http://www.ndc.scot.nhs.uk/National-Datasets/. Accessed 3 Jan 2020

John A, McGregor J, Fone D et al (2016) Case-finding for common mental disorders of anxiety and depression in primary care: an external validation of routinely collected data. BMC Med Inform Decis Mak 16:35. https://doi.org/10.1186/s12911-016-0274-7

JMDC (2020) JMDC Claims Database. https://www.jmdc.co.jp/en/jmdc-claims-database. Accessed 27 Jan 2020

Jurisson M, Vorobjov S, Kallikorm R et al (2015) The incidence of hip fractures in Estonia, 2005-2012. Osteoporos Int 26 (1):77–84

Kasteleyn MJ, Wezendonk A, Vos RC et al (2014) Repeat prescriptions of guideline-based secondary prevention medication in patients with type 2 diabetes and previous myocardial infarction in Dutch primary care. Fam Pract 31 (6):688–693

Kawasumi Y, Abrahamowicz M, Ernst P et al (2011) Development and validation of a predictive algorithm to identify adult asthmatics from medical services and pharmacy claims databases. Health Serv Res 46 (3):939–963

Kildemoes HW, Sorensen HT, Hallas J (2011) The Danish National Prescription Registry. Scand J Public Healt 39 (7 Suppl):38–41

Kelly JP, Rosenberg L, Kaufman DW et al (1990) Reliability of personal interview data in a hospital-based case-control study. Am J Epidemiol 131(1):79–90

Kim L, Kim JA, Kim S (2014) A guide for the utilization of health insurance review and assessment service national patient samples. Epidemiol Health 36:e2014008

Kimura S, Sato T, Ikeda S et al (2010) Development of a database of health insurance claims: standardization of disease classifications and anonymous record linkage. J Epidemiol 20. https://doi.org/10.2188/jea.JE20090066

Kimura T, Matsushita Y, Yang YHK et al (2011) Pharmacovigilance systems and databases in Korea, Japan, and Taiwan. Pharmacoepidemiol Drug Saf 20(12):1237–1245

Kulaylat AS, Schaefer EW, Messaris E et al (2019) Truven health analytics marketscan databases for clinical research in colon and rectal surgery. Clin Colon Rectal Surg 32 (1):54-60. https://doi.org/10.1055/s-0038-1673354

Kerr SJ, Mant A, Horn FE et al (2003) Lessons from early large-scale adoption of celecoxib and rofecoxib by Australian general practitioners. Med J Aust 179(8):403-407

Lynge E, Sandegaard JL, Rebolj M (2011) The Danish National Patient Register. Scand J Public Healt 39 (7 Suppl):30–33

Lu CY (2009) Pharmacoepidemiologic research in Australia: challenges and opportunities for monitoring patients with rheumatic diseases. Clin Rheumatol 28(4):371–377

Lyons RA, Jones KH, John G et al (2009) The SAIL databank: linking multiple health and social care datasets. BMC Med Inform Decis Mak 9:3–3

Manitoba Centre for Health Policy (2020) Manitoba Population Research Data Repository - Overview. http://www.umanitoba.ca/faculties/health_sciences/medicine/units/chs/departmen tal_units/mchp/resources/repository/index.html. Accessed 6 Jan 2020

Maggioni AP, Orso F, Calabria S et al (2016) The real-world evidence of heart failure: findings from 41 413 patients of the ARNO database. Eur J Heart Fail 18 (4):402–410. https://doi.org/10. 1002/ejhf.471

Marchesini G, Bernardi D, Miccoli R et al (2014) Under-treatment of migrants with diabetes in a universalistic health care system: The ARNO observatory. Nutr Metab Cardiovasc Dis 24 (4):393–399

Masclee GMC, Straatman H, Arfe A et al (2018) Risk of acute myocardial infarction during use of individual NSAIDs: A nested case-control study from the SOS project. PLoS One 13 (11):e0204746. https://doi.org/10.1371/journal.pone.0204746

National Health Insurance Research Database (2019) Background. https://nhird.nhri.org.tw/en/ index.htm. Accessed 17 Dec 2019

Newfoundland and Labrador Centre for Health Information (2020) HEALTHe NL: Better Care for Families. https://www.nlchi.nl.ca/. Accessed 6 Jan 2020

NHS digital (2020) Hospital Episode Statistics (HES) Database. https://www.hscic.gov.uk/hes. Accessed 3 Jan 2020

Nielen JTH, Boonen A, Dagnelie PC et al (2018) Disease burden of knee osteoarthritis patients with a joint replacement compared to matched controls: a population-based analysis of a dutch medical claims database. Osteoarthritis Cartilage 26 (2):202–210. https://doi.org/10.1016/j.joca. 2017.11.012

OPTUM (2013) Retrospective database analysis. https://www.optum.com/content/dam/optum/res ources/productSheets/Retrospective-Database-Analysis.pdf. Accessed 17 Dec 2019

Okamoto E (2014) Linkage rate between data from health checks and health insurance claims in the Japan National Database. J Epidemiol 24 (1):77–83

Oteri A, Trifiro G, Gagliostro MS et al (2010) Prescribing pattern of anti-epileptic drugs in an Italian setting of elderly outpatients: a population-based study during 2004-07. Brit J Clin Pharmaco 70(4):514–522

Oteri A, Mazzaglia G, Pecchioli S et al (2016) Prescribing pattern of antipsychotic drugs during the years 1996-2010: a population-based database study in Europe with a focus on torsadogenic drugs. Br J Clin Pharmacol 82 (2):487–497. https://doi.org/10.1111/bcp.12955

Petersen JL, Barron JJ, Hammill BG et al (2010) Clopidogrel use and clinical events after drug-eluting stent implantation: Findings from the HealthCore Integrated Research Database. Am Heart J 159 (3):462–470.e461

Pérez-Sáez MJ, Prieto-Alhambra D, Barrios C et al (2015) Increased hip fracture and mortality in chronic kidney disease individuals: The importance of competing risks. Bone 73(0):154–159

PHARMO Institute (2020) http://www.pharmo.nl/. Accessed 3 Jan 2020

Population Data BC (2020) Population Data BC (PopData). www.popdata.bc.ca. Accessed 6 Jan 2020

Pigeot I, Ahrens W (2008) Establishment of a pharmacoepidemiological database in Germany: methodological potential, scientific value and practical limitations. Pharmacoepidemiol Drug Saf 17 (3):215–223

Queensland Government Queensland Health (2019) Data linkage in Queensland. https://www.hea lth.qld.gov.au/hsu/link/datalink. Accessed 18 Dec 2019

QRESEARCH (2020) Generating new knowledge to improve patient care. http://www.qresea rch.org. Accessed 3 Jan 2020

Ramsay EN, Pratt NL, Ryan P et al (2013) Proton pump inhibitors and the risk of pneumonia: a comparison of cohort and self-controlled case series designs. BMC Med Res Methodol 13:82

Roos LL, Brownell M, Lix L et al (2008) From health research to social research: privacy, methods, approaches. Soc Sci Med 66(1):117–129

Ruigómez A, Brauer R, Rodríguez LAG et al (2014) Ascertainment of acute liver injury in two European primary care databases. Eur J Clin Pharmacol 70 (10):1227–1235. https://doi.org/10.1007/s00228-014-1721-y

SAIL Databank (2020) Secure Anonymised Information Linkage. https://www.saildatabank.com/. Accessed 3 Jan 2020

SA-NT Datalink (2019) Supporting health, social and economic research, education and policy in South Australia and the Northern Territory. https://www.santdatalink.org.au. Accessed 18 Dec 2019

Saltman DC, Sayer GP, Whicker SD (2005) Co-morbidity in general practice. Postgrad Med J 81 (957):474–480

Sayer GP, McGeechan K, Kemp A et al (2003) The General Practice Research Network: the capabilities of an electronic patient management system for longitudinal patient data. Pharmacoepidemiol Drug Saf 12 (6):483–489. https://doi.org/10.1002/pds.834

Seong JM, Choi NK, Jung SY et al (2011) Thiazolidinedione use in elderly patients with type 2 diabetes: with and without heart failure. Pharmacoepidemiol Drug Saf 20 (4):344–350

Schmidt M, Schmidt SAJ, Adelborg K et al (2019) The danish health care system and epidemiological research: from health care contacts to database records. Clin Epidemiol 11:563–591. https://doi.org/10.2147/clep.S179083

Schink T, Holstiege J, Kowalzik F et al (2014) Risk of febrile convulsions after MMRV vaccination in comparison to MMR or MMR+V vaccination. Vaccine 32(6):645–650

SIDIAP (2020) Sistema d'Informació per al desenvolupament de la Investigació en Atenció Primària. https://www.sidiap.org/. Accessed 29 Jan 2020

Sinnott SJ, Bennett K, Cahir C (2017) Pharmacoepidemiology resources in Ireland-an introduction to pharmacy claims data. Eur J Clin Pharmacol 73 (11):1449–1455. https://doi.org/10.1007/s00228-017-2310-7

Singhal M, Tan H, Coleman CI et al (2019) Effectiveness, treatment durability, and treatment costs of canagliflozin and glucagon-like peptide-1 receptor agonists in patients with type 2 diabetes in the USA. BMJ Open Diabetes Res Care 7 (1):e000704.https://doi.org/10.1136/bmjdrc-2019-000704

Socialstyrelsen (2020) The National patient register. https://www.socialstyrelsen.se/en/statistics-and-data/registers/register-information/the-national-patient-register. Accessed 3 Jan 2020

Smeets HM, Kortekaas MF, Rutten FH et al (2018) Routine primary care data for scientific research, quality of care programs and educational purposes: the Julius General Practitioners' Network (JGPN). BMC Health Serv Res 18(1):735. https://doi.org/10.1186/s12913-018-3528-5

Sorensen HT, Christensen T, Schlosser HK et al (2009) Use of medical databases in clinical epidemiology 2nd edn. Department of Clinical Epidemiology, Aarhus University Hospital

Suissa S, Henry D, Caetano P et al (2012) CNODES: the Canadian Network for Observational Drug Effect Studies. Open Med 6(4):e134–e140

Strom BL (2012) Overview of automated databases in pharmacoepidemiology. In: Strom BL, Kimmel SE, Hennessy S (eds) Pharmacoepidemiology, 5th edn. Wiley-Blackwell, Chichester, pp 118–122

Suissa S, Garbe E (2007) Primer: administrative health databases in observational studies of drug effects—advantages and disadvantages. Nat Clin Pract Rheumatol 3(12):725–732

Tanaka S, Seto K, Kawakami K (2015) Pharmacoepidemiology in Japan: medical databases and research achievements. J Pharm Health Care Sci 1(1):1–4.https://doi.org/10.1186/s40780-015-0016-5

Tamblyn R, Lavoie G, Petrella L et al (1995) The use of prescription claims databases in pharmacoepidemiological research: the accuracy and comprehensiveness of the prescription claims database in Québec. J Clin Epidemiol 48(8):999–1009

The Health Improvement Network (2020) What is THIN data? https://www.the-health-improvement-network.com/. Accessed 29 Jan 2020

Trinh L, Macartney K, McIntyre P et al (2017) Investigating adverse events following immunisation with pneumococcal polysaccharide vaccine using electronic General Practice data. Vaccine 35 (11):1524–1529. https://doi.org/10.1016/j.vaccine.2017.01.063

Thygesen LC, Daasnes C, Thaulow I et al (2011) Introduction to Danish (nationwide) registers on health and social issues: structure, access, legislation, and archiving. Scand J Public Healt 39 (7 Suppl):12–16

University of New Brunswick (2020) NB Institute for Research Data and Training (NB-IRDT). https://www.unb.ca/nbirdt/. Accessed 27 Jan 2020

University of Aberdeen (2020) Primary care clinical informatics unit http://www.abdn.ac.uk/pcciu/. Accessed 3 Jan 2020

University of Tasmania (2020) Tasmanian Data Linkage Unit (TDLU). https://www.menzies.utas. edu.au/research/research-centres/data-linkage-unit. Accessed 27 Jan 2020

US Department of Veterans Affairs (2019) Veterans Administration Information Resource Center. https://www.virec.research.va.gov/Index.asp. Accessed 18 Dec 2019

Valkhoff VE, Coloma PM, Masclee GMC et al (2014) Validation study in four health-care databases: upper gastrointestinal bleeding misclassification affects precision but not magnitude of drug-related upper gastrointestinal bleeding risk. J Clin Epidemiol 67 (8):921–931

Valkhoff VE, Schade R, t Jong GW et al (2013) Population-based analysis of non-steroidal anti-inflammatory drug use among children in four European countries in the SOS project: what size of data platforms and which study designs do we need to assess safety issues? BMC Pediatr 13:192. https://doi.org/10.1186/1471-2431-13-192

Venmans LM, Hak E, Gorter KJ et al (2009) Incidence and antibiotic prescription rates for common infections in patients with diabetes in primary care over the years 1995 to 2003. Int J Infect Dis 13 (6):e344–351

Victoria State Government (2019) The centre for victorian data linkage. https://www2.hea lth.vic.gov.au/about/reporting-planning-data/the-centre-for-victorian-data-linkage. Accessed 18 Dec 2019

Databases in Europe

Clinical Practice Research Datalink (CPRD)

Arlene M. Gallagher, Antonis A. Kousoulis, Tim Williams, Janet Valentine, and Puja Myles

Abstract The Clinical Practice Research Data link (CPRD) is the UK Government's preeminent research service providing anonymised NHS primary care and linked secondary data for retrospective and prospective research.

1 Database Description

1.1 Introduction

The UK's National Health Service (NHS) is a universal healthcare provider free at the point of use. Over 98% of the UK population is registered at one of 8875 general practices in the UK (NHS Digital 2020a; ISD Scotland 2019; HSC Business Services Organisation 2020; Public Health Wales NHS 2020), with general practitioners (GPs) functioning as gatekeepers to the UK healthcare system. Primary care records contain patient information gathered in general practice, as well as healthcare settings outside primary care, including data on demographics, symptoms, tests, diagnoses, treatments, behaviours and attendance in secondary care.

A patient can only be registered with one GP practice at any time. Upon registering for the first time, patients are assigned a unique patient identifier, the NHS number, which is used to identify a patient across all NHS healthcare settings. The existence of a cradle to grave healthcare patient primary care record, which can be linked to

A. M. Gallagher (✉) · T. Williams · J. Valentine · P. Myles
Clinical Practice Research Datalink (CPRD), Medicines and Healthcare Products Regulatory
Agency, 10 South Colonnade, Canary Wharf, London E14 4PU, UK
e-mail: arlene.gallagher@mhra.gov.uk

A. A. Kousoulis
Faculty of Epidemiology and Population Health, London School of Hygiene & Tropical
Medicine, London, UK

© Springer Nature Switzerland AG 2021
M. Sturkenboom and T. Schink (eds.), *Databases for Pharmacoepidemiological Research*, Springer Series on Epidemiology and Public Health,
https://doi.org/10.1007/978-3-030-51455-6_3

a range of secondary healthcare data sources, makes databases of UK primary care records rich sources of longitudinal population health data for research.

The Clinical Practice Research Datalink (CPRD) is the UK Government's preeminent research service providing anonymised NHS primary care and linked secondary data for retrospective and prospective research. CPRD services are designed to maximise the way anonymised NHS clinical data can be used to safeguard public health and improve the efficiency of clinical research. For more than 30 years, data provided by CPRD have supported a range of drug safety and epidemiological studies that have impacted on health care and resulted in over 2600 peer-reviewed publications (Clinical Practice Research Datalink 2020a).

1.2 Database Characteristics

CPRD receives all de-identified electronic health records from the patient population of consenting UK general practices, with the exception of individual patients who have opted-out of contributing data to CPRD. National opt-out statistics indicate that 2.75% of patients in England have opted out from the use of their health data for research or planning purposes (NHS Digital 2019). There are four main primary care patient management software systems in the UK and CPRD currently receives data from practices using Vision® and EMIS Health® systems. Data from practices using Vision® are curated into the CPRD GOLD database (Herrett et al. 2015) while data from practices using EMIS Health® are curated into the CPRD Aurum database (Wolf et al. 2019).

The CPRD databases are dynamic, in the sense that there is a continuing expansion in the volume of data available for research due to increasing numbers of GP practices opting to contribute data to CPRD, as well as the data collected by CPRD being updated on a daily basis. When a GP practice first signs up to CPRD, their entire patient population electronic healthcare records, including historic records, are onboarded into the CPRD databases, following which daily data updates are received by CPRD. Patients are included in the CPRD databases from when they first register with their GP practice until they transfer to another practice or death. Monthly snapshots of CPRD GOLD and CPRD Aurum databases (referred to as monthly builds) are generated and made available for observational research.

As of November 2020, the combined databases covered 59 million unique patients, of which over 16 million patients were currently registered, i.e. had not died or left the practice, representing 24% UK population coverage (https://www.cprd.com/data-highlights). CPRD is broadly representative of the diverse UK population, with a fairly even spread across deciles of age by gender compared to data from the Office of National Statistics (Wolf et al. 2019; Herrett et al. 2015), a very similar ethnicity profile compared to the UK Census (Mathur et al. 2014) and distribution across IMD 2015 deprivation deciles.

1.3 Available Data

Data are collected through the coded primary care records. These include basic demographic information (year of birth, sex, region, ethnicity), prescription details (see below), clinical events (symptoms and diagnoses), preventative care provided, tests (laboratory tests ordered and delivered in primary care with their results commonly added to the patient record via electronic links to laboratories), clinical tests performed (such as blood pressure or BMI measurements), immunisations, lifestyle indicators (BMI, smoking status, alcohol consumption), specialist referrals, hospital admissions and their major outcomes, and details relating to death.

Prescription details are only available for products prescribed by GPs but not for drugs administered in secondary care or dispensed over the counter. Prescribed medicines associated with consultations are automatically recorded with a product name and British National Formulary code, alongside the dosage instructions and quantity.

Diagnoses and other clinical data are largely coded by general practice staff using SNOMED CT (UK edition) (NHS Digital 2018b), Read version 2 (NHS Digital 2018a) and local EMIS Web® codes. UK general practices are currently transitioning to SNOMED CT as the single clinical terminology system and eventually, all prescription data will be coded using the Dictionary of Medicines and Devices (dm + d), which exists within the SNOMED CT terminological structure and is already available for CPRD Aurum (NHS Digital 2018b; NHS Business Services Authority 2018). CPRD provides data dictionaries and code browsers to researchers, and guidance on creating code lists is available to help identify codes of interest.

GPs in the UK are responsible for the general management of healthcare for women during pregnancy and will record any medical events in the GP files, as well as (where available) last menstrual period, delivery date, and delivery method. CPRD has developed a probabilistic mother-baby link algorithm based on data recorded in the primary care medical record contributing to CPRD GOLD. This identifies likely mother-baby pairs, based on family number plus maternity information from the mothers' primary care records and the month of birth of newly registered babies. Since the database is anonymised, it is not possible to do the same for fathers. A pregnancy register based on an algorithm that lists all pregnancies and associated details is also available for CPRD GOLD (Minassian et al. 2019).

GP practices in England contributing to CPRD also consent to their patient data being linked to secondary health-related datasets. Patient level data from consenting GP practices are linked via a trusted third party (TTP) using NHS number, exact date of birth, sex and patient residence postcode (Padmanabhan et al. 2019). CPRD does not receive or hold patient identifiers including name, full date of birth, postcode and NHS number. Identifiers are removed prior to transfer of data to CPRD to protect patient confidentiality. Personal identifiers are sent separately from GP practices to the TTP to enable linkage. Established linkages include Hospital Episode Statistics (hospitalisation data, including hospital admission and discharge dates, primary diagnosis for the admission using the ICD10 coding system, all clinically recorded data and all procedures performed, as well as Maternity, Critical and Augmented Care Data, but not in-hospital prescriptions) (Herbert et al. 2017), Office for National Statistics Death Registration Data (including date, place and causes of death) (Office for National Statistics 2018b), several measures of area-level deprivation [Index of Multiple Deprivation (Ministry of Housing C& LG 2015) and Townsend scores (Office for National Statistics 2018a)] as proxies of socioeconomic scores, and disease registries including the National Cancer Registration and Analysis Service (Public Health England 2017).

1.4 Strengths and Limitations

Key strengths of the CPRD databases are their size and coverage, longitudinal follow-up, representativeness, linkages to other healthcare datasets and data quality assurance processes. As of November 2020, CPRD received data from over 1750 practices, representing 24% UK population coverage (https://www.cprd.com/data-highlights). This high population coverage allows epidemiological associations to be investigated in more detail and estimated with a higher level of statistical precision than is possible with smaller data sources, which is of particular importance for the study of rare exposures and diseases (Dommett et al. 2013; Douglas et al. 2013). The length of patient follow-up [Median (25th and 75th percentile) 9.01 years (3.26–20.32) and 12.02 years (4.31–23.75) for currently registered patients in CPRD Aurum and CPRD GOLD respectively (Clinical Practice Research Datalink 2020b)] enables research into diseases with long latency and the study of long-term outcomes (Crooks et al. 2013; Cotton et al. 2013; Lalmohamed et al. 2012).

The General Medical Services Quality and Outcomes Framework contract which operates in primary care and was introduced in 2004, is an incentive payment programme for GPs which has facilitated accurate coding of key data items (for example, smoking status and the delivery of services in major disease area) (NHS Digital 2020b).

Although the primary care records in the CPRD database include data on primary diagnoses and referrals to specialist care in secondary care settings, the available data on disease management may be limited, as the patient's GP will only receive a summary of the care rather than the full secondary care record. The CPRD databases also do not currently include any data on medications prescribed in secondary care, either during a hospital stay or those prescribed by specialists in outpatient departments (for example, biologics for dermatological or rheumatological conditions).

Additional data may be available in free text entries or letters received by GPs from secondary care facilities, but this is not available to CPRD for data governance reasons. Despite these limitations, supplementary information on patient pathways can be obtained through linkage of primary care data to other data sources as described above and via CPRD's non-standard linkage service https://www.cprd.com/non-sta ndard-linkage. As with any routinely collected data sources, the data available within CPRD database have not been collected for research, but for clinical care and as such the recording and data completeness can vary across and within different GP practices.

1.5 Validation

Upon receipt of primary care data, CPRD implements various data quality checks covering the integrity, structure and format of the data, as well as further anonymisation measures before the data are incorporated into a research database. Validation of the CPRD primary care data has shown high positive predictive value of a number of diagnoses (including complex conditions and behavioural conditions) and, where evaluated, comparisons of incidence to other UK data sources are also broadly similar (van Staa et al. 2001; Ryan and Majeed 2002; Ronquist et al. 2004; Meier et al. 2000). Individual studies demonstrate a high level of validity across a range of conditions (Khan et al. 2010; Quint et al. 2014; Hagberg; Jick 2017; Jick et al. 2020; Persson et al. 2020) and a systematic review of the validity and validation of diagnoses in the primary care data found that overall, quantitative estimates of validity were high (median 89% of cases confirmed) and qualitative evidence from external rate comparisons and sensitivity analyses supported the validity of diagnoses (Herrett et al. 2010).

The quality of primary care data may be variable because data are entered by GPs during routine consultations, not for the purpose of research. CPRD undertakes various levels of validation and quality assurance on the daily GP data collection comprising of over 1000 checks covering the integrity, structure, and format of the data. Collection level validation ensures integrity by checking that a collection contains only expected data files. Structural checks at row-level are performed on the raw collection files to ensure that all data elements are of the correct type, length, and format. Duplicate records are identified and removed. Transformation level validation checks for referential integrity between records to ensure that there are no orphan records, for example that all event records link to a patient.

Research quality level validation is the final level of validation and covers the actual content of the data. CPRD provides GP practice and patient level data quality markers that may assist researchers as a first step to selecting research quality patients and defining periods where data recording was assessed as being up to standard. The patient level data quality metric is based on registration status, recording of events in the patient record, and valid age and gender. The practice-based quality metric is based on the continuity of recording and the number of recorded deaths. In addition, researchers are advised to undertake comprehensive data quality checks themselves before undertaking a study.

1.6 Governance and Ethical Issues

CPRD obtains annual research ethics approval from the UK's Health Research Authority (HRA) Research Ethics Committee (REC) to receive and supply patient data for public health research. All requests by researchers to access the data held by CPRD are reviewed by an expert review committee and data are only released for public health research subject to data governance requirements being met. A summary of all studies approved by the expert committee, including a non-technical description of the research, are published on the CPRD website in a searchable database. CPRD can facilitate collection of supplementary data to enhance the routinely collected data from the electronic healthcare record, validate recorded diagnoses via GP questionnaires or collect patient reported outcome data via patient questionnaires. The collection of these additional data may require separate ethical approval.

1.7 Documents and Publications

Data from CPRD (formerly GPRD) have been used in over 2600 published articles in peer-reviewed journals across all major therapeutic areas. A bibliography is maintained by CPRD and is available online (Clinical Practice Research Datalink 2020a). These publications cover a range of health-related research topics including pharmacoepidemiology, comparative effectiveness research, health services research, assessments of temporal trends in disease incidence, health economics, prognosis research, classical risk factor epidemiology and cluster randomised controlled trials (Ghosh et al. 2019). Key publications to date include studies showing the absence of an association between measles-mumps-rubella vaccine and autism (Smeeth et al. 2004a), cardiovascular risk after acute infection (Smeeth et al. 2004b), the lower risk of dementia associated with statin use (Jick et al. 2000), the risk of myocardial infarction in patients with psoriasis (Gelfand et al. 2006), the use of oral corticosteroids and fracture risk (van Staa et al. 2000), and the association between body mass index and cancer (Bhaskaran et al. 2014). Data from CPRD have also been used to inform clinical practice and public health policy e.g., providing evidence in a clinical guidance for the management of suspected cancer and demonstrating the safety of pertussis vaccination in pregnant women in the UK (Oyinlola et al. 2016; Donegan et al. 2014).

1.8 Data Access

Researchers can apply for a license to access CPRD data for public health research, subject to individual research protocols meeting CPRD data governance requirements. More details including the data specification, applications process, and access to linked data, are available on the CPRD website (https://www.cprd.com). Researchers can also request feasibility counts from CPRD to inform sample-size estimates and decisions regarding suitability of CPRD data for their proposed research. Any other queries including requests for the latest monthly database release notes describing the population coverage can be directed to CPRD Enquiries (enquiries@cprd.com).

References

Bhaskaran K, Douglas I, Forbes H et al (2014) Body-mass index and risk of 22 specific cancers: a population-based cohort study of 5.24 million UK adults. Lancet 384(9945):755–765. https://doi.org/10.1016/s0140-6736(14)60892-8

Clinical Practice Research Datalink (2020a) Bibliography. https://www.cprd.com/bibliography. Accessed 24 Jan 2020

Clinical Practice Research Datalink (2020b) CPRD GOLD and CPRD Aurum Release Notes. https://www.cprd.com/. Accessed 24 Jan 2020

Cotton SJ, Belcher J, Rose P et al (2013) The risk of a subsequent cancer diagnosis after herpes zoster infection: primary care database study. Br J Cancer 108(3):721–726. https://doi.org/10.1038/bjc.2013.13

Crooks CJ, Card TR, West J (2013) Excess long-term mortality following non-variceal upper gastrointestinal bleeding: a population-based cohort study. PLoS Med 10(4):e1001437. https://doi.org/10.1371/journal.pmed.1001437

Jick et al 2020 https://pubmed.ncbi.nlm.nih.gov/32222005/

NHS Digital (2018a) Read codes. https://digital.nhs.uk/services/terminology-and-classifications/read-codes. Accessed 19 Sept 2018

NHS Digital (2018b) SNOMED CT implementation in primary care. https://digital.nhs.uk/services/terminology-and-classifications/snomed-ct/snomed-ct-implementation-in-primary-care. Accessed 19 Sept 2018

NHS Digital (2019) National data opt-out. https://digital.nhs.uk/services/national-data-opt-out. Accessed 27 Jan 2020

NHS Digital (2020a) GP systems of choice. https://digital.nhs.uk/services/gp-systems-of-choice#more-information. Accessed 27 Jan 2020

NHS Digital (2020b) Quality and outcomes framework (QOF), enhanced services and core contract extraction specifications (business rules). https://digital.nhs.uk/data-and-information/data-collections-and-data-sets/data-collections/quality-and-outcomes-framework-qof. Accessed 24 Jan 2020

Dommett RM, Redaniel T, Stevens MC et al (2013) Risk of childhood cancer with symptoms in primary care: a population-based case-control study. Br J Gen Pract 63(606):e22-29. https://doi.org/10.3399/bjgp13X660742

Donegan K, King B, Bryan P (2014) Safety of pertussis vaccination in pregnant women in UK: observational study. BMJ 349:g4219. https://doi.org/10.1136/bmj.g4219

Douglas I, Evans S, Rawlins MD et al. (2013) Juvenile Huntington's disease: a population-based study using the General Practice Research Database. BMJ Open 3(4). https://doi.org/10.1136/bmjopen-2012-002085

Gelfand JM, Neimann AL, Shin DB et al (2006) Risk of myocardial infarction in patients with psoriasis. JAMA 296(14):1735–1741. https://doi.org/10.1001/jama.296.14.1735

Ghosh RE, Crellin E, Beatty S et al (2019) How Clinical Practice Research Datalink data are used to support pharmacovigilance. Ther Adv Drug Saf 10:2042098619854010. https://doi.org/10.1177/2042098619854010

Hagberg KW, Jick SS (2017) Validation of autism spectrum disorder diagnoses recorded in the Clinical Practice Research Datalink, 1990–2014. Clin Epidemiol 9:475–482. https://doi.org/10.2147/clep.S139107

Herbert A, Wijlaars L, Zylbersztejn A et al (2017) Data resource profile: hospital episode statistics admitted patient care (HES APC). Int J Epidemiol 46(4):1093–1093i. https://doi.org/10.1093/ije/dyx015

Herrett E, Thomas SL, Schoonen WM et al (2010) Validation and validity of diagnoses in the general practice research database: a systematic review. Br J Clin Pharmacol 69(1):4–14. https://doi.org/10.1111/j.1365-2125.2009.03537.x

Herrett E, Gallagher AM, Bhaskaran K et al (2015) Data resource profile: clinical practice research datalink (CPRD). Int J Epidemiol 44(3):827–836. https://doi.org/10.1093/ije/dyv098

HSC Business Services Organisation (2020) Northern Ireland GP Practice lists for professional use. https://www.hscbusiness.hscni.net/services/1816.htm. Accessed 27 Jan 2020

Jick H, Zornberg GL, Jick SS et al (2000) Statins and the risk of dementia. Lancet 356(9242):1627–1631. https://doi.org/10.1016/s0140-6736(00)03155-x

Khan NF, Harrison SE, Rose PW (2010) Validity of diagnostic coding within the general practice research database: a systematic review. Br J Gen Pract 60(572):e128-136. https://doi.org/10.3399/bjgp10X483562

Lalmohamed A, Bazelier MT, van Staa TP et al (2012) Causes of death in patients with multiple sclerosis and matched referent subjects: a population-based cohort study. Eur J Neurol 19(7):1007–1014. https://doi.org/10.1111/j.1468-1331.2012.03668.x

Mathur R, Bhaskaran K, Chaturvedi N et al (2014) Completeness and usability of ethnicity data in UK-based primary care and hospital databases. J Public Health (Oxf) 36(4):684–692. https://doi.org/10.1093/pubmed/fdt116

Meier CR, Napalkov PN, Wegmuller Y et al (2000) Population-based study on incidence, risk factors, clinical complications and drug utilisation associated with influenza in the United Kingdom. Eur J Clin Microbiol Infect Dis 19(11):834–842. https://doi.org/10.1007/s100960000376

Minassian C, Williams R, Meeraus WH et al (2019) Methods to generate and validate a pregnancy register in the UK Clinical Practice Research Datalink primary care database. Pharmacoepidemiol Drug Saf 28(7):923–933. https://doi.org/10.1002/pds.4811

Ministry of Housing C& LG (2015) English indices of deprivation 2015—GOV.UK. https://www.gov.uk/government/statistics/english-indices-of-deprivation-2015. Accessed 19 Sept 2018

NHS Business Services Authority (2018) Dictionary of medicines and devices (dm+d). https://www.nhsbsa.nhs.uk/pharmacies-gp-practices-and-appliance-contractors/dictionary-medicines-and-devices-dmd. Accessed 19 Sept 2018

Office for National Statistics (2018a) 2011 UK townsend deprivation scores. https://www.statistics.digitalresources.jisc.ac.uk/dataset/2011-uk-townsend-deprivation-scores. Accessed 19 Sept 2018

Office for National Statistics (2018b) Deaths registration data. https://www.ons.gov.uk/peoplepopulationandcommunity/birthsdeathsandmarriages/deaths. Accessed 27 Jan 2020

Oyinlola JO, Campbell J, Kousoulis AA (2016) Is real world evidence influencing practice? A systematic review of CPRD research in NICE guidances. BMC Health Serv Res 16:299. https://doi.org/10.1186/s12913-016-1562-8

Padmanabhan S, Carty L, Cameron E et al (2019) Approach to record linkage of primary care data from Clinical Practice Research Datalink to other health-related patient data: overview and implications. Eur J Epidemiol 34(1):91–99. https://doi.org/10.1007/s10654-018-0442-4

Persson et al 2020 https://pubmed.ncbi.nlm.nih.gov/32986901/

Public Health England (2017) National cancer registration and analysis service (NCRAS). https://www.gov.uk/guidance/national-cancer-registration-and-analysis-service-ncras. Accessed 27 Jan 2020

Public Health Wales NHS (2020) Health in Wales. https://www.wales.nhs.uk/statisticsanddata/typesofdata. Accessed 27 Jan 2020

Quint JK, Mullerova H, DiSantostefano RL et al (2014) Validation of chronic obstructive pulmonary disease recording in the Clinical Practice Research Datalink (CPRD-GOLD). BMJ Open 4(7):e005540. https://doi.org/10.1136/bmjopen-2014-005540

Ronquist G, Rodriguez LA, Ruigomez A et al (2004) Association between captopril, other antihypertensive drugs and risk of prostate cancer. Prostate 58(1):50–56. https://doi.org/10.1002/pros.10294

Ryan R, Majeed A (2002) Prevalence of treated hypertension in general practice in England and Wales, 1994 and 1998. Health Stat Q 16:14–18

ISD Scotland (2019) GP workforce and practice populations. https://www.isdscotland.org/Health-Topics/General-Practice/Workforce-and-Practice-Populations/. Accessed 27 Jan 2020

Smeeth L, Cook C, Fombonne E et al (2004) MMR vaccination and pervasive developmental disorders: a case-control study. Lancet 364(9438):963–969. https://doi.org/10.1016/s0140-6736(04)17020-7

Smeeth L, Thomas SL, Hall AJ et al (2004) Risk of myocardial infarction and stroke after acute infection or vaccination. N Engl J Med 351(25):2611–2618. https://doi.org/10.1056/NEJMoa041747

van Staa TP, Leufkens HG, Abenhaim L et al (2000) Use of oral corticosteroids and risk of fractures. J Bone Miner Res 15(6):993–1000. https://doi.org/10.1359/jbmr.2000.15.6.993

van Staa TP, Dennison EM, Leufkens HG et al (2001) Epidemiology of fractures in England and Wales. Bone 29(6):517–522. https://doi.org/10.1016/s8756-3282(01)00614-7

Wolf A, Dedman D, Campbell J et al (2019) Data resource profile: Clinical Practice Research Datalink (CPRD) Aurum. Int J Epidemiol 48(6):1740–1740g. https://doi.org/10.1093/ije/dyz034

IQVIA Medical Research Data (IMRD)

Melissa Myland, Caroline O'Leary, Bassam Bafadhal,
Mustafa Dungarwalla, Harshvinder Bhullar, Louise Pinder,
and James Philpott

Abstract IQVIA Medical Research Data (IMRD) are non-identified electronic
patient health records collected from UK General Practitioner (GP) clinical systems.
The IQVIA Medical Research Data currently incorporates data supplied from THIN,
a Cegedim database, which is licensed by IQVIA and data supplied by practices using
EMIS Health and contributing to IQVIA's Medical Research Extraction Scheme. The
data are generated from the daily record keeping of GPs and other staff within the
practice.

1 Database Description

1.1 Introduction

IQVIA Medical Research Data (IMRD) are non-identified electronic patient health
records collected from UK General Practitioner (GP) clinical systems. The IQVIA
Medical Research Data currently incorporates data supplied from THIN, a Cegedim
database, which is licensed by IQVIA and data supplied by practices using EMIS
Health and contributing to IQVIA's Medical Research Extraction Scheme. The data
are generated from the daily record keeping of GPs and other staff within the practice.

GP patient data collection software provides a means to render patient information non-identified. The collection software is automated and integrated within the
practice management systems meaning the data collection is unobtrusive and does
not affect any clinical use or updating of practice management systems. The non-
identified data are routinely collected from GP practices who agree to contribute
data.

M. Myland (✉) · C. O'Leary · B. Bafadhal · M. Dungarwalla · H. Bhullar · L. Pinder (✉) ·
J. Philpott
IQVIA, 210 Pentonville Road, London N1 9JY, UK
e-mail: louise.pinder@iqvia.com

© Springer Nature Switzerland AG 2021   67
M. Sturkenboom and T. Schink (eds.), *Databases for Pharmacoepidemiological
Research*, Springer Series on Epidemiology and Public Health,
https://doi.org/10.1007/978-3-030-51455-6_4

The practice management system holds complete clinical records for each patient. When a new practice is set up, the full non-identified data extract is collected and supplied. All subsequent collections are incremental, i.e., only those records that have been entered since the previous collection are extracted. In this way, retrospective data are always included with the first ever collection.

The research database was established to create a repository of UK real-world patient data for medical research to be conducted by academics, National Health Service (NHS), government, and industry across the life science sector. The use of IQVIA Medical Research Data for the purpose of medical research has been approved by the NHS Health Research Authority (NHS Research Ethics Committee ref. 18/LO/0441).

1.2   Database Characteristics

In the UK, the NHS provides centrally funded healthcare to UK residents which is free of charge at the point of delivery. The vast majority of UK residents are registered with a general practitioner (GP) near their home and consult their practice for routine health care. The system in the UK differs from some other parts of Europe in that a patient can only be registered with one GP practice at a time. Records are transferred electronically between practices in the event of a patient moving, which means a life-time record is held by the GP. The role of the UK GP is often described as a 'gatekeeper' as they decide on the patient's pathway through the health care system with regards to managing them in primary care or referring the patient to secondary care.

Patients are included in the research database when they register with a GP who contributes data and also when their practice signs up to data collection. When a practice joins the data collection scheme, a retrospective data collection is taken for all patients (including active, inactive or transferred-out) who have not opted out in order to obtain their complete medical history. When patients transfer out of their contributing practice, or die, their records up to that point remain in the database. Transferred-out patients are unable to be followed beyond their transfer. If the patient were to register with another practice who is a member of the data collection scheme, they would be given a new identifier. Patients can decide to opt out at any point by informing their practice, meaning that their data will no longer be collected from that time, with historical data kept in accordance with UK Medical Research Council (MRC) guidelines.

In summary, the data within the database includes:

- **Patient details**: Year of birth, sex, practice registration date, practice de-registration date, ethnicity
- **Morbidity data**: Symptoms, diagnoses with dates, referrals to hospitals
- **Prescribed medication**: All prescriptions with date issued, drug name, formulation, strength, quantity, dosing instructions

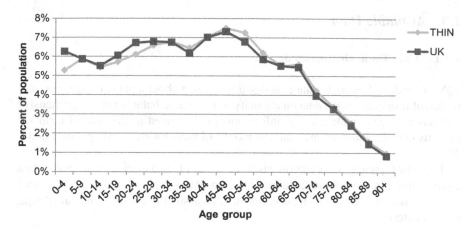

Fig. 1 Age of patients in the THIN component of the IQVIA Medical Research Data (version1805) compared to that of the rest of the UK in 2017

- **Immunisations:** All in-practice immunisations
- **Lab tests and other health data**: Smoking status, height, weight, blood pressure, pregnancy, birth, death.

Each year, three updated datasets of IQVIA Medical Research Data are released. These data are available to a range of groups including providers and commissioners of health care services (e.g., NHS England), academics and universities, life science industries, patient support groups and charities. IQVIA Medical Research Data may only be made available to external researchers for protocol-driven studies under specific Data Sharing Agreement (DSA) terms that restrict use of the data. At the time of writing the dataset contains patient data collected up to April 2019 for UK patients in England, Scotland, Wales, and Northern Ireland. In this dataset, there are a total of over 18 million patients from over 800 GP practices that can be used for research. Of these, around three million patients are currently active from 370 actively contributing practices. This represents about 4.5% of the total UK population.

Figure 1 shows the age distribution of the THIN[1] component of the IQVIA Medical Research Data compared with the UK, which is relatively similar.

Validation studies have been undertaken to examine how generalisable the THIN component of the IQVIA Medical Research Data is to the rest of the UK. Researchers have found these patients to be representative of the UK in terms of demographics (e.g., age, gender, socioeconomic status, and mortality), major Quality and Outcomes Framework (QOF) condition prevalence, and death rates (adjusted for demographics and deprivation). These patients generally reside in slightly more affluent areas compared to the rest of the UK, but the database is otherwise generalisable (Blak and Thompson 2009; Blak et al. 2011).

---

[1] A Cegedim database.

1.3   Available Data

1.3.1   Core Data: Demographics

IQVIA Medical Research Data contains information about a patient's age, sex, and region of residence. Some data on ethnicity are available but it is not comprehensive and has not been validated. Age information is restricted to the year of birth for patients over 15 and contains year and month of birth for paediatric patients under 15.

Important patient information such as date of registration with their data contributing practice and registration status (active, temporary resident, deceased) are also collected for research purposes such as assigning controls and calculating denominators.

1.3.2   Primary Care Data

Patients who consult with a GP will have a record of appointment details such as the date of consultation, symptoms, diagnoses, referrals, laboratory and physical tests, and diagnostic and therapeutic interventions. All these data (after excluding the patient identifiers) are part of the IQVIA Medical Research Data.

The Read clinical code system is used, which is a comprehensive clinical coding language including terms relating to observations (signs and symptoms), diagnoses, procedures and investigations. There are also codes for various administrative functions. The version used in the data is Version 2 which contains over 100,000 codes.

1.3.3   Prescription Data

Details of any prescriptions issued in primary care will appear in IQVIA Medical Research Data. Private prescriptions for GP prescribed medications not covered by NHS reimbursement (e.g., antimalarials, hepatitis A travel vaccination) may appear, but these medications are often prescribed in private medical travel clinics, in which case they will not appear. Over-the-counter pharmacy preparations bought by the patient are unlikely to appear in the IQVIA Medical Research Data (e.g., short term anti-diarrheal medications, laxatives, and low dose ibuprofen). Prescriptions issued by secondary care (specialists, hospitals) will not appear in the patient's electronic record and therefore will not be seen in the database. However, if secondary-initiated therapy requires continuation by the GP, these prescriptions will be in the patient's electronic record and therefore found in the IQVIA Medical Research Data. For example, if a drug for controlling hypertension (e.g., nifedipine) is prescribed in hospital then it will be continued by the GP. In contrast, if a patient is discharged on an anticoagulant like clexane for an additional, fixed four-week post-operative prophylaxis this is likely to be provided by the hospital pharmacy at discharge and will not appear in the GP record.

Drugs are mapped to system-specific codes which are in turn mapped to the British National Formulary (BNF) coded dictionary where the drug codes are organised into largely therapeutic chapters (i.e., anti-arrhythmics, anti-depressants, etc.). There is also a mapping to the international ATC classification system.

Prescription information will include the generic name of the drug, dosage, and quantity to be dispensed. The GP may also include information on how often the patient should take the drug. As each prescription has a date of issue, it is possible to track prescribing over time.

There is no direct indicator in the IQVIA Medical Research Data that identifies the specific clinical "indication" for which the drug was issued, although searching the concurrent GP visit diagnoses will commonly provide an indication. For example, a prescription for trimethoprim and a diagnosis of "urinary tract infection or pyelonephritis" will permit an inference to be made on the underlying cause. For chronic diseases, there is less likely to be a concurrent indication. For example, if a patient with a chronic history of back pain and dysmenorrhea is prescribed an NSAID. Both these indications will already be in the history and may not be re-entered.

1.3.4 Additional Health Data (AHD)

IQVIA Medical Research Data contains AHD information that includes lifestyle data, height and weight information, preventative healthcare measures, immunisations, laboratory test results (e.g., haemoglobin, lipids, renal function), and cause of death details. Identifying pregnancy within IQVIA Medical Research Data is possible through use of various algorithms, as GPs do not reliably code it as "pregnancy". Researchers at Nottingham University have undertaken extensive work on pregnancy outcomes and linkage to babies (using the household flag) in the THIN component of the IQVIA Medical Research Data.

1.3.5 Secondary Care Data

A referral to secondary care is recorded by the GP and will be seen in the IQVIA Medical Research Data. In the UK, almost all specialist care occurs in a secondary/tertiary care environment outside of the primary care centre. Once the patient has been seen in the hospital, the specialist is under obligation to provide the GP with a summary of the findings. Upon discharge from secondary care, a discharge summary will always be sent to the GP; increasingly the patient is also given a copy of the communication from the hospital. The GP will make an entry in the patient's record that such correspondence has been received; this can be seen in the IQVIA

Medical Research Data. The GP will code the important diagnoses (e.g., myocardial infarction, angioplasty) but may not code other "short-term resolved conditions" that occurred in hospital during the same episode (e.g., pneumonia, heart failure).

The level of detail available in the IQVIA Medical Research Data is dependent on the technology available at the practice. If a practice uses optical character recognition, then the content of the hospital correspondence can be seen; this may include diagnoses, length of stay, recommended prescribing, etc. If the correspondence is stored in scanned image format, then the content cannot be seen.

1.4   Strengths and Limitations

1.4.1   Strengths

The IQVIA Medical Research Data contains comprehensive recording of GP consultations and details including diagnoses, symptoms, and prescriptions issued, all in non-identified format. This provides high quality, longitudinal data on many diseases and a patient's general health. It is a repository of patient health information collected in a non-interventional manner reflecting a 'real-world' setting. As the UK population register with a GP who is the main contact for all health care, data recorded in IQVIA Medical Research Data are reflective of the general UK population and validation studies of the THIN component have confirmed this.

The IQVIA Medical Research Data is an invaluable research database as vast amounts of pre-collected data are readily available to use. The database also allows for researchers to select control subjects from the same source population as cases. Furthermore, the data format and coding systems allow researchers to develop and hone methodologies. It is also possible to study relatively rare exposures and outcomes due to IQVIA Medical Research Data's large patient population. Additionally, as the IQVIA Medical Research Data is continually updated, the effects of new treatments can also be assessed quickly.

1.4.2   Limitations

The main limitations of UK primary care databases are incomplete hospitalisation and secondary care records, and a lack of information regarding actual prescription dispensation compared with the prescribed drugs in IQVIA Medical Research Data. Such databases are also not appropriate for studies examining over-the-counter (OTC) medications as these are not routinely recorded by GPs. The data collected are primarily for the GP to manage a patient's care and not as a research tool. As such, only data the GP deems of relevance to their management of a patient's care are likely to be recorded and this should be considered in study design, e.g., a GP may not record the weight of patients where weight is not considered to be relevant. This may result in biased data.

1.5 Validation

Validation activities are undertaken both internally and externally to quantify the completeness of data within IQVIA Medical Research Data. Validation studies have been published on the THIN component of the database to examine how demographics, QOF condition prevalence, and death rates of patients compared to the rest of the UK; these were found to be similar, except slightly more patients in the THIN component were represented by the highest socioeconomic quintile (Blak et al. 2011).

Quality assurance measures are also performed at the practice level. Feedback reporting to practices identifies where data recording is not as accurate or complete as it should be. Previous feedback reports include the areas of diabetes, coronary heart disease, epilepsy, and asthma.

In addition, quality measures are undertaken and provided to researchers to inform their studies. For example, the date each practice's recording of death rates reached within three standard deviations of the regionally and demographically expected value is calculated and provided to researchers; This is known as the Acceptable Mortality Reporting (AMR) date.

1.6 Governance and Ethical Issues

The THIN data collection scheme and research database received NHS Health Research Authority [formerly known as the NHS Multi-Centre Research Ethics Committee (MREC)] approval in 2003.

In 2009, the independent Scientific Review Committees (SRCs) were established to review THIN database studies only. Studies that require patient involvement at some level (i.e., questionnaire completion) require individual approval from the NHS Health Research Authority (HRA) that covers each applicable GP practice.

In 2018, the NHS HRA approved the use of the SRC for review of IQVIA Medical Research Data incorporating data from THIN, a Cegedim database and data collected from comparable GP systems.

SRCs are composed of academic and industry researchers who are familiar with the IQVIA Medical Research Data and review studies on a volunteer basis. Each committee comprises three reviewers—one of which is the Chair and has the final verdict—and generally returns reviewed protocols to researchers within a three-week period.

Reviewers evaluate submitted protocols for scientific merit relating to IQVIA Medical Research Data and general feasibility; this process ensures that all studies conducted using IQVIA Medical Research Data that will be shared externally are well designed and use the data appropriately. The establishment of SRCs has simplified the application process for researchers and has led to a substantial decrease in the time required for scientific approval.

Contributing practices are required to display a notice in the practice waiting area detailing their involvement in the data collection scheme. Patients are able to opt out if they are uncomfortable with having their medical records used for research.

IQVIA Medical Research Data are used for research that falls into the following categories authorised by the NHS HRA:

- Epidemiology
- Pharmacoepidemiology
- Drug safety
- Public health research
- Drug utilisation studies
- Outcomes research
- Health economics research/Resource utilisation.

Small number restrictions are in place to ensure identification of patients is not possible. The identities of contributing GPs are also protected.

IQVIA Medical Research Data can be accessed via a sublicense, a 'cut' of the data, or commissioning IQVIA Real World Solutions (RWS) to conduct data analyses.

1.7 Documents and Publications

The bibliography contains over 700 publications and can be obtained on request to IQVIA. These publications show the potential scope of utilising a primary care database to investigate drug therapy risks, combine data across countries for rare events, analyse mother and baby linkage risks, investigate missed opportunities for earlier disease detection, and provide earlier signal detection of adverse drug events.

1.8 Administrative Information

The IQVIA Medical Research Data is maintained by IQVIA and funded via the provision of research services to commercial organisations, governmental institutions, and academic institutions.

Contact Details
Research: IQVIA Ltd., 210 Pentonville Road, London N1 9JY, +44 20 3075 5000
Website: https://www.iqvia.com/
Email: UKRWESDataScience@uk.imshealth.com

2 Practical Experience with the Database

Research on IQVIA Medical Research Data can involve a variety of methodologies depending on the researchers' experience, the format of the data they are using (i.e., a sublicense or extract), and the type of study they are performing. The following scenario represents an example of the criteria researchers would need to outline in order to effectively extract IQVIA Medical Research Data for research.

Example: A team of researchers would like to examine how the risk of experiencing first myocardial infarction (MI) differs between type 2 diabetics on anti-diabetic medication and type 2 diabetics who are not on anti-diabetic medication.

The researchers will be required to select a study period for the inclusion of cases and controls and to define appropriate baseline and follow-up periods. This will ensure quality and sufficient data content. They will also need to define their index date.

Study period: 1 January 2013–31 December 2018.

Index date: Date of first myocardial infarction.

Baseline: At least 1 year of data prior to index date.

Follow-up: At least 1 year of data following index date.

End date: The earliest of 31 December 2018 or death.

The researchers will then be required to define the population characteristics they would like to be included in the study, as well as exclusion criteria to remove unsuitable patients from the study.

Inclusion Criteria (case):

- *Age 45–65 years at index date*
- *First myocardial infarction between 1 January 2013–31 December 2017*
- *Prescription for study medication (would be defined) commencing ≥6 months prior to index date but not before 1 January 2013.*

Inclusion Criteria (control):

- *Age 45–65 years at index date*
- *First myocardial infarction between 1 January 2013–31 December 2017*
- *No prescription at any point in their medical record of study medication.*

Exclusion Criteria (both):

- *Prior myocardial infarction*
- *Type 1 diabetes diagnosis.*

The researchers may wish to stratify their results by looking at comorbidities that could be related (i.e., atherosclerosis).

As this information will all be coded in IQVIA Medical Research Data, the researchers will need to look up the relevant Read codes for diagnoses and drug codes for medications they would like to be included. Once these lists have been finalised, they can set to work on extracting their study population.

If the researchers had access to an IQVIA Medical Research Data sublicense, they would extract these patients on their own according to the criteria they had outlined as described above. In the case of a data extract, IQVIA would provide the researchers with a cut of the data including only the patients who fulfil the above criteria as approved by the researchers.

After outlining their study and population characteristics they would like to be included, the researchers would then commence the analysis of their choice. IQVIA Medical Research Data are available in CSV, SQL, and SAS formats to be analysed with a variety of statistical packages.

References

Blak BT, Thompson M (2009) How does the health improvement network (THIN) data on prevalence of chronic diseases compare with national figures? Value Health 12(7):A253. https://doi.org/10.1016/S1098-3015(10)74240-6

Blak BT, Thompson M, Dattani H et al (2011) Generalisability of The Health Improvement Network (THIN) database: demographics, chronic disease prevalence and mortality rates. Inform Prim Care 19(4):251–255. https://doi.org/10.14236/jhi.v19i4.820

The Health Service Executive—Primary Care Reimbursement Services Database (HSE-PCRS) in Ireland

Sarah-Jo Sinnott, Caitriona Cahir, and Kathleen Bennett

Abstract The Irish Health Service Executive-Primary Care Reimbursement Service (HSE-PCRS) database is a national repository of pharmacy claims data, representing dispensed prescriptions that were wholly or partially funded by public funds. It has been used in pharmacoepidemiology research, drug utilisation research, and health services research. This chapter provides a brief outline of how the Irish health care system operates, a description of the main features of the national dispensing database inclusive of information available and validity, examples of research using these data, and a comment on the future direction of the database.

1 Database Description

1.1 Introduction

The Irish Health Service Executive-Primary Care Reimbursement Service (HSE-PCRS) database is a national repository of pharmacy claims data, representing dispensed prescriptions that were wholly or partially funded by public funds. It has been used in pharmacoepidemiology research, drug utilisation research, and health services research. This chapter provides a brief outline of how the Irish health care system operates, a description of the main features of the national dispensing database inclusive of information available and validity, examples of research using these data, and a comment on the future direction of the database.

S.-J. Sinnott (✉)
Department of Non-Communicable Disease Epidemiology, London School of Hygiene and Tropical Medicine, London, UK
e-mail: sarah-jo.sinnott@lshtm.ac.uk; sarahjosinnott@gmail.com

C. Cahir · K. Bennett
Division of Population Health Sciences, Royal College of Surgeons in Ireland, Mercer Street, Dublin, Ireland

© Springer Nature Switzerland AG 2021
M. Sturkenboom and T. Schink (eds.), *Databases for Pharmacoepidemiological Research*, Springer Series on Epidemiology and Public Health,
https://doi.org/10.1007/978-3-030-51455-6_5

1.2 Brief Description of the Irish Health Care System

The Irish health care system is organised under the HSE; the public body responsible for the provision of publicly funded health and personal social services for everyone living in Ireland. The health system is predominantly tax funded and operates on a complex two-tiered basis (Connolly and Wren 2019). Across these public and private tiers, the majority of pharmaceutical expenditure is funded through the National Shared Services HSE-PCRS. Three principal community drug schemes exist under this system: (i) General Medical Services (GMS) scheme; (ii) Drug Payment (DP) scheme and (iii) Long Term Illness scheme (LTI). Other smaller specific schemes also exist, for example, the methadone treatment scheme for opioid dependence and a high technology drugs scheme which provides access to high cost innovative treatments, e.g., immunologics and cancer treatments, but these schemes are not discussed further here (Health Service Executive 2018).

1.2.1 General Medical Services Scheme

In 2018, almost 33% of the Irish population (1.6 million people) were in receipt of public health insurance or were covered by the GMS scheme (known locally as medical card holders) (Health Service Executive 2018). The GMS scheme entitles the individual to primary care services and hospital services free at the point of access. The exception to this is that prescription medications are subject to a flat copayment. The current copayment (as of January 2018) is €2.00 per item (capped at €20 per month per household) (Health Service Executive 2018). Copayment exemptions are extended to children in the care of the HSE, for example, in foster care and people living in emergency reception accommodation under the Irish Refugee Protection Programme. The supply of methadone for opiate dependence is also not subject to copayment. Eligibility for the GMS scheme is on the basis of income-related means-testing (Health Service Executive 2018). Automatic entitlement for those aged ≥70 years occurred between July 2001 and December 2008, however, since January 2009 means-testing was introduced for those aged ≥70 years but with a higher income threshold than those aged ≥66 years and those aged <66 years. Discretionary medical cards may be awarded in certain cases, for example, at diagnosis of cancer.

1.2.2 Drugs Payment Scheme

The remainder of the population ineligible for the GMS scheme is referred to as being in the "private" tier. Although hospital services are free to all individuals in Ireland, a proportion (approximately 43% in 2017) avail of private health insurance, the main advantage of which is more rapid access to secondary and tertiary specialist services (Connolly and Wren 2019; Health Insurance Authority 2017). For the most part, private health insurance does not cover primary care services, thus out of pocket payments for General Practitioner (GP) visits are standard practice. Individuals in the private health care system receive government-subsidised access to prescription medications through the DP scheme. Under the DP scheme, an individual or family pays up to a maximum of €134 per month (as of 2018) for their medications. Once this limit is reached, the individual or family incurs no further costs for the duration of the month (Health Service Executive 2018). In 2018, 6% of the population accessed medication under this scheme (Health Service Executive 2018). This reflects the proportion with medication costs $\geq$€134 per month.

1.2.3 Long Term Illness Scheme

Eligibility for the LTI scheme is independent of income and provided on the basis of individuals having been diagnosed with one of 16 chronic illnesses, for example, diabetes mellitus or epilepsy. Individuals in receipt of care on this scheme, approximately 4% of the population, are provided with prescription medicines relevant to the management of their chronic illness without any copayment (Health Service Executive 2018). However, individuals are responsible for GP consultation fees. Together, the LTI and GMS provide population-wide coverage for a number of chronic conditions, for example, diabetes and epilepsy.

1.3 Database Characteristics

All community pharmacists dispensing medications on the main drug schemes in Ireland submit their claims every month to the Irish Health Service Executive-Primary Care Reimbursement Service (HSE-PCRS) for reimbursement. The vast majority do so electronically (Health Information and Quality Authority 2019). The HSE-PCRS database thus captures data on every prescription filled in Ireland on the GMS scheme and the LTI scheme. However, data for medications dispensed on the DP scheme are incomplete because medications are paid for in full by the individual/family up to the monthly threshold. Hence, there is no requirement to submit a claim to the HSE-PCRS for medications already paid for by the individual. Drugs administered in hospital are not available in this database.

Individuals are eligible for inclusion in community drug scheme cohorts from the start of their eligibility for each scheme. Entry into the database occurs when a prescription is dispensed. Each individual can be followed for the duration of their eligibility and can be censored at the date on which eligibility is lost.

The majority of prescription claims in the HSE-PCRS derive from the GMS scheme, so the focus of this chapter is this scheme. The GMS population is approximately 33% of the Irish population (Health Service Executive 2018), but those who are socio-economically disadvantaged, women and those aged $\geq$70 years are over-represented, hence, there may be some limitations as regards generalisability in pharmacoepidemiological studies that rely solely on data from the GMS scheme

Table 1 Proportion of Irish men and women on GMS scheme in 2015

Age group (years)	% Men	% Women
0–15	36.2	35.5
16–24	35.1	39.6
25–34	24.4	30.2
35–44	27.0	31.2
45–54	29.9	31.0
55–64	33.2	34.8
65-69	43.4	51.5
70+	80.0	85.0
Total	35.6	39.2

Source Health Service Executive and Central Statistics Office (Central Statistics Office 2016)
Notes The % column represents the % men/women in the Irish population on the General Medical Services (GMS) scheme
GMS General Medical Services scheme

(Brown et al. 2015). For those aged ≥70 years, the database is representative of the Irish population at the same age, attributable to the fact that the majority of those aged ≥70 years are eligible for the GMS scheme (Central Statistics Office 2013). As of 2015, 80% of men and 85% of women aged ≥70 years were eligible (Central Statistics Office 2016). Therefore, studies in those aged ≥70 years have greater external validity than for other age-groups. For example, a study comparing the prevalence of potentially inappropriate prescribing (PIP) in the Republic of Ireland and Northern Ireland (which provides care via the UK National Health Service) found that PIP rates were similar between the two populations when restricted to those aged ≥70 years (Bradley et al. 2012).

However, less than 50% of the Irish population aged <70 years of age is eligible for the GMS scheme (Table 1). The impact of this limitation on generalisability was highlighted in a study comparing PIP between the Republic of Ireland and Northern Ireland in those aged 45–64 years; differences in the prevalence of potentially inappropriate prescribing between the settings were attributed to a larger proportion of socially-disadvantaged middle aged adults in the Irish database (Cooper et al. 2016). Additionally, greater proportions of those covered by the GMS scheme are smokers and women than in the general population (Brown et al. 2015). In studies of drug effects, care must be taken to ensure no prior evidence of confounding or effect modification by age, gender or smoking status. If no confounding or effect modification exists (or can be accounted for), one could reasonably assume that the effects of a drug in this population will be no different to a general population (Brown et al. 2015).

Within the HSE-PCRS pharmacy claims database, data are available from 1998 (Health Information and Quality Authority 2019). It is updated monthly due to the monthly processing of claims.

1.4 Available Data

1.4.1 Demographic Data

Information on age (age bands, e.g., 0–4; 5–11; 12–15;16–24, etc.) and gender at the individual level are available in the database, most complete for GMS and LTI eligible individuals. Information on the HSE region and one of nine community health organisations (CHOs) for each individual is also recorded. Unfortunately, clinical data and data on lifestyle behaviours are not available in this database. Due to the means-testing for GMS eligibility it is assumed that socio-economic status is lower than in the general population when restricted to <70 years. Deprivation can, however, be retrieved at the level of the prescribing GP (Cahir et al. 2014b). Data for date or cause of death are not routinely available although bespoke linkages have been constructed (see below section).

1.4.2 Drug Data

For each drug dispensed in Ireland and reimbursed by HSE-PCRS, data are available in the database for the date of dispensing, quantity of medication provided, strength, dosage form, route of administration, ingredient cost, community drug scheme on which drug was dispensed, and dispensing fees to the pharmacist. Prescriptions are coded using the World Health Organisation Anatomical Therapeutic Chemical (WHO-ATC) classification system and corresponding Daily Defined Dose (DDD) (WHO Collaborating Centre for Drug Statistics Methodology 2019). Missing data are negligible for all medication-related fields.

1.4.3 Other Data

The majority of drugs reimbursed and available in the HSE-PCRS database are from prescriptions written by GPs in primary care. Some prescriptions, however, may have been initiated by hospital consultant physicians including those on the high tech drugs scheme, e.g., interferon for multiple sclerosis or oral anti-cancer drugs. Data on diagnoses, procedures, laboratory results, and similar are not available because it is primarily a pharmacy claims database.

1.4.4 Linkages

The National Cancer Registry Ireland (NCRI), a population-based cancer registry, has been linked with HSE-PCRS data, so that detailed information on medication use is available for those with GMS eligibility and a diagnosis of cancer. This linked database facilitates detailed and high quality pharmacoepidemiological studies of cancer survival with drug exposure data available in combination with comprehensive clinical data on type and staging of cancer (Spillane et al. 2014; Flahavan et al. 2014). A second linkage has been established with The Irish Longitudinal Study of Ageing (TILDA), a nationally representative cohort study of over 8000 adults aged >50 years (Kearney et al. 2011). This linkage has permitted the conduct of high quality health services research, in particular of potentially inappropriate prescribing (Moriarty et al. 2015a, 2016). Linkages have also been established for hospital data (McMahon et al. 2014), central treatment lists for methadone users (Cousins et al. 2016), bespoke cohorts, for example, a cohort admitted to hospital with an adverse drug event (Cahir et al. 2017) or a community dwelling cohort (Cahir et al. 2014a, c; Kim et al. 2018; McLoughlin et al. 2019), and mortality data (Moore et al. 2017).

1.5 Strengths and Limitations

The national HSE-PCRS pharmacy claims database in Ireland is large and accurate. Although it is limited by its' generalisability in those aged less than 70 years, it is almost completely representative of those aged ≥70 years. This is significant because older people will make up more than 20% of Ireland's population by 2040 (McGill 2010). Furthermore, older people use the most medications in the population (Kaufman et al. 2002). Thus, the ability to carry out pharmacoepidemiological research in this population is of paramount importance. For pharmacoepidemiological research seeking to make associations between drug causes and effects (adverse events, effectiveness) the generalisability to the younger population is of concern if gender, age, and smoking are confounding variables or effect modifiers of the medication under study.

There are no clinical or outcome data in the HSE-PCRS database, but linkages to other databases are possible where patient consent is available.

Other limitations are common to all international databases of prescription claims (Schneeweiss and Avorn 2005). For example, information on medications not reimbursable by the HSE-PCRS is not available in the database. This is somewhat ameliorated in the Irish database due to a comprehensive reimbursable medications list. The relatively low copayment also means that those eligible for the GMS scheme may opt to get a prescription for an item that can be bought over the counter, if the copayment is less than the item cost. There is no information on the indication for the medication or on outcomes of any medications.

Despite these limitations, the HSE-PCRS database represents the largest source of drug exposure data in Ireland and has been demonstrated to be of good quality. It has contributed significantly to national policy-making. Additionally, universal knowledge and understanding are amplified through pharmacoepidemiology studies in cancer, health service research in inappropriate prescribing, and pharmacoeconomic analyses at the end of life stage.

1.6 Validation

Pharmacy claims databases are thought to be highly accurate because the data collected must be complete, correct, and up-to-date for reimbursement purposes (Schneeweiss and Avorn 2005). In a study of 97 patients in two Irish hospitals, it was found that the HSE-PCRS database was the most accurate method of medicine reconciliation relative to GP records and records from individual community pharmacies (Grimes et al. 2013). Considering difficulties relating to patient recall found in a study comparing self-reported drug data to dispensed drugs in HSE-PCRS in 2641 patients aged over 50 years (Richardson et al. 2013), the HSE-PCRS database represents the most accurate and complete source of information on drug utilisation in the GMS/LTI populations (Grimes et al. 2013; Richardson et al. 2013).

Furthermore, prior research indicates an association between drug exposure measured through dispensed drug records and clinical outcomes (Franklin et al. 2015; Lo-Ciganic et al. 2016). Thus, pharmacoepidemiological studies using pharmacy claims data can reasonably attempt to establish associations between causes (medications) and outcomes (for example, side effects or medication effectiveness). One limitation of HSE-PCRS data for assessing exposure to medications is worth noting. At present, there is no number of days' supply or duration of use variable, which is common in some other international prescription claims databases (Sinnott et al. 2016a). There are two workarounds to this limitation. First, the date on which a medication is dispensed along with the quantity provided can be used to estimate a duration of use. Secondly, the number of defined daily doses (DDDs) can be calculated as a proxy for days' supply by multiplying the strength of the medication dispensed by the quantity dispensed and then dividing this number by the DDD. For example, if a person is dispensed 112 tablets of 500 mg metformin, which has a DDD of 2000 mg, the person received 28 DDDs [i.e., (112 * 500)/2000]. This method has been shown to be generally accurate for drugs such as anti-hypertensive agents, proton pump inhibitors (PPIs), and cyclo-oxygenase-2 inhibitor anti-inflammatory painkillers (Sinnott et al. 2016a). However, the method can overestimate exposure for statins, atypical anti-psychotic agents, and warfarin and can underestimate for sporadically used agents such as non-selective non-steroidal anti-inflammatory drugs (Sinnott et al. 2016a).

1.7 Governance and Ethical Issues

The HSE-PCRS database falls under the remit of the HSE National Services Division. Overall responsibility and accountability for this Division lies with the HSE National Director of National Services. Requests for aggregate data can be made to the HSE-PCRS Analysis and Reporting Unit, however, there is no standard policy in place for handling such requests (Health Information and Quality Authority 2019).

1.8   The Future

The Health Information and Quality Authority (HIQA) is a statutory body that has regulatory functions in the provision of health and social services in Ireland and also has responsibilities for supporting sustainable improvements. HIQA has acknowledged that the continual development of the Irish health system is dependent on the availability of good quality data to facilitate monitoring, evaluation, and improvement. HIQA has also recognised the power and promise of the HSE-PCRS database in addressing research and policy questions of relevance and importance to the domestic and the global population. With this in mind, HIQA has made a series of recommendations to the HSE-PCRS focusing on governance and use of information. A core recommendation is that the HSE-PCRS should develop an over-arching long-term strategy that deals with data governance and quality improvement, for example, on how HSE-PCRS data can be used to generate information that in turn can be used to improve the health service. A second key recommendation is that accessibility to the data should be improved to all relevant stakeholders, e.g., patients, clinicians, policy-makers, researchers (Health Information and Quality Authority 2019).

The foundations for acting upon the HIQA recommendations have been partially laid already. The recent legislation for a unique health identifier in Ireland will assist in the development of a more complete clinical-medication database (Oireachtas Eireann 2014). Moreover, the current move to incorporate an electronic health record for each individual in Ireland presents a new paradigm for pharmacoepidemiological research in Ireland, within a framework of anonymity, consent, and appropriate governance (eHealth Ireland 2020). The availability of electronic health record data and the potential for linkages to other databases via a unique health identifier present unparalleled opportunities to carry out much needed research related to national health policies, drug effectiveness, and drug safety in large and heterogeneous populations.

Given the current era of big-data, rapidly advancing software technology, and an emphasis on making data-driven decisions it is now essential for government/public bodies, the regulator, and all invested stakeholders to align on a set of strategic priorities for this most valuable data source.

2   Practical Experience with the Database

2.1   Chronic Disease Epidemiology

Methods to calculate burden of disease metrics frequently require weighting of the data to reflect underlying population trends that cannot be detected in sample-based surveys or cohort studies. The HSE-PCRS database allows calculation (rather than estimation) of disease prevalence in specific populations such as those aged ≥ 70 years and those with specific diseases. For example, Naughton et al. calculated the prevalence of chronic disease in those aged >70 years (Naughton et al. 2006). Sinnott et al.

and Murphy et al. have relied on GMS and LTI data, which when combined provide data on every diabetes medication dispensed in Ireland thus capturing all treated individuals with diabetes, to examine the epidemiology of diabetes and geographic variation in prescribing (Sinnott et al. 2017a; Murphy et al. 2017). A limitation of the data is that without codes for diagnosis/indication some misclassification is possible, for example, women with polycystic ovary syndrome who are prescribed metformin may be included in the diabetes numerator (Sinnott et al. 2017a).

2.2   Health Services Research

The availability of the HSE-PCRS database has enabled the conduct of high quality drug utilisation research, research into adherence to medicines, and also pharmaceutical policy analysis.

2.2.1   Drug Utilisation Research

Drug utilisation research refers to the study of the use of medicines in populations with special emphasis on the resulting medical, social, and economic consequences (World Health Organisation 2003). Trends in the prescribing of (1) psychotropic medicines and antibiotics in paediatric populations (Boland et al. 2015; Keogh et al. 2012), (2) pyschoactive and sedative medicines in both a general and an older population (Byrne et al. 2018; Cadogan et al. 2018), (3) vitamin-D supplementation in a breast cancer population (Madden et al. 2018), and (4) the prevalence of polypharmacy (≥ 5 concurrent prescribed medications) have all been explored (Boland et al. 2015; Keogh et al. 2012; Moriarty et al. 2015b). The effectiveness of randomised interventions designed to improve prescribing of (i) antibiotics and (ii) preventive therapies in cardiovascular disease was evaluated using data held in the HSE-PCRS database for each GP practice involved in each of the trials (Naughton et al. 2007, 2009). Drug utilisation studies are an essential tool in evaluating the effect of prescribing interventions and provide an important resource for the conduct of pragmatic trials. This is contingent upon the availability of an up-to-date claims database and consent of involved parties.

The Health Products Regulatory Authority, the regulatory agency for medicines and medical devices in Ireland, frequently publishes drug safety warnings (Health Products Regulatory Authority 2020). A recent examination of domperidone dispensing after a 2014 safety warning revealed no decline in dispensing nor any change in the co-prescribing of drugs interacting with domperidone (Teeling et al. 2018). In 2010, Irish pharmacists were issued formal guidance to restrict the sale of over-the-counter codeine containing products. An analysis of dispensing data demonstrated that in the years after the implementation of this guidance there was some growth in the prescribing/dispening of the restricted products indicating that individuals who had been using codeine over-the-counter had started accessing the product via their GPs as an alternative route of access (Kennedy et al. 2019).

The practical value of the database in making predictions for future costs to government has recently been explored. The demographic structure of Irish society is rapidly changing owing mostly to an aging population (McGill 2010). The impact of this demographic change on medication costs on the GMS scheme has been forecast using current HSE-PCRS data and Central Statistics Office population projections. It is estimated that the GMS medications bill will rise from €1.3 billion in 2016 to €1.9 billion in 2026 (Conway et al. 2014). A related study using HSE-PCRS data found that proximity to death may be a more important driver of pharmaceutical cost than age alone (Moore et al. 2017).

2.2.2 Adherence and Medication Taking Behaviour

Pharmacy records or pharmacy claims data offer one tool for assessing medication taking behaviour in patients with chronic diseases, amongst others, and are particularly useful for the evaluation of drugs intended for long-term therapy. Medication taking behaviour can be defined in terms of two distinct variables: (1) adherence which is acting in accordance with the agreed prescribed interval and dosage of the treatment and (2) persistence which is continuing the treatment for the prescribed duration of time (Osterberg and Blaschke 2005). The HSE-PCRS has been used successfully to describe treatment adherence, persistence, initiation, and switching (Grimes et al. 2015). It has also been used to make comparisons of adherence to chronic illness medicines with other countries (Menditto et al. 2018; Sinnott et al. 2017b). A linkage to the TILDA cohort study has facilitated an examination of adherence to anti-hypertensive therapy and the role it plays in health service utilisation (Walsh et al. 2019). It is important to acknowledge, however, that adherence and persistence measures based on dispensed drug data reflect drug availability as opposed to true exposure.

2.2.3 Pharmaceutical Policy Analysis

After the global economic recession in 2008, several policy measures were implemented in Ireland to help reduce expenditure on publicly reimbursed medications. First, a copayment on the GMS scheme was introduced in October 2010 at 50 cents per prescription item. Using HSE-PCRS data to evaluate the impact of this policy Sinnott et al. found that adherence to less-essential medicines was affected to a greater degree than adherence to essential medicines. The exception to this pattern was that adherence to anti-depressant medicines was reduced substantially after the introduction of the copayment and its subsequent increase to €1.50 (Sinnott et al. 2016b). Second, reference pricing, generic substitution, and preferred drug initiatives have all been evaluated using HSE-PCRS data relying on dispensing trends and associated cost data (Spillane et al. 2015; McDowell et al. 2018).

2.2.4 Pharmacoeconomics and Health Technology Assessment (HTA)

Pharmacoeconomic analyses are used to decide whether the use of a new drug is likely to represent value for money for the health care system. Such analyses are generally comparative in nature, requiring information on the costs and utilisation of alternative treatments in specific indications (Tilson and Barry 2010). Real-world pharmacy claims data are also helpful in establishing whether evidence from the highly selected populations in phase III randomised controlled trials are transferrable to the unselected populations of everyday clinical practice (Grimes et al. 2016). The numbers of eligible recipients of new drugs can be calculated from existing pharmacy claims data to provide an estimate of the likely budget impact of introducing or reimbursement of these new medicines (Sinnott et al. 2017a).

Acknowledgements This chapter is based on an article the authors published in 2017 (Sinnott et al. 2017c). All statistics have been updated, as has the reference list.

References

Boland F, Galvin R, Reulbach U et al (2015) Psychostimulant prescribing trends in a paediatric population in Ireland: a national cohort study. BMC Pediatr 15(1):118

Bradley MC, Fahey T, Cahir C et al (2012) Potentially inappropriate prescribing and cost outcomes for older people: a cross-sectional study using the Northern Ireland Enhanced Prescribing Database. Eur J Clin Pharmacol 68(10):1425–1433

Brown C, Barron TI, Bennett K et al (2015) Generalisability of pharmacoepidemiological studies using restricted prescription data. Ir J Med Sci: 1–5

Byrne CJ, Walsh C, Cahir C et al (2018) Anticholinergic and sedative drug burden in community-dwelling older people: a national database study. BMJ Open 8(7):e022500

Cadogan CA, Ryan C, Cahir C et al (2018) Benzodiazepine and Z-drug prescribing in Ireland: analysis of national prescribing trends from 2005 to 2015. Br J Clin Pharmacol 84(6):1354–1363

Cahir C, Bennett K, Teljeur C et al (2014a) Potentially inappropriate prescribing and adverse health outcomes in community dwelling older patients. Br J Clin Pharmacol 77(1):201–210

Cahir C, Curran C, Byrne C et al (2017) Adverse drug reactions in an Ageing PopulaTion (ADAPT) study protocol: a cross-sectional and prospective cohort study of hospital admissions related to adverse drug reactions in older patients. BMJ Open 7(6):e017322

Cahir C, Fahey T, Teljeur C et al (2014b) Prescriber variation in potentially inappropriate prescribing in older populations in Ireland. BMC Fam Pract 15(1):1

Cahir C, Moriarty F, Teljeur C et al (2014c) Potentially inappropriate prescribing and vulnerability and hospitalization in older community-dwelling patients. Ann Pharmacother 48(12):1546–1554

Central Statistics Office (2013) Ireland: persons with a medical card in 2013. http://www.cso.ie/en/releasesandpublications/ep/p-wamii/womenandmeninireland2013/healthlist/health/#d.en.65619. Accessed 2 Feb 2020

Central Statistics Office (2016) Women and Men in Ireland 2016. https://www.cso.ie/en/releasesandpublications/ep/p-wamii/womenandmeninireland2016/health/. Accessed 11 Feb 2020

Connolly S, Wren M-A (2019) The 2011 proposal for Universal Health Insurance in Ireland: potential implications for healthcare expenditure. Health Policy 120(7):790–796. https://doi.org/10.1016/j.healthpol.2016.05.010

Conway A, Kenneally M, Woods N et al (2014) The implications of regional and national demographic projections for future GMS costs in Ireland through to 2026. BMC Health Serv Res 14(1):1

Cooper JA, Moriarty F, Ryan C et al (2016) Potentially inappropriate prescribing in two populations with differing socio-economic profiles: a cross-sectional database study using the PROMPT criteria. Eur J Clin Pharmacol 72(5):583–591

Cousins G, Boland F, Courtney B et al (2016) Risk of mortality on and off methadone substitution treatment in primary care: a national cohort study. Addiction 111(1):73–82

eHealth Ireland (2020) Electronic health record (EHR). http://www.ehealthireland.ie/Strategic-Programmes/Electronic-Health-Record-EHR-/. Accessed 2 Feb 2020

Flahavan E, Bennett K, Sharp L et al (2014) A cohort study investigating aspirin use and survival in men with prostate cancer. Ann Oncol 25(1):154–159

Franklin JM, Krumme AA, Tong AY et al (2015) Association between trajectories of statin adherence and subsequent cardiovascular events. Pharmacoepidemiol Drug Saf 24(10):1105–1113. https://doi.org/10.1002/pds.3787

Grimes RT, Bennett K, Canavan R et al (2016) The impact of initial antidiabetic agent and use of monitoring agents on prescription costs in newly treated type 2 diabetes: a retrospective cohort analysis. Diabetes Res Clin Pract 113:152–159. https://doi.org/10.1016/j.diabres.2015.12.020

Grimes RT, Bennett K, Tilson L et al (2015) Initial therapy, persistence and regimen change in a cohort of newly treated type 2 diabetes patients. Br J Clin Pharmacol 79(6):1000–1009

Grimes T, Fitzsimons M, Galvin M et al (2013) Relative accuracy and availability of an Irish national database of dispensed medication as a source of medication history information: observational study and retrospective record analysis. J Clin Pharm Ther 38(3):219–224. https://doi.org/10.1111/jcpt.12036

Health Information and Quality Authority (2019) Review of information management practices in the HSE primary care reimbursement service (PCRS). https://www.hiqa.ie/sites/default/files/2019-03/Review-of-information-management-practices-in-the-hse-Primary-Care-Reimburse ment-Service-(PCRS).pdf. Accessed 2 Feb 2020

Health Insurance Authority (2017) A review of private health insurance in Ireland, 2017. https://www.hia.ie/sites/default/files/Consumer%20Survey%20on%20the%20private%20health%20i nsurance%20market%20in%20Ireland%202017.pdf. Accessed 2 Feb 2020

Health Products Regulatory Authority (2020) Find a medicine. http://www.hpra.ie/. Accessed 2 Feb 2020

Health Service Executive (2018) Primary Care Reimbursement Service. Statistical Analysis of Claims and Payments 2018. https://www.hse.ie/eng/staff/pcrs/pcrs-publications/annual-report-2018.pdf. Accessed 2 Feb 2020

Kaufman DW, Kelly JP, Rosenberg L et al (2002) Recent patterns of medication use in the ambulatory adult population of the united states: The slone survey. JAMA; 287(3): 337–44.

Kearney PM, Cronin H, O'Regan C et al (2011) Cohort profile: the Irish longitudinal study on ageing. Int J Epidemiol 40(4):877–884

Kennedy C, Duggan E, Bennett K et al (2019) Rates of reported codeine-related poisonings and codeine prescribing following new national guidance in Ireland. Pharmacoepidemiol Drug Saf 28(1):106–111

Keogh C, Motterlini N, Reulbach U et al (2012) Antibiotic prescribing trends in a paediatric subpopulation in Ireland. Pharmacoepidemiol Drug Saf 21(9):945–952

Kim S, Bennett K, Wallace E et al (2018) Measuring medication adherence in older community-dwelling patients with multimorbidity. Eur J Clin Pharmacol 74(3):357–364

Lo-Ciganic WH, Donohue JM, Jones BL et al (2016) Trajectories of diabetes medication adherence and hospitalization risk: a retrospective cohort study in a large state medicaid program. J Gen Intern Med 31(9):1052–1060. https://doi.org/10.1007/s11606-016-3747-6

Madden JM, Duffy MJ, Zgaga L et al (2018) Trends in vitamin D supplement use in a general female and breast cancer population in Ireland: a repeated cross-sectional study. PLoS One 13(12). https://doi.org/10.1371/journal.pone.0209033

McDowell R, Bennett K, Moriarty F et al (2018) An evaluation of prescribing trends and patterns of claims within the preferred drugs initiative in Ireland (2011–2016): an interrupted time-series study. BMJ Open 8(4):e019315

McGill P (2010) Ilustrating aging in Ireland North and South: key facts and figures. Centre for Aging Research and Development in Ireland. http://www.cardi.ie/userfiles/Master%20CARDI%20Statistical%20Paper_%28web%29.pdf

McLoughlin A, Bennett K, Cahir C (2019) Developing a model of the determinants of medication nonadherence in older community-dwelling patients. Ann Behav Med 53(11):942–954

McMahon CG, Cahir CA, Kenny RA et al (2014) Inappropriate prescribing in older fallers presenting to an Irish emergency department. Age Ageing 43(1):44–50

Menditto E, Cahir C, Aza-Pascual-Salcedo M et al (2018) Adherence to chronic medication in older populations: application of a common protocol among three European cohorts. Patient Prefer Adherence 12:1975

Moore PV, Bennett K, Normand C (2017) Counting the time lived, the time left or illness? Age, proximity to death, morbidity and prescribing expenditures. Soc Sci Med 184:1–14. https://doi.org/10.1016/j.socscimed.2017.04.038

Moriarty F, Bennett K, Cahir C et al (2016) Potentially inappropriate prescribing according to STOPP and START and adverse outcomes in community-dwelling older people: a prospective cohort study. Br J Clin Pharmacol 82(3):849–857. https://doi.org/10.1111/bcp.12995

Moriarty F, Bennett K, Fahey T et al (2015a) Longitudinal prevalence of potentially inappropriate medicines and potential prescribing omissions in a cohort of community-dwelling older people. Eur J Clin Pharmacol 71(4):473–482. https://doi.org/10.1007/s00228-015-1815-1

Moriarty F, Hardy C, Bennett K et al (2015b) Trends and interaction of polypharmacy and potentially inappropriate prescribing in primary care over 15 years in Ireland: a repeated cross-sectional study. BMJ Open 5(9):e008656

Murphy ME, Bennett K, Fahey T et al (2017) Geographical variation in anti-diabetic prescribing in Ireland in 2013 and 2014: a cross-sectional analysis. Fam Pract 34(5):587–592. https://doi.org/10.1093/fampra/cmx036

Naughton C, Bennett K, Feely J (2006) Prevalence of chronic disease in the elderly based on a national pharmacy claims database. Age Ageing 35(6):633–636

Naughton C, Feely J, Bennett K (2007) A clustered randomized trial of the effects of feedback using academic detailing compared to postal bulletin on prescribing of preventative cardiovascular therapy. Fam Pract 24(5):475–480

Naughton C, Feely J, Bennett K (2009) A RCT evaluating the effectiveness and cost-effectiveness of academic detailing versus postal prescribing feedback in changing GP antibiotic prescribing. J Eval Clin Pract 15(5):807–812

O'Mahony L, Liddy AM, Barry M et al (2015) Hormonal contraceptive use in Ireland: trends and co-prescribing practices. Br J Clin Pharmacol 80(6):1315–1323

Oireachtas Eireann (2014) Health Identifiers Act 2014. http://www.irishstatutebook.ie/eli/2014/act/15/enacted/en/pdf. Accessed 2 Feb 2020

Osterberg L, Blaschke T (2005) Adherence to medication. N Engl J Med 353(5):487–497

Richardson K, Kenny RA, Peklar J et al (2013) Agreement between patient interview data on prescription medication use and pharmacy records in those aged older than 50 years varied by therapeutic group and reporting of indicated health conditions. J Clin Epidemiol 66 (11):1308–1316. https://doi.org/10.1016/j.jclinepi.2013.02.016

Schneeweiss S, Avorn J (2005) A review of uses of health care utilization databases for epidemiologic research on therapeutics. J Clin Epidemiol 58(4):323–337

Sinnott S-J, McHugh S, Whelton H et al (2017a) Estimating the prevalence and incidence of type 2 diabetes using population level pharmacy claims data: a cross-sectional study. BMJ Open Diabetes Res Care 5(1):e000288. https://doi.org/10.1136/bmjdrc-2016-000288

Sinnott S-J, Polinski JM, Byrne S et al (2016a) Measuring drug exposure: concordance between defined daily dose and days' supply depended on drug class. J Clin Epidemiol 69:107–113

Sinnott S-J, Whelton H, Franklin JM et al (2017b) The international generalisability of evidence
    for health policy: a cross country comparison of medication adherence following policy change.
    Health Policy 121(1):27–34
Sinnott SJ, Bennett K, Cahir C (2017c) Pharmacoepidemiology resources in Ireland-an introduction
    to pharmacy claims data. Eur J Clin Pharmacol 73(11):1449–1455. https://doi.org/10.1007/s00
    228-017-2310-7
Sinnott SJ, Normand C, Byrne S et al (2016b) Copayments for prescription medicines on a public
    health insurance scheme in Ireland. Pharmacoepidemiol Drug Saf 25(6):695–704. https://doi.org/
    10.1002/pds.3917
Spillane S, Bennett K, Sharp L et al (2014) Metformin exposure and disseminated disease in patients
    with colorectal cancer. Cancer Epidemiol 38(1):79–84
Spillane S, Usher C, Bennett K et al (2015) Introduction of generic substitution and reference
    pricing in Ireland: early effects on state pharmaceutical expenditure and generic penetration, and
    associated success factors. J Pharm Policy Pract 8(1):1
Teeling M, MacAvin MJ, Bennett K (2018) Impact of safety warnings on domperidone prescribing
    in Ireland. Ir J Med Sci 187(2):281–285. https://doi.org/10.1007/s11845-017-1657-1
Tilson L, Barry M (2010) Recent developments in pharmacoeconomic evaluation in Ireland. Expert
    Rev Pharmacoecon Outcomes Res 10(3):221–224. https://doi.org/10.1586/erp.10.33
Walsh CA, Cahir C, Bennett KE (2019) Association between adherence to antihypertensive medi-
    cations and health outcomes in middle and older aged community dwelling adults; results from
    the Irish longitudinal study on ageing. Eur J Clin Pharmacol 75(9):1283–1292
WHO Collaborating Centre for Drug Statistics Methodology (2019) ATC/DDD Index 2020. http://
    www.whocc.no/atc_ddd_index/. Accessed 2 Feb 2020
World Health Organisation (2003) Introduction to drug utilization research. Chapter 1: What is drug
    utilisation research and why is it needed? Available from http://apps.who.int/medicinedocs/en/d/
    Js4876e/

Pharmacoepidemiological Research Data Sources in the Nordic Countries—Administrative Registers in Finland, Sweden, and Norway

Tuire Prami, Rosa Juuti, and Ilona Iso-Mustajärvi

Abstract From a pharmacoepidemiological point of view, administrative real-world register data originating from routine medical practice are essential in post-approval observational studies. Finland, Sweden, and Norway are located in the north of Europe, and their combined population is around 20 million people.

1 Database Description

1.1 Introduction

From a pharmacoepidemiological point of view, administrative real-world register data originating from routine medical practice are essential in post-approval observational studies. Finland, Sweden, and Norway are located in the north of Europe, and their combined population is around 20 million people. The Nordic countries have a common history and strong cultural ties, including similar political systems. The social structure is similar, and free education and health care cover the whole population. In addition to Finland, Sweden, and Norway, the Nordic countries include Denmark and Iceland, but this chapter concentrates on the three countries firstly mentioned.

T. Prami (✉) · R. Juuti · I. Iso-Mustajärvi
EPID Research, Espoo, Finland
e-mail: phd.prami@gmail.com

T. Prami
Oriola Corporation, Espoo, Finland

R. Juuti
Health and Social Data Permit Authority Findata, Helsinki, Finland

I. Iso-Mustajärvi
MedEngine, Helsinki, Finland

© Springer Nature Switzerland AG 2021
M. Sturkenboom and T. Schink (eds.), *Databases for Pharmacoepidemiological Research*, Springer Series on Epidemiology and Public Health,
https://doi.org/10.1007/978-3-030-51455-6_6

1.2 Database Characteristics

The Nordic national health registers have population-wide coverage within each country. Inclusion is not based on incomes, insurances or other social statuses, and the overall quality of the registers is high. All Nordic citizens have unique personal identification numbers (IDs), which makes linkage of different registers possible. The main Finnish, Swedish, and Norwegian administrative registers used in pharmacoepidemiological studies are described below.

1.2.1 Prescription Registers

The prescription registers contain information on outpatient medication purchases. In Finland, the data have been electronically available since 1994, in Sweden since 2005, and in Norway since 2004 (Table 1). The prescription-only medicines are sold exclusively in pharmacies, and for dispensing, a prescription issued by a physician or

Table 1 Personal level data availability in the selected Nordic health registers

Register	Finland	Sweden	Norway
Prescriptions	1994	2005	2004
Hospital Care	1956 1967[a] 1998[b]	1964 1987[a] 1997[c] 2001[d]	2008
Primary Care	2011	-	2017
Cancers	1952	1958	1952
Medical Births	1987	1973	1967
Causes of Death	1969	1961	1951

[a]Nationwide coverage
[b]Outpatient hospital visits and day surgeries
[c]Day surgeries
[d]Outpatient hospital visits

a dentist is required. The data in the prescription registers are updated continuously (at least monthly), but the final data for the particular year are available during the first quarter of the following year.

In Norway, the prescription register is a so-called pseudonymous register (Furu 2008). In practice, this results in a few limitations in using the data for register-based research where data linkage is required. It is, for example, not possible to form a study cohort in the Norwegian prescription register and deliver the IDs of this population to other registers for data extraction. Instead, another register must form the cohort and deliver the ID information to the prescription register for further prescription data extraction and linkage.

Apart from the prescription registers, there are separate vaccination registers in each country. Adequate data have been available only since the 2010s, and they cover mainly children vaccinations and vaccinations given under national immunization programs. In recent years, the aim has been to include other sectors in the data too to cover self-imposed vaccinations as well as vaccinations administered via the private sector and occupational health care. In Finland, the responsible authority for registering vaccinations is the Finnish Institute for Health and Welfare, in Sweden the Public Health Agency and in Norway the Norwegian Institute for Public Health.

1.2.2 Patient Registers

Nationwide data on all inpatient and outpatient visits to hospitals are recorded in all Nordic countries. A hospital discharge register was established in Finland in 1956 (nationwide coverage from 1967 onwards), in Sweden in 1964 (nationwide coverage from 1987 onwards) and in Norway in 1997 (Table 1) (Lovdata 2020; Ludvigsson et al. 2011; Sund 2012). The Finnish Care Register for Health Care is one of the oldest in the world. The Finnish register was supplemented with data on day surgeries and outpatient hospital visits in 1998, and the Swedish register in 1997 and in 2001, respectively (Ludvigsson et al. 2011; Sund 2012). In addition to this, data on primary care has been available through a separate register in Finland since 2011 (Sund 2012) and in Norway since 2017 (Bakken et al. 2019).

Data within the Norwegian patient register have been documented at individual patient level since 2007 and were linked with IDs and names only after that (Lovdata 2020). This means that in the Norwegian patient register, a single person could be identified only ever since the law came into effect in 2007.

Hospital care registers in all countries are updated regularly. The Swedish register is updated monthly and the Finnish and Norwegian registers once a year. In Finland, the data for the previous year are available in September, and in Norway between March and June as the different health care sectors update their data at different times.

1.2.3 Cancer Registers

Finland, Sweden, and Norway all have a long history of cancer registration (Table 1). The Nordic cancer registries are among the oldest population-based registries in the world with more than 60 years of complete coverage (Pukkala et al. 2018). Notification is compulsory for all health care providers in these countries (Finnish Cancer Registry 2019; Larsen et al. 2009; Nilsson et al. 2014). In Finland and Norway, information from death certificates is by default reported to the cancer registers, whereas in Sweden a separate notification is needed to transfer autopsy-related cancer diagnoses to the register (Barlow et al. 2009; Nilsson et al. 2014).

Lag time of the Finnish Cancer Registry is somewhat longer than in other health registers because of the delays in notification: approximately two years (Korhonen et al. 2002). In Norway and Sweden, the lag time is approximately one year.

1.2.4 Medical Birth Registers

Finland, Sweden, and Norway have been keeping medical birth registers (MBRs) for an extensive period of time (Table 1), and notification to the registers is compulsory (Langhoff-Roos et al. 2014). For example, in Norway, the MBR was founded partly because of the thalidomide catastrophe (Irgens 2000). All live and stillbirths are reported to the registers. In these registers, the new-born child is usually followed-up until discharge from the hospital or until the end of the first week of life, whichever comes first (Gissler 2010). In Finland, additional data are collected on premature infants. Congenital anomalies are either recorded in the MBR as in Norway, or reported to a specific malformations register as in Finland and Sweden (Finnish Institute for Health and Welfare 2020a; Källén 2015). Data lag times of the registers are between 9 and 12 months.

In all three countries, the MBR data of labours originate from maternity wards in public hospitals where in practise all children are born. These data are supplemented by birth and death certificates (Finnish Institute for Health and Welfare 2020b). For example, information on perinatal deaths (stillbirths or deaths during the first week of life) is revised and supplemented from the cause of death registers. This cross-linking of the medical birth registers' data with those in population and cause of death registers increases the quality and completeness of the birth data (Gissler 2010).

In Finland, Sweden, and Norway, planned home births represent between 0.01 and 0.15% of all births (Gissler 2010). Finland and Norway have separate statistics on unplanned home births and births during transportation to hospital. They represent 0.2 and 0.7% of the births in these countries, respectively. The Nordic medical birth registers cover even these cases.

1.2.5 Cause of Death Registers

Statistics on all deceased people who live in a particular country or live abroad but are registered in that country are recorded in the cause of death registers in the Nordic countries (Norwegian Institute of Public Health 2020b; Socialstyrelsen 2020a; Statistics Finland 2020a). Nationwide cause of death registers were established in the 1950s–1960s (Table 1). The lag time for data updates varies from 8 months in Sweden to 13 months in Finland.

1.3 Available Data

The Nordic registers share many similarities such as common data content and structure. In each country, it is possible to collect the population-wide information without informed consent from the individuals. There are, however, some differences in coding systems and general processes (Furu et al. 2010). Lifestyle factors such as smoking habits and alcohol consumption, as well as detailed clinical data, such as blood pressure measurements, are lacking in these registers or are only recorded sporadically. Some of the quality registers include this kind of data with better coverage.

1.3.1 Prescription Registers

In Sweden and Norway, all prescribed medicines purchased in pharmacies are included in the prescription registers (Norwegian Institute of Public Health 2019; Socialstyrelsen 2019). The data on non-prescription over-the-counter (OTC) medicine sales are not in the prescription databases. As an exception, prescribed and dispensed OTC drugs, e.g., for chronic diseases are included.

In Finland, the information in the prescription register contains purchases made by outpatients in pharmacies, but is limited to those purchases of prescribed medicines reimbursed by the government. This excludes, for instance, most contraceptives. Since 2011, electronic prescriptions irrespective of the reimbursement status have been recorded in a separate e-prescription register.

This Finnish electronic prescription system has been compulsory in public health care since April 2013, in private health care since January 2015, and in small private clinics that write less than 5000 prescriptions per year since January 2017. It is possible for the patient to refuse the e-prescription and have a traditional paper prescription instead, in which case the information is not recorded in the e-prescription register but in the traditional prescription register instead.

In all countries, the prescription register data include, for example, information on the prescriber, ID of the patient (revealing the date of birth and sex of the patient), generic name of the drug, anatomical therapeutic chemical classification of the drug

(ATC code), brand name, formulation and package size, amount in defined daily doses (DDD), and date of purchase.

In general, indication for or intended duration of drug use as such are not available in prescription registers. The indication (as well as the exact prescribed dose) is available only as free text, which cannot be easily utilized for research purposes. The reimbursement code may, however, function as a proxy for diagnosis in some cases (Furu et al. 2007). In Finland, information on chronic diseases can be obtained from a separate register on special reimbursements for treatment of chronic diseases.

1.3.2 Patient Registers

All Nordic countries have a hospital care register (including both in- and outpatient visits), and they include demographic variables as well as data on time and place of treatment, duration of hospitalizations, primary and secondary diagnoses, and surgical procedures performed. Data on drugs administered during hospital care are widely underreported and this variable is thus considered unusable. The diagnoses have been recorded using the 10th revision of the International Classification of Diseases (ICD-10) in all hospital care registers in Nordic countries since the late 1990s. Procedures are recorded using NOMESCO classification for surgical procedures (NCSP) in all three countries.

In Finland, there has been a nationwide register for public primary care available since 2011 (Sund 2012) and in Norway since 2017 (Bakken et al. 2019; Helsedirektoratet 2020b). In general, these registers include similar data to the hospital care registers, but in the primary care setting. In both registers, the diagnoses are coded with the 2nd edition of International Classification of Primary Care (ICPC-2) codes. Sweden does not have a nationwide primary care register with data available for research due to problems with data integrity and data volumes, but they have a nationwide quality system through which aggregate data can be viewed (Swedish Association of Local Authorities and Regions 2020b).

Data from occupational health care organized often in the private sector are not available in nationwide registers. In Finland, information on occupational health care service usage is available from the hospital care register from 2019 onwards, but without patient-level information on, e.g., diagnoses (Terveyden ja hyvinvoinnin laitos 2020a).

1.3.3 Cancer Registers

In all three countries, malignant cancers are recorded in the cancer registers. Many *in situ* tumours are also reported, though there have been some temporal and anatomical site-related changes in the registration of these as well as in their inclusion in the national statistics (Pukkala et al. 2018). The variable contents are basically similar in the three countries. The registers include data on socio-demographic details of the patient, time of the diagnosis, topography and morphology of the tumour, and clinical stage of the disease (Finnish Cancer Registry 2019; Larsen et al. 2009; The National Board of Health and Welfare 2020). In Finland and Norway, the cancer treatment is also available, although only the treatment given and planned at the time of reporting is recorded (Finnish Cancer Registry 2019; Larsen et al. 2009).

1.3.4 Medical Birth Registers

Some variation between the medical birth registers exists, but they all include background information (e.g., marital and smoking statuses) and diagnoses (ICD codes) of the mother as well as information on previous pregnancies and deliveries. Details of the current pregnancy and delivery, including the course and possible interventions taken, and details on the health of the newborn are also recorded in all three countries (Gissler 2010).

There have been changes to the data content of the MBRs over the years in order to improve reliability of the register. In addition, updates of the notification forms have been carried out to bring the collected information more in line with current care practices.

1.3.5 Cause of Death Registers

Cause of death registers include demographic variables as well as data on cause (ICD codes), time, and place of death. Data, for example, on underlying causes of death, nature of injury, and information on surgery within four weeks before death or intent in cases of injury or poisoning are also available from the registers.

1.4 Strengths and Limitations

Finland, Sweden, and Norway have well-developed population-wide register systems with tens of years of longitudinal data (Table 1). In each Nordic country, all residents have a unique personal ID that encodes date of birth and sex. Based on similar legislation, use of different health registers is allowed for research purposes in all countries, and data linkage between different registers is possible at the individual level by using the IDs. This is an important factor behind the long tradition of register-based epidemiological studies in the Nordic countries. In general, the data are free of charge but moderate costs occur for administrative tasks and data mining. Pooling data from several countries enables running a powerful study with an international but homogenous population.

Main challenges in using these registers for research lie in the need of knowledge of local health care systems, local language, and the inherent limitations of the data collection in each country. In the data management phase, in-depth understanding of differences between coding and variable structure in different countries is required.

Thus, it is very important to have collaborators in each country with experience on working with the registers.

In Sweden and Norway, there are, in addition to administrative registers, several regional and nationwide quality registers, which can be used for research purposes in different therapy areas (Cancer Registry of Norway 2020; Swedish Association of Local Authorities and Regions 2020a). In Finland, national development for set-up of quality registers has begun in 2018 (Terveyden ja hyvinvoinnin laitos 2020b). Quality registers often gather data from different health registers, but they also collect data from patients with surveys. In general, data linkage between different individuals, e.g., family members, is not possible if not embedded into the original data (e.g., maternal and new-born information in MBRs). In Sweden and Norway, there are, however, separate generation databases (the Swedish Multi-generation Register; Generation Database held by Statistics Norway) that enable the linkage of family members.

1.5 Validation

1.5.1 Prescription Registers

Quality of the data in the Finnish Prescription Register has been estimated very high. Quality assessments performed by the register holder can be found since 2006 (Kansaneläkelaitos 2019). Coverage of the Finnish Prescription Register containing information on all reimbursed drug purchases of all permanent residents in Finland is about 97% of the prescriptions. Missing data includes, e.g., relatively inexpensive packages with no reimbursement.

The Swedish Prescribed Drug Register was evaluated in 2007 and in 2016 (Wallerstedt et al. 2016; Wettermark et al. 2007). A dropout from the register can occur, e.g., due to a misrecorded ID or protected identity of the patient. The rate of missingness varies between recorded variables, being nowadays approximately 0% for the most important variables (Socialstyrelsen 2020f).

The quality of the Norwegian Prescription Database was evaluated in 2008 (Furu 2008). The proportion of prescriptions having invalid ID information was approximately 2% in 2007. In order to detect possible inconsistencies, the register holder runs frequent routine checks on the data before transferring it to the actual register. Overall, the quality of the data is high.

1.5.2 Patient Registers

The quality of the patient registers in general is very good. The validity of the documented data varies between different types of diagnoses in all countries. The positive predictive value (PPV) for rare diagnoses is lower than for common diseases.

In Finland, the data coverage in recent years has been reported to be 95% of the visits. Among the recorded visits, 8% of outpatient visits and 0.1% of inpatient visits were lacking diagnosis data (Finnish Institute for Health and Welfare 2020c). In Sweden, the PPV of documented diagnoses is generally 85–95%, but sensitivity varies between different diagnoses (Ludvigsson et al. 2011). Diagnosis data was lacking in approximately 1% of all visits between 1988-2016 (Socialstyrelsen 2020d). In Norway, the data coverage is presented in comparison to various disease-specific quality registers by dividing the number of observations in the patient register by the combined number of observations in the patient register and the quality register in question. This way, the coverage percentage per specific disease varies between 84 and 100% (Helsedirektoratet 2020a).

1.5.3 Cancer Registers

The accuracy of the data in the Finnish Cancer Registry was regarded good when the records were checked by specialists. The total false-positive discrepancy rates varied from 2.4 to 10.7% for eight major cancer sites (including, e.g., lung, prostate, stomach, and pancreatic cancers) (Korhonen et al. 2002). Between 2009 and 2013, the record completeness was estimated at 96 and 86% for solid tumours and non-solid tumours, respectively (Leinonen et al. 2017). Underreporting was most prominent for hematological malignancies and other tumours not histologically verified.

A quality study published in 2009 compared data from the Swedish Cancer Register to that of the patient register and found the underreporting rate to be approximately 4% (Barlow et al. 2009). The differences were highly dependent on the cancer site and age of the patient.

Sweden is the only Nordic country with no legal basis to routinely use cancer information from the death certificates to supplement the national cancer registry (Pukkala et al. 2018). This reduces the completeness of registration particularly for poorly investigated cases, and the validity of incident cancer cases becomes incomplete. Due to this, the proportion of underreporting of cancer cases is higher in Sweden than in the other Nordic countries.

Underreporting in the Cancer Registry of Norway was estimated to be 2.2% in 2005 (Larsen et al. 2009). This was especially evident in hematologic and central nervous system malignancies. In another Norwegian study, patient register data was compared with data from the Cancer Registry of Norway and was found to differ for different cancer diagnoses (Bakken et al. 2012). For the studied diagnoses the compliance rate was between 81 and 97%.

The core characteristics of the Nordic cancer registers were recently described and compared by a multinational research team including members from all five Nordic cancer registers (Pukkala et al. 2018). This publication explains differences in cancer incidence rates across the countries. Even though the information in the Nordic cancer registries can be in general considered very similar, there are many differences in registration routines, classification systems and inclusion of some tumours. These differences are important to be aware of when comparing trends between the countries.

1.5.4 Medical Birth Registers

The statistical coverage of birth cases as such is up to 100% in the Nordic countries. Validation of the medical birth registers has been conducted in each country, but only in relation to certain outcomes or variables and for different periods of time (Baghestan et al. 2007; Gissler and Shelley 2002; Mattsson et al. 2016). The results from the validation studies have been used to improve notification and quality control routines (Langhoff-Roos et al. 2014). In Finland and Sweden, the registers publish yearly quality descriptions of the data (Finnish Institute for Health and Welfare 2020b; Socialstyrelsen 2020c).

1.5.5 Cause of Death Registers

Data coverage in causes of death registers is extremely high. In all three countries, the coverage of the register is very close to 100% because all deaths are verified against the population register. In recent years, the number of missing death certificates from the yearly statistics has been 0.9% in Finland, 1–2% in Sweden and less than 2% in Norway (Pedersen and Ellingsen 2015; Socialstyrelsen 2020b; Statistics Finland 2020b). The greatest source of uncertainty is the reporting doctor's determination and further the proper recording of the cause of death.

1.6 Governance and Ethical Issues

1.6.1 Legal Issues

Strict laws about confidentiality of data in health registers apply in all Nordic countries. National regulations set limits on the disclosure of data that may lead to identification of individuals. By default the register holders of health registers are prohibited from disclosing information of specific individuals when personal identification is possible. In general, only aggregated or de-identified data can be delivered from the original register holders to the applicant. Through an exception identifiable data can be, however, provided for research purposes.

Personal level data—even with the possibility to identify a particular person—can be used for scientific purposes in certain circumstances. This applies to specific research projects that are described in detail, and in which there is a need for individual level data in order for the results to be purposeful. The data may be disclosed if it is clear that no damage or harm will be caused for the individual or someone close to him/her. The researchers need to be experienced enough and have feasible resources to handle confidential register data.

As the Nordic countries have long traditions of strict personal data legislation, the European Union (EU) General Data Protection Regulation (GDPR), valid since 2016 and put into effect in the member states in 2018, did not substantially alter the underlying premise for performing research based on register data or register linkage, or the movement of data within EU countries (Privacy Europe 2019). This can be stated at least from a northern European point of view, where the issue remains for close monitoring.

1.6.2   Ethics Committee Review

An ethical committee evaluates the purpose of the study and whether it can be considered ethically unobjectionable. In all Nordic countries, independent ethics committees (ECs) evaluate whether studies have been planned in an ethically acceptable manner. No unnecessary harm or risks must be caused to potential research subjects. Particular emphasis is given to safety, legality, and rights of the subjects. Ethics committees are not responsible for granting licenses or permits to carry out the planned study.

There are several ethics committees within each Nordic country, but an application must be sent to only one of the boards, usually to the regional ethics committee based on the principal investigator's location. In principal, this is the case also among different countries within the European Union. EC permit processes are liable to a fee. In each Nordic country, the applicant receives the EC decision within two months of submission of a complete application.

In Sweden, there has been a law (2003:460) in force since January 1, 2004, which deals with vetting the ethics of all studies that involve humans and handling sensitive personal level data. Also in Norway, ethics committee approval is needed for pharmacoepidemiological studies if identifiable personal information from one or several health registers is used.

According to the Finnish legislation (488/1999), approval from an ethics committee is required for medical research that intervenes with the integrity of human subjects. This act does not apply solely to document- or statistics-based register studies. It is then possible to run a pure register-based study without vetting issued by an EC. An EC approval can, however, be requested for these types of studies if considered applicable by the researchers.

1.6.3   Data Permit Processes

Data from health registers can be accessed after a study permit process. In case of pharmacoepidemiological studies, the application is based on a detailed study protocol with scientific aims. The procedure for applying for data is separately described in detail for each data holder in different countries. The application processes are usually carried out in the local languages.

Commonly in all Nordic countries, many of the data holders are responsible for more than one register. In these cases, the data from all the registers under one organization can be applied for with one permit. These permit processes are handled by the particular register holder, as is the case with data permit processes including one source register only.

If data are requested from different register holders, a separate application is needed for all of them in Sweden and in Norway. This used to be the case in Finland too, but since January 1, 2020, the new Health and Social Data Permit Authority Findata is responsible for handling the data permit processes for studies with several data holders in Finland, and thus only one data permit is required.

Data from different sources can be linked with the IDs. In Sweden and in Norway, this data linkage phase is usually performed by one of the register holders involved in the data delivery. This limits the transfer of the highly confidential data. In Finland, Findata is responsible for linking data originating from different register holders. Based on the new processes, this type of Finnish data is not in prinicple delivered to the researchers anymore but Findata stores them and gives researchers remote access to them.

For register studies, the permit processes take 3–6 months in Sweden (Social-styrelsen 2020e). Also in Norway, the permit processes are well described and scheduled. Depending on the level of data linkage, the data are delivered 30–60 days after submission of an approved application (Norwegian Institute of Public Health 2020a). In Finland, this study phase has been unpredictable and unnecessarily time-consuming. One purpose of Findata is to speed up the permit process.

1.6.4 Governance and Data Protection Authorities

The informed consent of an individual to participate in a study is usually not needed in scientific studies where all information originates from registers and individuals are not contacted, and where the information collected does not affect the treatment of the individual.

When collecting data from health registers, a new register will eventually be formed. The research organization is responsible for lawful management of personal data as data controller. According to the GDPR, the data controller must be able to prove its GDPR compliance. This means, for example, ability to demonstrate a designated data protection officer, train the research staff for secure data handling, and document the data collection, storage and handling processes. The data protection authorities regulating personal data handling are the Office of the Data Protection Ombudsman (in Finland), the Swedish Data Protection Authority, and the Norwegian Data Protection Authority.

1.7 Documents and Publications

A number of articles published in peer-reviewed journals reflect the contribution of Nordic registers to pharmacoepidemiological studies. Wettermark *et al.* found that from 2005 to 2010 a total of 245 studies were performed in Finland, Sweden, and Norway using prescription databases (Wettermark et al. 2013). These studies were found in PubMed in English. In addition to the internationally published studies, surveys reported in local languages are numerous.

Of the 245 studies mentioned above, 97 were performed in Finland, 61 in Sweden, and 87 in Norway. At the same time, Denmark contributed to the field with 262 studies (Wettermark et al. 2013). More than half of the studies from Finland (55%) were drug effectiveness or safety studies whereas drug utilization studies were highlighted in Sweden (80%) and Norway (69%). This reflects the fact that in the Finnish studies, it was more common to link data from other registers to the exposure data (70%, 52%, and 31%, respectively). Drug utilization studies from Sweden concentrated on polypharmacy, quality of prescribing, physicians' adherence to clinical guidelines, as well as on patients' compliance. The drug utilization studies on abuse were mainly performed in Norway.

Less than 10% of the studies reviewed by Wettermark *et al.* covered all drug groups (2013). Most commonly studied medication therapy areas were the nervous system (ATC class N; 42%), the cardiovascular system (ATC class C; 20%), and the alimentary tract and metabolism (ATC class A; 13%). Studies in children originated most commonly from Finland (12 studies) and Norway (10 studies) and studies in the elderly from Sweden (19 studies).

To date, the review on the topic by Wettermark *et al.* is still the most recent (2013). In general, the number of pharmacoepidemiological studies has been increasing including multinational studies.

One example involves all five Nordic countries. Its cohort originating from nation-wide registers covers the whole Nordic population (Furu et al. 2015). The subject of this study handles the association between maternal drug exposure and birth defects—an aspect often studied particularly in Nordic countries.

A recent study describes anti-diabetic treatment patterns in four Nordic countries. All type 2 diabetes mellitus patients treated with glucose-lowering drugs between 2006 and 2015 were identified in prescription registers in Denmark, Finland, Norway, and Sweden (Persson et al. 2018). The data were linked with national patient registers and cause of death registers.

1.7.1 Nordic Research Network

The Nordic PharmacoEpidemiological Network (NorPEN) is a network of researchers in the five Nordic countries. Its purpose is to facilitate research within the field of pharmacoepidemiology. The core activity of NorPEN relates to annual/bi-annual scientific meetings which include educational elements.

NorPEN was created by ten pharmacoepidemiology research groups in 2008. Since then, a number of collaborative international research projects have been conducted, and several scientific publications have derived from the network. A list of these is published on the NorPEN web site (NorPEN 2019).

1.8 Administrative Information

1.8.1 Prescription Registers

In Finland, the register is run by the Social Insurance Institution, in Sweden by the National Board of Health and Welfare and in Norway by the Norwegian Institute for Public Health.

1.8.2 Patient Registers

Patient registers in Finland, Sweden, and Norway are run by the Finnish Institute for Health and Welfare, the National Board of Health and Welfare, and the Norwegian Directorate of Health, respectively.

1.8.3 Cancer Registers

Responsible authorities for cancer registers in Finland, Sweden, and Norway are the Cancer Society of Finland, the National Board of Health and Welfare, and the Institute of Population-based Cancer Research, respectively.

1.8.4 Medical Birth Registers

Medical birth registers in Finland, Sweden, and Norway are run by the Finnish Institute for Health and Welfare, the National Board of Health and Welfare, and the Norwegian Institute of Public Health, respectively.

1.8.5 Cause of Death Registers

The cause of death registers in Finland, Sweden, and Norway are run by Statistics Finland, the National Board of Health and Welfare, and the Norwegian Institute of Public Health, respectively.

References

Baghestan E, Børdahl PE, Rasmussen SA et al (2007) A validation of the diagnosis of obstetric sphincter tears in two Norwegian databases, the Medical Birth Registry and the Patient Administration System. Acta Obstet Gynecol Scand 86(2):205–209. https://doi.org/10.1080/000163406 01111364

Bakken IJ, Ariansen AMS, Knudsen GP et al (2019) The Norwegian Patient Registry and the Norwegian Registry for Primary Health Care: research potential of two nationwide health-care registries. Scand J Public Health 1403494819859737. https://doi.org/10.1177/1403494819859737

Bakken IJ, Gystad SO, Christensen ØOS et al (2012) Comparison of data from the Norwegian Patient Register and the Cancer Registry of Norway. Tidsskrift for Den Norske Lægeforening: Tidsskrift for Praktisk Medicin, Ny Række 132(11):1336–1340. https://doi.org/10.4045/tidsskr. 11.1099

Barlow L, Westergren K, Holmberg L et al (2009) The completeness of the Swedish Cancer Register: a sample survey for year 1998. Acta Oncologica (Stockholm, Sweden) 48(1):27–33. https://doi.org/10.1080/02841860802247664

Cancer Registry of Norway (2020) Clinical registries. https://www.kreftregisteret.no/en/The-Reg istries/Clinical-Registries/. Accessed 6 Jan 2020

Finnish Cancer Registry (2019) Description of statistics and their quality. https://cancerregistry.fi/ statistics/statistical-descriptions-quality-reports/. Accessed 31 Dec 2019

Finnish Institute for Health and Welfare (2020a) Congenital anomalies—quality description. https://thl.fi/en/web/thlfi-en/statistics/information-on-statistics/quality-descriptions/congen ital-anomalies. Accessed 17 Jan 2020

Finnish Institute for Health and Welfare (2020b) Medical birth register—quality description. https://thl.fi/en/web/thlfi-en/statistics/information-on-statistics/quality-descriptions/partur ients-delivers-and-newborns. Accessed 6 Jan 2020

Finnish Institute for Health and Welfare (2020c) Trends in access to specialised health care—quality description. https://thl.fi/en/web/thlfi-en/statistics/information-on-statistics/quality-descriptions/ trends-in-access-to-specialised-health-care. Accessed 2 Jan 2020

Furu K (2008) Establishment of the nationwide Norwegian prescription database (NorPD)—new opportunities for research in pharmacoepidemiology in Norway. Norsk epidemiologi 18(2):129–136

Furu K, Kieler H, Haglund B et al (2015) Selective serotonin reuptake inhibitors and venlafaxine in early pregnancy and risk of birth defects: population based cohort study and sibling design. BMJ 350(apr17 3):h1798. https://doi.org/10.1136/bmj.h1798

Furu K, Skurtveit S, Langhammer A et al (2007) Use of anti-asthmatic medications as a proxy for prevalence of asthma in children and adolescents in Norway: a nationwide prescription database analysis. Eur J Clin Pharmacol 63(7):693–698. https://doi.org/10.1007/s00228-007-0301-9

Furu K, Wettermark B, Andersen M et al (2010) The Nordic countries as a cohort for pharmacoepidemiological research. Basic Clin Pharmacol Toxicol 106(2):86–94. https://doi.org/10.1111/j. 1742-7843.2009.00494.x

Gissler M (2010) Registration of births and induced abortions in the Nordic countries. Finn Yearb Popul Res XLV:171–178

Gissler M, Shelley J (2002) Quality of data on subsequent events in a routine medical birth register. Med Inform Internet Med 27(1):33–38. https://doi.org/10.1080/14639230110119234

Helsedirektoratet (2020a) Norwegian Patient Registry—contents and quality (In Norwegian: Innhold og kvalitet i NPR). https://www.helsedirektoratet.no/tema/statistikk-registre-og-rap porter/helsedata-og-helseregistre/norsk-pasientregister-npr/innhold-og-kvalitet-i-npr. Accessed 5 Jan 2020 (in Norwegian)

Helsedirektoratet (2020b) Norwegian Registry for Primary Health Care (in Norwegian: Kommunalt pasient- og brukerregister (KPR). https://www.helsedirektoratet.no/tema/statistikk-registre-og-rapporter/helsedata-og-helseregistre/kommunalt-pasient-og-brukerregister-kpr. Accessed 5 Jan 2020 (in Norwegian)

Irgens LM (2000) The Medical Birth Registry of Norway. Epidemiological research and surveillance throughout 30 years. Acta Obstet Gynecol Scand 79(6):435–439. https://doi.org/10.1034/j.1600-0412.2000.079006435.x

Källén B (2015) Registration of congenital malformations in the Swedish Health Registers. Report of The Swedish National Board of Health and Welfare

Kansaneläkelaitos (2019) Finnish prescription register: quality description. (in Finnish: Laatuseloste: Tilasto korvatuista resepteistä). https://www.kela.fi/laatuseloste15. Accessed 23 Dec 2019 (in Finnish)

Korhonen P, Malila N, Pukkala E et al (2002) The Finnish cancer registry as follow-up source of a large trial cohort–accuracy and delay. Acta Oncologica (Stockholm, Sweden) 41(4):381–388

Langhoff-Roos J, Krebs L, Klungsøyr K et al (2014) The Nordic medical birth registers–a potential goldmine for clinical research. Acta Obstet Gynecol Scand 93(2):132–137. https://doi.org/10.1111/aogs.12302

Larsen IK, Småstuen M, Johannesen TB et al (2009) Data quality at the cancer registry of Norway: an overview of comparability, completeness, validity and timeliness. Eur J Cancer (Oxford, England: 1990) 45(7):1218–1231. https://doi.org/10.1016/j.ejca.2008.10.037

Leinonen MK, Miettinen J, Heikkinen S et al (2017) Quality measures of the population-based Finnish cancer registry indicate sound data quality for solid malignant tumours. Eur J Cancer 77:31–39. https://doi.org/10.1016/j.ejca.2017.02.017

Lovdata (2020) Regulations on the collection and treatment of health information in the Norwegian Patient Register (in Norwegian: Forskrift om innsamling og behandling av helseopplysninger i Norsk pasientregister). https://lovdata.no/dokument/SF/forskrift/2007-12-07-1389. Accessed 17 Jan 2020 (in Norwegian)

Ludvigsson JF, Andersson E, Ekbom A et al (2011) External review and validation of the Swedish national inpatient register. BMC Public Health 11:450. https://doi.org/10.1186/1471-2458-11-450

Mattsson K, Källén K, Rignell-Hydbom A et al (2016) Cotinine validation of self-reported smoking during pregnancy in the Swedish Medical Birth Register. Nicotine Tob Res: Official J Soc Res Nicotine Tob 18(1):79–83. https://doi.org/10.1093/ntr/ntv087

Nilsson M, Tavelin B, Axelsson B (2014) A study of patients not registered in the Swedish Cancer Register but reported to the Swedish Register of Palliative Care 2009 as deceased due to cancer. Acta Oncologica (Stockholm, Sweden) 53(3):414–419. https://doi.org/10.3109/0284186X.2013.819115

NorPEN (2019) Nordic PharmacoEpidemiological Network. http://www.norpen.org/pages/publications.html. Accessed 3 Jan 2019

Norwegian Institute of Public Health (2019) Norwegian prescription database. https://www.fhi.no/hn/helseregistre-og-registre/reseptregisteret/. Accessed 30 Dec 2019

Norwegian Institute of Public Health (2020a) How to apply for access to data. http://www.fhi.no/en/op/data-access-from-health-registries-health-studies-and-biobanks/data-access/applying-for-access-to-data/. Accessed 17 Jan 2020

Norwegian Institute of Public Health (2020b) Norwegian Cause of Death Registry. http://www.fhi.no/en/hn/health-registries/cause-of-death-registry/. Accessed 17 Jan 2020

Pedersen AG, Ellingsen CL (2015) Data quality in the causes of death registry. Tidsskrift for Den Norske Lægeforening: Tidsskrift for Praktisk Medicin, Ny Række 135(8):768–770. https://doi.org/10.4045/tidsskr.14.1065

Persson F, Bodegard J, Lahtela JT et al (2018) Different patterns of second-line treatment in type 2 diabetes after metformin monotherapy in Denmark, Finland, Norway and Sweden (D360 Nordic): a multinational observational study. Endocrinol, Diabetes Metab 1(4):e00036. https://doi.org/10.1002/edm2.36

Privacy Europe (2019) General Data Protection Regulation (GDPR). https://gdpr.eu/. Accessed 7 Jan 2019

Pukkala E, Engholm G, Højsgaard Schmidt LK et al (2018) Nordic cancer registries—an overview of their procedures and data comparability. Acta Oncologica (Stockholm, Sweden) 57(4):440–455. https://doi.org/10.1080/0284186X.2017.1407039

Socialstyrelsen (2019) The Swedish prescribed drug register (in Swedish: Läkemedelsregistret). https://www.socialstyrelsen.se/statistik-och-data/register/alla-register/lakemedelsregistret/. Accessed 30 Dec 2019 (in Swedish)

Socialstyrelsen (2020a) Cause of death register (in Swedish: Dödsorsaksregistret). https://www.socialstyrelsen.se/statistik-och-data/register/alla-register/dodsorsaksregistret/. Accessed 17 Jan 2020 (in Swedish)

Socialstyrelsen (2020b) Cause of death register: missing information and quality (in Swedish: Dödsorsaksregistret: Bortfall och kvalitet). https://www.socialstyrelsen.se/statistik-och-data/register/alla-register/dodsorsaksregistret/bortfall-och-kvalitet/. Accessed 6 Jan 2020 (in Swedish)

Socialstyrelsen (2020c) Medical birth register: missing information and quality (in Swedish: Bortfall och kvalitet om medicinska födelseregistret). https://www.socialstyrelsen.se/statistik-och-data/register/alla-register/medicinska-fodelseregistret/bortfall-och-kvalitet/. Accessed 6 Jan 2020 (in Swedish)

Socialstyrelsen (2020d) The national patient register—Socialstyrelsen. https://www.socialstyrelsen.se/en/statistics-and-data/registers/register-information/the-national-patient-register/. Accessed 5 Jan 2020

Socialstyrelsen (2020e) Order data and statistics (in Swedish: Beställa data och statistik). https://bestalladata.socialstyrelsen.se/data-for-forskning/tid-och-kostnader/. Accessed 17 Jan 2020 (in Swedish)

Socialstyrelsen (2020f) The Swedish prescribed drug register—missing information and quality (In Swedish: Läkemedelsregistret - Bortfall och kvalitet). https://www.socialstyrelsen.se/statistik-och-data/register/alla-register/lakemedelsregistret/bortfall-och-kvalitet/. Accessed 2 Jan 2020

Statistics Finland (2020a) Causes of death in 2018. http://www.stat.fi/til/ksyyt/2018/ksyyt_2018_2019-12-16_kat_001_en.html. Accessed 17 Jan 2020

Statistics Finland (2020b) Quality description: causes of death 2017. https://www.stat.fi/til/ksyyt/2017/ksyyt_2017_2018-12-17_laa_001_en.html. Accessed 6 Jan 2020

Sund R (2012) Quality of the Finnish hospital discharge register: a systematic review. Scand J Public Health 40(6):505–515. https://doi.org/10.1177/1403494812456637

Swedish Association of Local Authorities and Regions (2020a) National quality registers in Sweden (in Swedish: Nationella Kvalitetsregister). www.kvalitetsregister.se. Accessed 6 Jan 2020 (in Swedish)

Swedish Association of Local Authorities and Regions (2020b) Primary care quality Sweden. https://skr.se/tjanster/englishpages/activities/primarycarequality.10073.html. Accessed 5 Jan 2020

Terveyden ja hyvinvoinnin laitos (2020a) Collection of data in occupational healthcare (in Finnish: Työterveyshuollon tietojen tiedonkeruu). https://thl.fi/tilastot-ja-data/ohjeet-tietojen-toimittamiseen/tyoterveyshuollon-tietojen-tiedonkeruu. Accessed 6 Jan 2020 (in Finnish)

Terveyden ja hyvinvoinnin laitos (2020b) National healthcare quality registers (in Finnish: Terveydenhuollon kansalliset laaturekisterit). https://thl.fi/web/sote-uudistus/arviointi-ja-tietoikkuna/terveydenhuollon-kansalliset-laaturekisterit. Accessed 6 Jan 2020 (in Finnish)

The National Board of Health and Welfare (2020) Swedish cancer registry. https://www.socialstyrelsen.se/en/statistics-and-data/registers/register-information/swedish-cancer-register/. Accessed 6 Jan 2020

Wallerstedt SM, Wettermark B, Hoffmann M (2016) The first decade with the Swedish Prescribed drug register—a systematic review of the output in the scientific literature. Basic Clin Pharmacol Toxicol 119(5):464–469. https://doi.org/10.1111/bcpt.12613

Wettermark B, Hammar N, Fored CM et al (2007) The new Swedish prescribed drug register–opportunities for pharmacoepidemiological research and experience from the first six months. Pharmacoepidemiol Drug Saf 16(7):726–735. https://doi.org/10.1002/pds.1294

Wettermark B, Zoëga H, Furu K et al (2013) The Nordic prescription databases as a resource for pharmacoepidemiological research—a literature review. Pharmacoepidemiol Drug Saf 22(7):691–699. https://doi.org/10.1002/pds.3457

PHARMO Database Network

Marina Bakker and Ron Herings

Abstract The first linkage of healthcare databases that laid the basis for the PHARMO Database Network dates back to the first quarter of 1989 and was an initiative of Prof. Dr. B.Ch. Stricker and Dr. R.M.C. Herings. Drug exposure files of community pharmacies (now the Out-patient Pharmacy Database) were linked to the hospital administration records of the national Hospital Database creating the PHARmacoMOrbidity linkage. With these linked data, questions on the use, effectiveness, and safety of drugs in daily clinical practice could be answered.

1 Database Description

1.1 Introduction

The first linkage of healthcare databases that laid the basis for the PHARMO Database Network dates back to the first quarter of 1989 and was an initiative of Prof. Dr. B.Ch. Stricker and Dr. R.M.C. Herings. Drug exposure files of community pharmacies (now the Out-patient Pharmacy Database) were linked to the hospital administration records of the national Hospital Database creating the PHARmacoMOrbidity linkage. With these linked data, questions on the use, effectiveness, and safety of drugs in daily clinical practice could be answered. Since then, many other healthcare databases were linked, creating the PHARMO Database Network.

M. Bakker (✉) · R. Herings (✉)
PHARMO Institute for Drug Outcomes Research, Van Deventlaan 30-40, 3528 AE Utrecht, The Netherlands
e-mail: ron.herings@pharmo.nl

© Springer Nature Switzerland AG 2021
M. Sturkenboom and T. Schink (eds.), *Databases for Pharmacoepidemiological Research*, Springer Series on Epidemiology and Public Health,
https://doi.org/10.1007/978-3-030-51455-6_7

1.2   Database Characteristics

The PHARMO Database Network is a population-based network of electronic health-care databases and combines anonymous data from different primary and secondary healthcare settings in the Netherlands (see Fig. 1).

These different data sources, including data from general practitioners (GP), in- and out-patient pharmacies, clinical laboratories, hospitals, the cancer registry, pathology registry, and perinatal registry, are linked on a patient level through validated algorithms. To ensure the privacy of the data in the PHARMO Database Network, the collection, processing, linkage, and anonymisation of the data is performed by STIZON. STIZON is an independent, ISO/IEC 27001 certified foundation, which acts as a Trusted Third Party (TTP) between the data sources and the PHARMO Institute. Caregivers join the PHARMO Database Network so that they can improve their quality of care via scientific research and feedback information (benchmarking information and feedback on quality indicators). Detailed information on the methodology and the validation of the used record linkage method can be found elsewhere (van Herk-Sukel et al. 2010; Herings and Pedersen 2012). It is possible to link additional data collections to the existing database network, such as data collected from chart reviews, patient-reported outcomes (PRO), or data from an interventional trial among patients in the GP setting. The additional data is collected by the healthcare provider who reports the additional information back to STIZON, including patient identifiable information that allows linkage to the data in

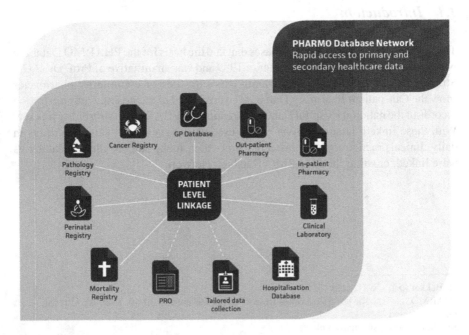

Fig. 1 PHARMO database network

the PHARMO Database Network. The additional data collections are anonymised before they are shared with PHARMO for research purposes.

The longitudinal nature of the PHARMO Database Network system enables the patient-centric follow-up of more than 9 million persons of a well-defined population in the Netherlands for an average of twelve years. In 2018, the PHARMO Database Network covered 6 million active persons out of 17 million inhabitants of the Netherlands. Data collection period, catchment area, and overlap between data sources differ. Therefore, the final cohort size for any study will depend on the data sources included. As data sources are linked on an annual basis, the average lag time of the data is one year.

1.3   Available Data

All electronic patient records in the PHARMO Database Network include information on age, sex, socioeconomic status (based on zip code), and mortality (only date of death). Other available information depends on the data source. Two types of databases can be distinguished in the PHARMO Database Network. The in-house databases are collected and processed by STIZON. The core partnership databases are collected and processed by other parties.

1.3.1   PHARMO In-House Databases

The PHARMO in-house databases include the GP Database, the Out-patient Pharmacy Database, the In-patient Pharmacy Database, and the Clinical Laboratory Database.

The GP Database comprises data from electronic patient records registered by GPs from 2003 onwards. The records include information on diagnoses and symptoms, laboratory and (physical) examination test results, referrals to specialists, lifestyle factors, and healthcare product/drug prescriptions. The prescription records include information on type of product, indication, prescription date, brand name/code, dosage regimen, quantity and route of administration as well as prescriber information. Drug prescriptions are coded according to the WHO Anatomical Therapeutic Chemical (ATC) Classification System. Diagnoses and symptoms are coded according to the International Classification of Primary Care (ICPC) but can also be entered as free text. ICPC codes can be mapped to ICD codes. GP data cover a catchment area representing 3.2 million residents (~20% of the Dutch population).

The Out-patient Pharmacy Database comprises GP or specialist prescribed healthcare products dispensed by the out-patient pharmacy, irrespective of reimbursement. The In-patient Pharmacy Database comprises drug dispensings from the hospital pharmacy, given during a hospitalisation. The dispensing records of both the Out-patient and the In-patient Pharmacy Database (1985 onwards) include information on the type of product, date, dosage regimen, quantity, route of administration, and for the Out-patient Pharmacy Database also prescriber specialty and costs. Drug dispensings are coded according to the ATC Classification System. The Out-patient Pharmacy Database covers a catchment area representing 4.2 million residents (~25% of the Dutch population). The In-patient Pharmacy Database covers a catchment area representing 2.0 million residents (~10% of the Dutch population).

The Clinical Laboratory Database comprises more than 3 billion results of tests performed on clinical specimens. These laboratory tests are requested by GPs, medical specialists or other healthcare providers in order to get information concerning diagnosis, treatment or prevention of disease. The electronic records include information on date and time of testing, test result, unit of measurement, and type of clinical specimen. Laboratory tests are coded according to the Dutch WCIA Coding System. Clinical laboratory data cover a catchment area representing 3 million residents (~20% of the Dutch population).

1.3.2 Core Partnership Databases

For research purposes, the PHARMO Database Network is yearly, or on an ad hoc basis, linked to core partnership databases including the National Hospital Database, National Cancer Registry (NKR), Pathology Registry, and Perinatal Registry via the TTP.

The Hospital Database comprises datasets containing data on hospital admissions, ambulatory consultations, and high budget impact medication. The Hospital Database is collected and maintained by the Dutch Hospital Data Foundation (www.dhd.nl) and comprises records from nearly all hospitals in the Netherlands. The hospital admissions dataset comprises hospital admissions for more than 24 h and admissions for less than 24 h for which a bed is required (i.e., in-patient records). The records include information on hospital admission and discharge dates, discharge diagnoses, and procedures. The ambulatory consultations dataset comprises all ambulatory consultations (i.e., out-patient records). The records include information on each contact, including date, diagnoses, and procedures. The high budget impact medication dataset comprises all dispensed high budget impact medication, which is dispensed through hospitals. The records include information on date of dispensing, type of medication, number of units, indication of use, and prescriber. Diagnoses are coded according to the International Classification of Diseases (ICD 9 and ICD 10) and procedures are coded according to the Dutch Hospital Data Foundation registration system for procedures, which links to the Dutch declaration codes. Drug dispensings are coded according to the Dutch Z-index code. The Dutch Hospital Data Foundation has been collecting hospitalization records from nearly all hospitals in the Netherlands since 1963. Permission for use of the data is obtained from each hospital and PHARMO has data on hospital admissions from over 80% of the hospitals. Data on ambulatory contacts and high budget impact medication are available from 2017 onwards from over 50% of the hospitals.

The Cancer Registry is maintained by the Netherlands Comprehensive Cancer Organisation (IKNL 2020) and comprises information on newly diagnosed cancer patients in the Netherlands, including cancer diagnosis, tumour staging (according to the TNM-classification), tumour site (topography), and morphology (histology) [according to the WHO International Classification of Diseases for Oncology (ICD-O-3)], co-morbidity at diagnosis, and treatment received directly after diagnosis.

The nationwide network and registry of histopathology and cytopathology in the Netherlands is maintained by the PALGA foundation (PALGA 2020) and comprises excerpts of histological, cytological, and autopsy examinations. Electronic records include a summary of the pathology report and the so-called PALGA diagnosis which is structured along five classification axes: topography, morphology, function, procedure, and diseases.

The Netherlands Perinatal Registry (PRN) is maintained by Perined (PRN 2020) and comprises data on pregnancies, births, and neonatal outcomes of births in the Netherlands. All data is voluntarily collected by perinatal caregivers, mainly for benchmarking. Records include information on mothers (e.g., maternal age, obstetric history, parity), pregnancy (e.g., mode of conception, mode of delivery), and children (e.g., birth weight, gestational age, Apgar score). Pregnancies resulting in miscarriage or abortion are included as long as the mother already has visited a midwife or gynecologist. Mothers and children (and other family members) are linked using address data. Diagnoses and symptoms are coded according to the Perinatal Registry code lists.

1.4 Strengths and Limitations

The major strength of the PHARMO Database Network is that it provides unprecedented rich and detailed information of more than 9 million residents of a well-defined population in the Netherlands for an average of twelve years. Through yearly updates, the longitudinal follow-up of individuals in the network increases. Tailor-made and disease-specific cohorts are created from the PHARMO Database Network which are based on the cradle to grave principle. Moreover, individual medical information may even be available from before birth through linkage with the PRN or by identifying mother-child relationships in the PHARMO databases. Through linkages with various healthcare databases, a complete profile of an individual's medical history throughout life can be created, giving a complete overview of a patient's journey. If required, additional patient data can be collected by reaching out to the treating physicians in reported outcomes studies.

The GP Database is representative for the Netherlands in terms of sex and age distribution. All patients in the Netherlands should be registered with a GP as this is a requirement of the mandatory health insurance in the Netherlands. The representativeness of the pharmacy databases enables the study of real-life drug use in the Netherlands. All drug use by patients, excluding OTC drugs, will be captured; with the In-patient Pharmacy Database capturing all drug use administered in-hospital (e.g., intravenously administered chemotherapies) and the Out-patient Pharmacy Database capturing all drugs dispensed outside the hospital.

As with any healthcare database, identification of medical events is limited to data that are captured as part of the medical record or other linked data sources. These data are not primarily collected for research purposes and will rely on recording of appropriate diagnostic codes to detect these events. Furthermore, reporting of events depends on the information deemed relevant by the treating physician to record in the system. This applies specifically for information regarding lifestyle (e.g., exercise habits, alcohol consumption, and cigarette smoking). Also, mild adverse events may be underreported for that reason. On the other hand, completeness of information in the GP Database has increased in recent years as health insurance companies reimburse higher amounts to GPs with more complete data (benchmarking), providing an extra incentive to improve completeness. Serious adverse events leading to hospital admissions are more likely to be detected because all admissions are captured in the Hospital Database.

Selecting the optimal data source for a specific study question is important. For example, the biometric data recorded in the GP Database are to some extent not complete and may be biased to include more information of patients with a higher risk profile (higher HbA1c, higher BMI, higher blood pressure) than the overall population, while in the Clinical Laboratory Database all results of tests performed on clinical specimens are recorded, regardless of the test results.

1.5 Validation

The PHARMO Database Network consists of different healthcare databases which are linked on a patient level through validated algorithms. Detailed information on the methodology and the validation of the used record linkage method can be found elsewhere (van Herk-Sukel et al. 2010; Herings and Pedersen 2012). For each study, it is determined per patient from which time point onwards the patient is registered in the different databases and from which time point the patient is lost to follow-up (due to, for example, death or moving out of the database catchment area). Patients are regarded eligible to be included in a study if they are registered and can be followed in all required databases. Furthermore, specific study checks on the linked data are performed. These partially depend on the specific databases required for the study and on their importance to the selection of patients or outcomes. For example, for the dispensing records, dosage regimen and dispensed quantity are checked and extremely high dosages and quantities for the specific type of drug are regarded as missing values. PHARMO can apply for chart review to extract additional information about a case at the corresponding healthcare provider. However, approval is needed from the individual healthcare providers.

1.6 Governance and Ethical Issues

Since 2012, the PHARMO Database Network has been created by STIZON (Stichting Informatievoorziening voor Zorg en Onderzoek). STIZON is an independent, ISO/IEC 27001 certified foundation which acts as a Trusted Third Party (TTP) between the data sources and the PHARMO Institute. STIZON is authorised by the data providers to manage and process the identifiable patient data. STIZON collects and maintains the identifiable patient data retrieved from the various data providers (e.g., general practitioners and pharmacists) and links the data on a patient level. Before the PHARMO Database Network can be used for research by the PHARMO Institute, the data is depleted of personal information that may be traced back to persons (such as date of birth). The use of the PHARMO Database Network of the PHARMO Institute is controlled by an independent compliance committee, which consists of representatives of the participating data providers and an independent privacy expert. Access to the PHARMO Database Network is granted only in the context of approved research projects. Researchers from the PHARMO Institute as well as academics from universities or research institutes are granted the opportunity to perform scientific studies using the anonymised data from the PHARMO Database Network. This endeavour is in line with the policy and mission of the PHARMO Institute to contribute to a better understanding of the use, safety, effectiveness, and cost of pharmaceuticals as used in real life.

Each data request is checked against the policies that apply for use of data from the PHARMO Database Network and the agreements with the relevant data providers. The PHARMO Institute conducts research according to the latest directives regarding privacy and handling of data. A study using solely the PHARMO Database Network is a retrospective, non-interventional study and therefore does not pose any risks for patients. Confidentiality of patient records is maintained at all times. All study reports contain aggregate data only and will not identify individual patients, healthcare providers, and institutes. PHARMO is not allowed to disclose any information that may be traced back to identifiable persons or that is on a patient level. However, aggregated data may be shared with research partners, e.g., for pooled analyses.

Because of the use of de-identified data from existing databases without any direct enrolment of subjects or breach of confidentiality with regards to personal identifiers or health information, ethical approval or informed consent is not necessary according to the Dutch law regarding human medical scientific research [Wet medisch-wetenschappelijk onderzoek met mensen (WMO)], which is enforced by the Central Committee on Research involving Human Subjects (Centrale Commissie Mensgebonden Onderzoek, CCMO).

Additional data collections, such as data collected from chart reviews or patient-reported outcomes (PRO) require PHARMO's compliance committee approval, ethics review board approval, healthcare provider approval, and, if needed, informed consent. De-identification algorithms need to be reversed by STIZON (the same party responsible for de-identification of the databases) to obtain original patient id numbers that allow access to the patient (charts). After obtaining the required information for research, all personal information will be removed again by STIZON before researchers are allowed to access the data and perform their research. Reporting of the chart review information will never disclose information traceable to individual patients, in accordance with WMO.

1.7 Documents and Publications

To date, over 500 publications of studies using data from the PHARMO Database Network have appeared in peer-reviewed journals. These mostly concern drug utilisation studies describing the pattern, persistence, and/or determinants of drug use, studies on the effectiveness of drugs, and studies on the safety of drugs. Publications describing the PHARMO Database Network include a general description of the PHARMO Database Network (Herings and Pedersen 2012) and a publication focused on the linkage with the Cancer Registry (van Herk-Sukel et al. 2010). Recent examples of drug utilisation studies include the use of topical tacrolimus and primecolimus in four European countries (Kuiper et al. 2018), the treatment of type 2 diabetes across Europe (Overbeek et al. 2017), chemotherapy in patients with ovarian cancer (Houben et al. 2017), the use of oral contraceptives in three European countries (Bezemer et al. 2016b), and anticoagulant treatment for VTE (Bezemer et al. 2016a). Examples of publications on drug effectiveness include a comparison of liraglutide and basal insulin regarding glycemic and weight control (Overbeek et al. 2018), LDL-C goal attainment following lipid-modifying therapy (Kuiper et al. 2017b), survival related to chemotherapy exposure in patients with Chronic Lymphoid Leukaemia (Kuiper et al. 2017a), and an evaluation of smoking cessation drugs(Penning-van Beest et al. 2011).

Relevant papers on drug safety include studies on the association between coumarin use, renal function and serious bleeding events (Houben et al. 2018b), the risk of lymphoma and skin cancer in users of topical tacrolimus, pimecrolimus and corticosteroids (Castellsague et al. 2018), safety outcomes in children using proton pump inhibitors or histamine-2 receptor antagonists (Houben et al. 2018a), a PASS comparing quetiapine to risperidone and olanzapine (Heintjes et al. 2016), and the association between pioglitazone and bladder cancer in patients with type 2 diabetes (Korhonen et al. 2016). Finally, publications particularly highlighting the linkages with our partnership databases, including the Hospital Database, Cancer Registry, Pathology Registry and Perinatal Registry, include a study in which the Hospital Database was used to determine the rate of prostate surgery and acute urinary retention in men treated with dutasteride or finasteride (Kuiper et al. 2016), a study using the Cancer Registry for identification of breast cancer patients and staging (Overbeek et al. 2019), a study in which the Pathology Registry was used to select patients with lung cancer (van Herk-Sukel et al. 2013), and a study on the risk of morbidities and healthcare utilisation in children born following preterm labour compared to full-term labour using data from the Perinatal Registry (Houben et al. 2019).

1.8 Administrative Information

The PHARMO Database Network is maintained by STIZON (Stichting Infor-matievoorziening voor Zorg en Onderzoek) and funded by own resources.

Contact Details

Organisation/affiliation: PHARMO Institute and STIZON, Van Deventerlaan 30-40, 3528 AE Utrecht, The Netherlands

Administrative Contact: Heleen van Engeland, Office Manager, pharmo@pharmo.nl/stizon@stizon.nl, +31 30 7440 800

Website: www.pharmo.nl/www.stizon.nl

References

Bezemer ID, van der Berg EJ, Herings R et al (2016) Anticoagulant treatment after VTE in the Netherlands: a retrospective cohort study. Jacobs J Hematol 2(2):030

Bezemer ID, Verhamme KM, Gini R et al (2016) Use of oral contraceptives in three European countries: a population-based multi-database study. Eur J Contracept Reprod Health Care 21(1):81–87. https://doi.org/10.3109/13625187.2015.1102220

Castellsague J, Kuiper JG, Pottegard A et al (2018) A cohort study on the risk of lymphoma and skin cancer in users of topical tacrolimus, pimecrolimus, and corticosteroids (Joint European Longitudinal Lymphoma and Skin Cancer Evaluation—JOELLE study). Clin Epidemiol 10:299–310. https://doi.org/10.2147/clep.S146442

Heintjes EM, Overbeek JA, Penning-van Beest FJ et al (2016) Post authorization safety study comparing quetiapine to risperidone and olanzapine. Hum Psychopharmacol 31(4):304–312. https://doi.org/10.1002/hup.2539

Herings RMC, Pedersen L (2012) Pharmacy-based medical record linkage systems. In: Strom BL, Kimmel SE, Hennessy S (eds) Pharmacoepidemiology, 5th edn. Wiley, Chichester, pp 271–286

Houben E, van Haalen HG, Sparreboom W et al (2017) Chemotherapy for ovarian cancer in the Netherlands: a population-based study on treatment patterns and outcomes. Med Oncol 34(4):50. https://doi.org/10.1007/s12032-017-0901-x

Houben E, Johansson S, Nagy P et al (2018) Observational cohort study: safety outcomes in children using proton pump inhibitors or histamine-2 receptor antagonists. Curr Med Res Opin 34(4):577–583. https://doi.org/10.1080/03007995.2017.1407302

Houben E, Smits E, Overbeek JA et al (2018) No evidence for an association between renal function and serious bleeding events in patients treated with coumarins: a population-based study. Ann Pharmacother 52(3):221–234. https://doi.org/10.1177/1060028017735340

Houben E, Smits E, Pimenta JM et al (2019) Increased risk of morbidities and health-care utilisation in children born following preterm labour compared with full-term labour: a population-based study. J Paediatr Child Health 55(4):446–453. https://doi.org/10.1111/jpc.14225

IKNL-Netherlands Comprehensive Cancer Organisation (2020) https://www.iknl.nl/. Accessed 17 Jan 2020

Korhonen P, Heintjes EM, Williams R et al (2016) Pioglitazone use and risk of bladder cancer in patients with type 2 diabetes: retrospective cohort study using datasets from four European countries. BMJ 354:i3903. https://doi.org/10.1136/bmj.i3903

Kuiper JG, Bezemer ID, Driessen MT et al (2016) Rates of prostate surgery and acute urinary retention for benign prostatic hyperplasia in men treated with dutasteride or finasteride. BMC Urol 16(1):53. https://doi.org/10.1186/s12894-016-0170-6

Kuiper J, Musingarimi P, Tapprich C et al (2017) Chemotherapy exposure and outcomes of chronic lymphoid leukemia patients. J Clin Intensive Care Med 2:025–033

Kuiper JG, Sanchez RJ, Houben E et al (2017) Use of lipid-modifying therapy and LDL-C goal attainment in a high-cardiovascular-risk population in the Netherlands. Clin Ther 39(4):819–827.e811. https://doi.org/10.1016/j.clinthera.2017.03.001

Kuiper JG, van Herk-Sukel MPP, Castellsague J et al (2018) Use of topical tacrolimus and topical pimecrolimus in four European countries: a multicentre database cohort study. Drugs Real World Outcomes 5(2):109–116. https://doi.org/10.1007/s40801-018-0133-1

Overbeek JA, Heintjes EM, Prieto-Alhambra D et al (2017) Type 2 diabetes mellitus treatment patterns across Europe: a population-based multi-database study. Clin Ther 39(4):759–770. https://doi.org/10.1016/j.clinthera.2017.02.008

Overbeek JA, Heintjes EM, Huisman EL et al (2018) Clinical effectiveness of liraglutide vs basal insulin in a real-world setting: evidence of improved glycaemic and weight control in obese people with type 2 diabetes. Diabetes Obes Metab 20(9):2093–2102. https://doi.org/10.1111/dom.13335

Overbeek JA, van Herk-Sukel MPP, Vissers PAJ et al (2019) Type 2 diabetes, but not insulin (analog) treatment, is associated with more advanced stages of breast cancer: a national linkage of cancer and pharmacy registries. Diabetes Care 42(3):434–442. https://doi.org/10.2337/dc18-2146

PALGA (2020) The nationwide network and registry of histopathology and cytopathology. https://www.palga.nl/. Accessed 17 Jan 2020

Penning-van Beest FJ, Overbeek JA, Smulders M et al (2011) Evaluation of smoking cessation drug use and outcomes in the Netherlands. J Med Econ 14(1):124–129. https://doi.org/10.3111/13696998.2010.551165

PRN-The Netherlands Perinatal Registry (2020) Perined. https://www.perined.nl/, 17 Jan 2020

van Herk-Sukel MP, van de Poll-Franse LV, Lemmens VE et al (2010) New opportunities for drug outcomes research in cancer patients: the linkage of the Eindhoven Cancer Registry and the PHARMO Record Linkage System. Eur J Cancer 46(2):395–404. https://doi.org/10.1016/j.ejca.2009.09.010

van Herk-Sukel MP, Shantakumar S, Penning-van Beest FJ et al (2013) Pulmonary embolism, myocardial infarction, and ischemic stroke in lung cancer patients: results from a longitudinal study. Lung 191(5):501–509. https://doi.org/10.1007/s00408-013-9485-1

German Pharmacoepidemiological Research Database (GePaRD)

Ulrike Haug and Tania Schink

Abstract The German Pharmacoepidemiological Research Database (GePaRD) is an administrative database based on claims data from statutory health insurance providers in Germany. It was set up for research on the utilization and safety of drugs and vaccines in the real-world setting, but is also used for other purposes such as the utilization of screening tests.

1 Database Description

1.1 Introduction

The German Pharmacoepidemiological Research Database (GePaRD) is an administrative database based on claims data from statutory health insurance providers in Germany. It was set up for research on the utilization and safety of drugs and vaccines in the real-world setting, but is also used for other purposes such as the utilization of screening tests. In Germany, about 90% of the general population are covered by statutory health insurance (Statista 2020). Membership in statutory health insurance is compulsory but there are exceptions, e.g., for persons with a very high income and for civil servants. These persons can choose private health insurance, i.e., they belong to the 10% of the population not covered by statutory health insurance. Around 75% of these higher-income patients, however, remain voluntary members of statutory health insurance. The health insurance system in Germany is characterized by uniform access to all levels of care and free choice of providers. An advantage of data from German health insurance providers is the stability of their membership which makes long-term follow-up studies feasible. In a pilot database of more than

U. Haug (✉) · T. Schink
Leibniz Institute for Prevention Research and Epidemiology – BIPS, Achterstrasse 30, 28359 Bremen, Germany
e-mail: haug@leibniz-bips.de

© Springer Nature Switzerland AG 2021
M. Sturkenboom and T. Schink (eds.), *Databases for Pharmacoepidemiological Research*, Springer Series on Epidemiology and Public Health,
https://doi.org/10.1007/978-3-030-51455-6_8

3.5 million insurants from three statutory health insurance providers, membership was stable in about 75% of all subjects over four years (Pigeot and Ahrens 2008).

1.2 Database Characteristics

GePaRD is based on claims data from four statutory health insurance providers and currently (as of January 2020) includes information on about 25 million persons who have been insured with one of the participating health insurances since 2004 or later. Per data year, there is information on approximately 17% of the German population and all geographical regions of the country are represented. The four health insurance providers participating in GePaRD are not equal in size; two of them cover the majority of persons in GePaRD. In previous analyses, the data has been shown to be representative with respect to drug prescriptions (Fassmer and Schink 2014; Schink and Garbe 2010). All persons insured with one of the four health insurance providers contributing to GePaRD entered the database on January 1, 2004 or at the start of insurance with the respective provider (whichever came first) and are followed up until the end of insurance or death. Usually, the database is updated annually and the lag time is about two years.

1.3 Available Data

GePaRD contains demographic information such as year of birth, sex, and region of residence as well as information on hospitalizations, outpatient visits, and outpatient drug prescriptions.

Information on hospitalizations includes the date of admission, the admission diagnosis, diagnostic and surgical/medical procedures during the hospital stay, the discharge date, main and secondary discharge diagnoses, and the reason for discharge (incl. death).

Outpatient data include diagnoses as well as outpatient diagnostic and therapeutic procedures and services. Physicians in the outpatient setting are expected to code the disease(s) for which they treat their patients once per quarter (GBA 2019; KBV 2011). Additionally, it is mandatory in the outpatient setting to code the diagnostic certainty. This coding differentiates between "confirmed", "suspected", "status post", and "excluded" diagnoses. Outpatient diagnosis codes are thus available on a quarterly basis only. However, given that an exact date is available for outpatient visits, the diagnosis can be assigned to the date of the visit if there was only one outpatient visit in the respective quarter, i.e., the exact date of diagnosis can partly be determined indirectly.

Hospital and outpatient diagnoses are coded using the International Classification of Diseases, version 10 in the German Modification (ICD-10-GM) with at least four digits; diagnostic and surgical/medical procedures are coded using the Operations and

Procedures Coding System (OPS) and outpatient treatment/diagnostic procedures as well as immunizations are coded using claim codes for outpatient services and procedures (*Einheitlicher Bewertungsmaßstab*, EBM).

GePaRD contains information on all drugs prescribed by physicians that were dispensed in a pharmacy and were reimbursed by the health insurance provider. Information on drugs is coded based on the German modification of the Anatomical Therapeutic Chemical (ATC) Classification System. Information on drugs that are purchased over the counter (OTC) is not available in the database. Furthermore, there is no information on medication administered in the hospital, but there are a few exceptions regarding expensive drugs (e.g., monoclonal antibodies).

Outpatient drug data include the dates of the prescription and dispensation, the number of prescribed packages, the specialty of the prescribing physician, and the central pharmaceutical number of the drug. Based on the central pharmaceutical number, information on the generic and brand name of the drug, packaging size, strength, the defined daily dose (DDD), and further pharmaceutical information (e.g., route of administration) is linked to GePaRD.

If lab tests and physical exams were performed, the related information including the date is available in the database provided that they are reimbursable. The results of these examinations or lab tests are not available, but can partly be derived indirectly if specific ICD-10 diagnoses or treatments are coded subsequently to the test or the exam.

There is no lifestyle information in GePaRD. Certain subgroups that have developed diseases due to an unhealthy lifestyle may be identified through diagnosis codes (e.g., obesity, liver diseases due to alcohol abuse) or specific treatments. There is also an ICD-10 code for heavy smoking but it is expected that this information is only in the database if the person was treated for this condition. The socioeconomic status can be approximated through information on the educational level for the majority of persons in GePaRD.

There is information in GePaRD allowing for research on drug safety during pregnancy. Based on the respective codes, algorithms to identify pregnancies and classify pregnancy outcomes (Mikolajczyk et al. 2013; Wentzell et al. 2018), to estimate the beginning of pregnancy (Schink et al. 2020) and to link mothers with their offspring (Garbe et al. 2011) have been developed.

Linkage of GePaRD to other data sources such as cancer registries is possible for specific research questions if approved by the health insurance providers and the responsible authorities but the required data flow is complex due to strict regulations for data protection (see Sect. 1.5). It is not possible to access patient records for case validation or to contact patients, e.g., for the collection of bio-samples unless the health insurance provider is willing to do this within a research project approved by an ethics committee.

1.4   Strengths and Limitations

A major strength of the GePaRD database is its large sample size allowing, for example, investigation of rare exposures and outcomes. In addition, millions of individuals can be followed up over a long period of time given that only a minority of persons in Germany switches between health insurance providers. In the outpatient setting, the data cover the care provided by general practitioners and specialists. While in databases recording only the prescription of drugs it is uncertain whether prescriptions were actually filled, GePaRD only contains information on drugs that were actually dispensed, i.e., this part of primary non-adherence is not an issue in GePaRD. In terms of drug safety in pregnancy, it is advantageous that the beginning of pregnancy can be estimated very precisely and that the majority of newborns can be followed up for many years, i.e., outcomes occurring later in life can also be studied.

There are limitations inherent to the fact that GePaRD is based on claims data. This includes the lack of information on lifestyle factors, lab values, and other measurements (e.g., lung function), overall frailty, the severity of diseases, cause of death, and OTC medication. Particularly in the outpatient setting, miscoding or unspecific coding of diseases may occur, i.e., algorithms combining different types of information are typically applied to define cases. Furthermore, information on the prescribed daily dose is not available in GePaRD; thus the dose and intended duration have to be estimated and sensitivity analyses have to be performed to check the robustness of the results.

1.5   Validation

As mentioned before, direct validation by linking GePaRD to other data sources for specific research questions is possible but the required data flow is complex due to strict regulations for data protection. Such linkages have successfully been conducted, e.g., to validate the vital status and the date of death in GePaRD (Langner et al. 2019; Ohlmeier et al. 2016).

Other options typically used to plausibilize algorithms developed for the definition of diseases include the comparison of prevalences and incidences with other data sources (indirect validation), e.g., disease registries (Czwikla et al. 2017). Furthermore, for certain outcomes such as acute liver injury, the positive predictive values of algorithms developed based on claims have been determined by applying the algorithm to data from a hospital information system (Timmer et al. 2018). Finally, there is the option of reviewing a random sample of patient profiles including all codes available in GePaRD by clinical experts blinded to the classification of the algorithm.

1.6   Governance and Ethical Issues

Although GePaRD is maintained by BIPS, the data contained in GePaRD are legally still owned by the respective statutory health insurance providers. Access to the database is granted only at BIPS in the context of approved research projects. Third parties may only access the data in cooperation with BIPS and after signing an agreement for guest researchers at BIPS.

In Germany, the utilization of health insurance data for scientific research is regulated by the Code of Social Law. All involved health insurance providers as well as the Federal Office for Social Security (formerly German Federal (Social) Insurance Office) and the Senator for Science, Health, and Consumer Protection in Bremen as their responsible authorities have to approve the use of GePaRD data for specific research questions. Informed consent for studies based on claims data is required by law unless obtaining consent appears unacceptable and would bias results, which is typically the case in pharmacoepidemiological studies. According to the Ethics Committee of the University of Bremen studies based on GePaRD are exempt from institutional review board review.

1.7   Administrative Information

The database is maintained by BIPS and has been established by own resources.

Contact Details

Organization/affiliation: Leibniz Institute for Prevention Research and Epidemiology – BIPS GmbH, Achterstrasse 30, 28359 Bremen, Germany

　　Administrative Contact: gepard@leibniz-bips.de

　　Website: https://www.bips-institut.de/en/research/research-infrastructures/gepard.html

References

Czwikla J, Jobski K, Schink T (2017) The impact of the lookback period and definition of confirmatory events on the identification of incident cancer cases in administrative data. BMC Med Res Methodol 17(1):122. https://doi.org/10.1186/s12874-017-0407-4

Fassmer A, Schink T (2014) Repräsentativität von ambulanten Arzneiverordnungen in der German Pharmacoepidemiological Research Database (GePaRD). Paper presented at the 9. Jahrestagung der Deutschen Gesellschaft für Epidemiologie (DGEpi), Ulm, 17–20 Sept 2014

Garbe E, Suling M, Kloss S et al (2011) Linkage of mother-baby pairs in the German Pharmacoepidemiological Research Database. Pharmacoepidemiol Drug Saf 20(3):258–264. https://doi.org/10.1002/pds.2038

GBA (2019) Richtlinie des Gemeinsamen Bundesausschusses zu Untersuchungs- und Behandlungsmethoden der vertragsärztlichen Versorgung (Richtlinie Methoden vertragsärztliche Versorgung). Bundesanzeiger Nr 48 (S 1 523) vom 9 März 2006, zuletzt geändert am 20 Juni 2019 veröffentlicht im Bundesanzeiger (BAnz AT 04092019 B2) in Kraft getreten am 5 Sept 2019

KBV (2011) Ambulante Kodierrichtlinien – Definition der Behandlungsdiagnose. Dtsch Arztebl International 108(4):165–167

Langner I, Ohlmeier C, Zeeb H et al (2019) Individual mortality information in the German Pharmacoepidemiological Research Database (GePaRD): a validation study using a record linkage with a large cancer registry. BMJ Open 9(7):e028223. https://doi.org/10.1136/bmjopen-2018-028223

Mikolajczyk RT, Kraut AA, Garbe E (2013) Evaluation of pregnancy outcome records in the German Pharmacoepidemiological Research Database (GePaRD). Pharmacoepidemiol Drug Saf 22(8):873–880. https://doi.org/10.1002/pds.3467

Ohlmeier C, Langner I, Garbe E et al (2016) Validating mortality in the German Pharmacoepidemiological Research Database (GePaRD) against a mortality registry. Pharmacoepidemiol Drug Saf 25(7):778–784. https://doi.org/10.1002/pds.4005

Pigeot I, Ahrens W (2008) Establishment of a pharmacoepidemiological database in Germany: methodological potential, scientific value and practical limitations. Pharmacoepidemiol Drug Saf 17(3):215–223. https://doi.org/10.1002/pds.1545

Schink T, Garbe E (2010) Assessment of the representativity of in-patient hospital diagnoses in the German Pharmacoepidemiological Research Database. In: Abstracts of the 26th international conference on pharmacoepidemiology & therapeutic risk management, 19–22 Aug 2010. Brighton, United Kingdom. Pharmacoepidemiol Drug Saf 19(s1):S178–S179. https://doi.org/10.1002/pds.2019

Schink T, Wentzell N, Dathe K et al (2020) Estimating the beginning of pregnancy in German claims data: development of an algorithm with a focus on the expected delivery date. Front Public Health 8:350. https://doi.org/10.3389/fpubh.2020.00350

Statista (2020) Anzahl der Mitglieder und Versicherten der gesetzlichen und privaten Krankenversicherung in den Jahren 2013 bis 2019. https://de.statista.com/statistik/daten/studie/155823/umfrage/gkv-pkv-mitglieder-und-versichertenzahl-im-vergleich/. Accessed 3 Jan 2020

Timmer A, Kappen S, de Sordi D et al (2018) Validity of hospital ICD-10 GM codes to identify acute liver injury. In: Abstract of the 34th international conference on pharmacoepidemiology & therapeutic risk management, 22–26 Aug 2018. Prague, Czech Republic. Pharmacoepidemiol Drug Saf 27. https://doi.org/10.1002/pds.4629

Wentzell N, Schink T, Haug U et al (2018) Optimizing an algorithm for the identification and classification of pregnancy outcomes in German claims data. Pharmacoepidemiol Drug Saf 27(9):1005–1010. https://doi.org/10.1002/pds.4588

Institute for Applied Health Research Berlin (InGef) Database

Frank Andersohn and Jochen Walker

Abstract The InGef (former: Health Risk Institute; HRI) database is an anonymized administrative database consisting of claims information from more than 60 German statutory health insurances (SHIs). Primary aim of the InGef is to perform health services research in cooperation with external research teams and SHIs.

1 Database Description

1.1 Introduction

The InGef (former: Health Risk Institute; HRI) database is an anonymized administrative database consisting of claims information from more than 60 German statutory health insurances (SHIs). Primary aim of the InGef is to perform health services research in cooperation with external research teams and SHIs.

1.2 Database Characteristics

In Germany, about 85% of the population (70 million inhabitants) are insured in an SHI while the remaining persons are insured in private health insurances. The InGef database currently (December 2019) includes longitudinal data from approximately nine million SHI members insured in one of the contributing SHIs (mainly company

F. Andersohn (✉)
Frank Andersohn Consulting & Research Services, Mandelstr. 16, 10409 Berlin, Germany
e-mail: info@pharmacoepi-consulting.com

J. Walker
Institute for Applied Health Research Berlin (InGef) GmbH, Spittelmarkt 12, 10117 Berlin, Germany
e-mail: jochen.walker@ingef.de

© Springer Nature Switzerland AG 2021
M. Sturkenboom and T. Schink (eds.), *Databases for Pharmacoepidemiological Research*, Springer Series on Epidemiology and Public Health, https://doi.org/10.1007/978-3-030-51455-6_9

or guild health insurances) and covers all geographic regions of Germany. The type and structure of claims data submitted by health care providers to German SHIs is regulated by law in Germany. As a consequence, data from different SHIs can be pooled without problems related to coding, etc.

The claims data that are used to establish the database are collected in a specialized data center owned by SHIs, providing data warehouse and IT services. All data entered into the InGef database are anonymized by the data center, acting as a trust center for this anonymization process. The anonymization process ensures that an identification of individual insurance members, physicians (or other health care providers), or SHIs is not possible. Access to the anonymized data is strictly controlled. No person level data is allowed to be transmitted for analysis, i.e., all data analyses have to be performed in-house by InGef employees or trained associated researchers.

To comply with the InGef data protection concept, the available calendar time for analyses is limited to a look-back period of six years. Project-related data sets may be stored for longer time periods if required (e.g., to comply with good research principles or regulatory requirements) but shall only be used to clarify requests on the results of the specific research project. The persistence (membership over time) is rather high in the InGef database: During a period of five years (2009–2013), 70.6% of insurance members survived and remained insured with the same SHI without any gap in their observational time (Andersohn and Walker 2016). Persons leaving one of the participating SHIs and entering another participating SHI, can be linked during yearly database consistency updates and are thus not lost over time. The InGef database is dynamic in nature, i.e., claims data are updated in an ongoing process and SHIs may join or leave the database. The lag-time (i.e., delay of data being available in the database) is approximately 3–9 months, depending on the type of data (e.g., hospital data is usually available before ambulatory data).

1.3   Available Data

German SHI claims data available in the InGef database include information on demographics (quarter of birth, gender, quarter of death if applicable, region of residence on administrative district level), hospitalizations, outpatient services (diagnoses, treatments, specialities of physicians), dispensings of drugs, dispensings of remedies and aids, and sick leave and sickness allowance times. In addition, costs or cost estimates from the SHI perspective are available for all important costs of all healthcare sectors. All diagnoses in Germany are coded using the International Classification of Diseases, version 10 in the German Modification (ICD-10-GM).

Content and coding of hospitalization data are strictly formalized in Germany, as hospitalizations are reimbursed based on diagnosis-related groups (DRGs). Important data elements to be submitted by hospitals include dates of admission and discharge, admission diagnosis and type of admission (e.g., normal or emergency), primary, secondary, and ancillary discharge diagnoses, procedures performed during the in-hospital stay (e.g., surgery), and the reason for discharge. In addition, the claimed DRG number and the associated costs are included in the dataset. With the exception of some very expensive medications, data on in-hospital drug treatment is usually not available. Some treatments (such as anti-cancer chemotherapy) may, however, be identified via related procedure codes.

All ambulatory physicians providing services to SHI insurance members are required to record and code diagnoses related to these services on a quarterly level. In contrast, services are coded on day level. Coding of services is crucial for the physician to receive payment, i.e., each service is related to a certain number of service points that are afterwards converted into actual Euro values.

Drug dispensings by pharmacies only include those that are reimbursed within the German SHI system. Drugs that are not reimbursable by SHI are, for instance, those categorized as lifestyle medications, e.g., oral contraceptives used by adults ≥20 years of age. With some exceptions, drugs available over the counter (OTC) are also not reimbursable in Germany and are thus not contained in the database. Data on the product dispensed include a unique identifier (central pharmaceutical number = *Pharmazentralnummer*, PZN) that can be used to exactly identify, e.g., the actual package dispensed with important characteristics such as brand name, tablet strength, number of tablets, etc. In addition, data on the day of prescribing, day of dispensing, number of packages dispensed, an anonymized identifier of the prescribing physician and the dispensing pharmacy, and costs are included in the data set.

Sick leave periods are also included in the InGef database and usually include information on the start and end of the respective sick leave period, as well as related diagnoses. In Germany, sickness allowance is paid by SHIs after a sick-leave period of six weeks (i.e., the first six weeks have to be covered by the employer, the following times, in principle, by the SHI). Sickness allowance times are thus also included in the data with similar data elements as for sick leave periods in addition to the costs from SHI perspective.

1.4 Strengths and Limitations

Strengths of the InGef database include the large number of insurants in the database, allowing analyses on rather rare exposures and outcomes. A maximum follow-up period of six years is usually sufficient for most research questions. A randomly selected research subset of approximately four million insurants that exactly matches the age- and sex structure of the German SHI population is available. The rather short delay of data being available in the database (3–9 months) is certainly a strength if the availability of very recent data is required to answer the research question. The data source has been used for several observational studies, e.g., in the areas of drug utilization (Schmedt et al. 2019b; Viniol et al. 2019), disease epidemiology (Haas et al. 2016; Ohlmeier et al. 2019), health economics (Bode et al. 2017; Lonnemann et al. 2017), and comparative drug safety and effectiveness (Hohmann et al. 2019; Schmedt et al. 2019a).

The InGef database shares disadvantages of claims data with other administrative databases, such as missing or incomplete data on socioeconomic factors, lifestyle, lab values, physical examinations, quality of life, and drugs dispensed outside the SHI system. Drug exposure times needs to be estimated from dispensings only, i.e., without having data on the prescribed daily dose. Due to the anonymized nature of the database, no case validation using medical charts, patient/physician interview is possible. In Germany, ambulatory diagnoses are only available on a quarterly basis which often needs to be considered already by the study design (e.g., definition of the start of observation).

1.5   Validation

Before entering the InGef database, the data elements are checked with respect to data format, completeness, and plausibility. Due to the anonymized nature of the database, no direct validation of the data (e.g., using medical charts as the gold standard) is possible. However, indirect validation by comparison of important measures of morbidity and overall mortality with respective reference values from the underlying population from national statistics was performed. Results for hospitalization rates, overall mortality, and drug dispensing rates of the 20 most often reimbursed drug classes were in good accordance with national reference data (Andersohn and Walker 2016, Fig. 1).

1.6   Governance and Ethical Issues

All data in the anonymized InGef database are owned by the respective SHIs and approval for each research project by the SHIs is necessary. As it would be infeasible to request approval from all SHIs for each project, the decision about acceptance of a study is made by the internal InGef scientific research group. As all research projects with the InGef database utilize completely anonymized data only, no additional permissions from authorities are necessary. It is not allowed to transmit any patient level data of the InGef database, i.e., all analyses have to be performed in-house. All variables that may allow de-identification of individuals are anonymized and coarsened if necessary. As a consequence, the data can be considered anonymized in accordance with German law (§ 67 SGB X), i.e., de-anonymization is not possible or requires an unreasonably high amount of time, effort, and costs. Informed consent of SHI members or approval by an ethics committee is not required for studies using these anonymized data sets.

1.7 Administrative Information

The database is maintained by InGef.

Contact Details

Organization/affiliation: Institute for Applied Health Research Berlin (InGef) GmbH, Spittelmarkt 12, 10117 Berlin, Germany.

Administrative Contact: Dr. Jochen Walker, jochen.walker@ingef.de, +49 (0) 30 586 945-444.

Website: https://www.ingef.de

References

Andersohn F, Walker J (2016) Characteristics and external validity of the German Health Risk Institute (HRI) Database. Pharmacoepidemiol Drug Saf 25(1):106–109. https://doi.org/10.1002/pds.3895

Bode K, Vogel R, Walker J et al (2017) Health care costs of borderline personality disorder and matched controls with major depressive disorder: a comparative study based on anonymized claims data. Eur J Health Econ 18(9):1125–1135. https://doi.org/10.1007/s10198-016-0858-2

Haas J, Braun S, Wutzler P (2016) Burden of influenza in Germany: a retrospective claims database analysis for the influenza season 2012/2013. Eur J Health Econ 17(6):669–679. https://doi.org/10.1007/s10198-015-0708-7

Hohmann C, Hohnloser SH, Jacob J et al (2019) Non-vitamin K oral anticoagulants in comparison to phenprocoumon in geriatric and non-geriatric patients with non-valvular atrial fibrillation. Thromb Haemost 119(6):971–980. https://doi.org/10.1055/s-0039-1683422

Lonnemann G, Duttlinger J, Hohmann D et al (2017) Timely referral to outpatient nephrology care slows progression and reduces treatment costs of chronic kidney diseases. Kidney Int Rep 2(2):142–151. https://doi.org/10.1016/j.ekir.2016.09.062

Ohlmeier C, Saum KU, Galetzka W et al (2019) Epidemiology and health care utilization of patients suffering from Huntington's disease in Germany: real world evidence based on German claims data. BMC Neurol 19(1):318. https://doi.org/10.1186/s12883-019-1556-3

Schmedt N, Andersohn F, Walker J et al (2019) Sodium-glucose co-transporter-2 inhibitors and the risk of fractures of the upper or lower limbs in patients with type 2 diabetes: a nested case-control study. Diabetes Obes Metab 21(1):52–60. https://doi.org/10.1111/dom.13480

Schmedt N, Schiffner-Rohe J, Sprenger R et al (2019) Pneumococcal vaccination rates in immuno-compromised patients—a cohort study based on claims data from more than 200,000 patients in Germany. PLoS ONE 14(8):e0220848. https://doi.org/10.1371/journal.pone.0220848

Viniol A, Ploner T, Hickstein L et al (2019) Prescribing practice of pregabalin/gabapentin in pain therapy: an evaluation of German claim data. BMJ Open 9(3):e021535. https://doi.org/10.1136/bmjopen-2018-021535

National Health Insurance Claims Database in France (SNIRAM), Système Nationale des Données de Santé (SNDS) and Health Data Hub (HDH)

Nicholas Moore, Patrick Blin, Régis Lassalle, Nicolas Thurin, Pauline Bosco-Levy, and Cécile Droz

Abstract SNIIRAM (*Système National d'Informations Inter-Régimes de l'Assurance Maladie*) is the French National claims database from the health insurance system. The SNIIRAM database includes information from the three main claims systems *Caisse nationale de l'assurance maladie des travailleurs salariés* (CNAMTS), *Régime social des indépendants* (RSI) now merged with CNAM, and *Mutualité sociale agricole* (MSA) and an increasing number of the smaller systems.

1 Database Description

1.1 Introduction

SNIIRAM (*Système National d'Informations Inter-Régimes de l'Assurance Maladie*) is the French National claims database from the health insurance system. The SNIIRAM database includes information from the three main claims systems *Caisse nationale de l'assurance maladie des travailleurs salariés* (CNAMTS), *Régime social des indépendants* (RSI) now merged with CNAM, and *Mutualité sociale agricole* (MSA) and an increasing number of the smaller systems. SNIIRAM is linked to the national hospital discharge database (PMSI) and the national death registry (CepiDC) to form the Système National des Données de Santé (SNDS), now part of the Health Data Hub since January 2020.

The purpose of the SNDS is to provide a tool for researchers to explore all aspects of the French health care system at a population level.

N. Moore (✉) · P. Blin · R. Lassalle · N. Thurin · P. Bosco-Levy · C. Droz (✉)
INSERM CIC1401, Bordeaux PharmacoEpi, University of Bordeaux, 33076 Bordeaux Cedex, France
e-mail: nicholas.moore@u-bordeaux.fr

C. Droz
e-mail: cecile.droz@u-bordeaux.fr

© Springer Nature Switzerland AG 2021
M. Sturkenboom and T. Schink (eds.), *Databases for Pharmacoepidemiological Research*, Springer Series on Epidemiology and Public Health,
https://doi.org/10.1007/978-3-030-51455-6_10

1.2   The French Health Care System

The French health care system features a mix of public and private services. General practitioners (GPs) and most specialists are in private practices. Secondary care is offered by private clinics and local hospitals, tertiary care by public university hospitals.

Patients have the freedom of choice when consulting a GP or specialist, but must be registered with a primary physician. The primary physician is supposed to refer the patient to specialists and hospitals (except for gynaecology, ophthalmology, paediatrics or psychiatry, or in an emergency).

The health care system is universal and covers, to various degrees, most medical expenses through a public system called Social Security (*Sécurité sociale*), which is complemented by public mutual funds and private insurance companies. Coverage includes the vast majority of drugs.

When incurring a medical expense, or upon admission to a hospital, the patient presents a smartcard (*carte Vitale*) which is used to transmit reimbursement information to the health care system's insurance system, which is in charge of the reimbursement.

There are several dozen different health care insurance systems with similar characteristics, based on mutual insurance. There is no relevant difference between the systems in coverage. The three main systems for salaried persons (CNAMTS), for self-employed professionals (RSI, now merged with CNAM), and for farmers (MSA) cover over 95% of the population. There are other smaller systems that share the same general principles and coverage.

Hospitals are reimbursed trough diagnosis-related groups for diseases and through cost modifiers, such as concomitant diseases or organ failures, and duration of stay. In addition, there are payments covering the hospitals' costs for a restricted list of expensive drugs and medical devices.

1.3   Database Characteristics

Claims information is systematically retrieved at the source of the claims (e.g., in pharmacies, in physician offices) using a patient smartcard to retrieve and identify data, linked to a patients' unique identifier. Data from local centres are transferred to regional concentrators and then to the national database.

The SNDS database includes all claims information for over 99% of the French population (68 Million persons).

All French citizens enter the database at birth when the national identification number is attributed. During childhood, attribution of claims can be to the child's or the parents' identification number, but this is usually solved at data entry. Only a person's own identification number is used beyond the age of 18.

Exit is by death or expatriation. Patients changing jobs or health care insurance systems (e.g., from the salaried workers to the independents or farmers) retain the same identification number, allowing continuous data acquisition. Patients remain in the database even in the absence of any health-related activity.

For repatriates, re-entry (using the same identification number) can occur when patients are reintegrated into the national health care system.

Data in SNIIRAM are available from 2003 for CNAMTS and from 2009 for RSI and MSA. No end of the data collection is envisioned. Follow-up of patients in the SNIIRAM database is potentially lifelong.

Data in SNIIRAM are continuously updated. Claims data are considered to be 99% complete within six months after the event. Some paper-based claims can be submitted up to two years after the event. Hospital data is updated in the third quarter of the year following the year of interest (i.e., September 2015 for 2014 data).

1.4 Available Data

1.4.1 Core Data

Core demographic data include age, sex, and region of residence. No data on ethnicity is available. Salaried and independent (self-employed) persons as well as students and several other specific statuses can be identified through their health care insurance plan. Unemployed people can also be identified directly through the presence of CMU (*Couverture Maladie Universelle*), which indicates joblessness. The CMU is a public system of health insurance coverage in France for those who are not otherwise covered through business or employment. Poverty (i.e., low social economic status) can also be identified through the CMU. Other databases exist including socioeconomic information, but these are not linked to the SNDS databases yet.

The national death registry includes the dates of deaths. Causes of death are available in the national death registry and are starting to be included from 2014 with a 3-year lag time.

1.4.2 Diagnoses

The SNIIRAM data include the presence of outpatient chronic diseases and their dates of first registration. Chronic diseases are registered according to a list of 30 disease areas along with 3,448 ICD-10 codes.

The PMSI database contains data on all hospital admissions, including main, secondary, and associate diagnoses, which are coded in ICD-10.

1.4.3   Medication

All reimbursed outpatient prescription medication is recorded as dispensed preparations packs, including a unique registration code (CIP), as well as ATC and European Pharmaceutical Market Research Association (EPhMRA) codes. The description of the packs includes the number of tablets, the strength, the number of packs dispensed, the date of prescription, the nature of the prescriber, the date of dispensing, and the dispensing pharmacy (anonymized).

Drugs that are sold over-the-counter (OTC), but can also be prescribed and then are reimbursed (OTC strength drugs), such as ibuprofen or paracetamol, may be found in the database if they were prescribed. True OTC and prescription drugs that are not covered are not recorded.

There is no information available about in-hospital prescriptions, except for expensive drugs on a specific list. This concerns essentially public hospitals. Private clinics may provide more information.

1.4.4   Procedures

The date and the nature of physician as well as paramedical (nurses, physiotherapists, etc.) interventions are recorded in the database, including procedures such as endoscopy.

In-hospital procedures and devices and outpatient devices are recorded as LPP (*Liste des produits et prestations*) codes in the PMSI database.

The date and nature of medical transports are also available in the database.

1.4.5   Laboratory Results

The date and nature of all laboratory tests are recorded. The results of laboratory tests are not available, except in case they are the indication for a hospital admission. Physical examination results are not available.

1.4.6   Other Information

The number of days a patient was on paid sick leave as well as certain lifestyle interventions or aids, such as wheelchairs or crutches, are available in the database.

1.4.7   Cost Information

All of the above-mentioned information is accompanied by costing information including total costs, the amount reimbursed by the main health care insurance and by possible complementary mutual funds or private insurances. This information though is often complex to decrypt and difficult to understand without expertise.

1.4.8 Hospitalisation Data (PMSI)

The claims database is linked to the national hospital information database PMSI. The PMSI database contains data from both public and private hospitals. It includes hospital admissions in medical, surgical, and obstetrical wards. Psychiatric hospitalisations are included as well as treatment in rehabilitation centres. In addition to admission data and length of stay, it includes information such as the source of the admission and the destination of discharge, which may be another department of the same hospital or another hospital, in addition to discharge for home or death.

1.4.9 Death

The third component of SNDS is the linkage to the national death registry, which provides date of death. Cause of death is available for 2013–2015.

1.4.10 Linkage

Family members (e.g., mothers with children) can be identified in the database if the children are registered with the mother's insurance number and upon specific request.

Other linkages are still under study (e.g., linkage to a tax database which includes income levels).

The development of the national health data hub should include linkable hospital data repositories and GP databases, including clinical data and lab test results or other information such as biomarkers or tumour pathology.

It is not possible to re-identify subjects and to gather additional information or re-contact the patient, e.g., for bio samples. It is, however, possible to link from the patient to the database using either determinist matching with the national health ID number (NIR) with ethical and data protection committee approval and written consent, or probabilistic matching after data protection committee approval. This matching allows the pairing of clinical data (from primary data collection or pre-existing cohort data) to the health care claims data.

1.5 Strengths and Limitations

One major strength of the database is its exhaustiveness of documented medical events; all prescribed reimbursed medical activities, all prescribed drugs, all hospital admissions (to public or private hospitals), and all deaths are recorded.

Another major strength is its size and representativeness for the French population. The database includes all claims information for over 99% of the entire French population.

Internationally applied coding systems, such as ICD-10 and ATC are used. In addition, the hospital diagnoses undergo audits by the health care insurance system and cross audits between hospitals.

On the other hand, the whole data array represents over a hundred tables, with an extremely complex architecture. The main source data was developed to ensure the reimbursement of individual medical expenses and claims, not for medical research. Using these data to follow individual patients over time and across different types of information and linking the data to the two other databases can be challenging. Considerable work is being done to facilitate the use of the database for research purposes and to develop compatibility with common data models (OHDSI, EHDEN, EU-ADR).

1.6 Validation

Data are checked on an ad-hoc basis for outliers, as part of the usual data management before analysis.

Validation of specific hospital diagnoses from the PMSI database has shown a high validity of main diagnostic codes (>75% PPV) (Bezin et al. 2015), in addition to the systematic quality assurance process of the hospital coding systems (Gilleron et al. 2018). Researchers cannot identify individuals from the anonymised database, and so no direct revalidation is possible from the general database. Methods of internal validation are being developed (Thurin et al. 2018, 2019).

Diagnostic certainty has been shown to be reasonably good for outpatient chronic diseases. The sensitivity for chronic diseases is potentially lower. Some chronic diseases are not registered because of social stigma issues (psychiatric diseases, epilepsy), or because disease treatment is already covered (e.g., registration for hypertension if heart failure or ischemic heart disease is already present).

1.7   Governance and Ethical Issues

The SNDS database is owned by the national health care system and the French state.

Access to the data is regulated by law. SNDS is directly accessible to the health care insurance system and to a number of public institutions such as the French medicines agency (ANSM) or to regional health agencies. For researchers, the access is authorised on a per-protocol basis by the *Institut National des Données de Santé* (INDS). A request for data access, including a full protocol and the source of the financing, is submitted to INDS, reviewed by a scientific committee for pertinence and public health interest. After approval the protocol is transmitted to the national data protection agency (*Commission Nationale de l'Informatique et des Libertés*, CNIL). There are a number of variables that cannot be accessed simultaneously, such as date of birth, place of residence, date of hospital admission, date of death. After approval, the CNAM which is the data curator needs to sign a convention for data access. Data can be accessed on a reserved space on the CNAM servers, or can be transferred to a security referential compliant computer system.

Further information on this evolving process and the impact of the Health Data Hub can be found on their websites (Health Data Hub 2020; Plateforme des Données de Santé 2020).

The time-frame for study approval is two months for INDS and scientific approval, 2–4 months for the CNIL, and 2–6 months for the CNAM convention. Despite much improvement the time to access the data is still 9–12 months.

Data cannot be exported outside the authorised structure, but studies can be redone upon request, or data extraction can be re-requested from the same source for study validation purposes.

All persons desiring to access SNDS need to attend formal training (3 days) in accessing the database to obtain accreditation. Access is authorised on a per-study basis.

The three databases (SNIIRAM, PMSI, and the national death registry) are linked through a unique personal identification number (*numéro d'inscription au repertoire des personnes physiques*, NIR), which is de-identified using two successive hash scrambling operations (Quantin et al. 1998a, b; Quantin et al. 1996, 1997). This one-way scrambling algorithm allows the linkage of the different databases but does not permit to go back to the original NIR or to the patients. The national death registry is maintained by the national institute for statistics and economic studies (*Institut national de la statistique et des études économiques*, INSEE). The hospital database (PMSI) is maintained by regional health authorities (ARS) and the agency for hospital information (ATIH), which transfers it on a yearly basis to SNIIRAM.

Due to the anonymous nature of the data, patient consent is not required. Patients have no possibility to opt out from the database.

1.8 Documents and Publications

The SNDS database and their potentials for epidemiological, pharmacoepidemiological, and health economics studies have been described (Tuppin et al. 2010; Moulis et al. 2015; Bezin et al. 2017).

Many studies have used the National health care system data on drug related risks, including benfluorex and valvular disease (Weill et al. 2010), pioglitazone and cancer of the bladder (Neumann et al. 2012), olmesartan and malabsorption (Basson et al. 2016), Glargine and cancer (Fagot et al. 2013), on the comparative effectiveness of statins (Neumann et al. 2014), and on the risk of bleeding after oral anticoagulants (Maura et al. 2015).

The pharmacoepidemiology unit of the university hospital in Bordeaux has performed a series of studies concerning, for instance, the identification of rheumatoid arthritis (Bernard et al. 2012), treatment patterns in Parkinson's disease (Blin et al. 2015), utilisation of 'over-the-counter' and prescription-strength NSAIDs (Duong et al. 2014), Insulin glargine and cancer (Blin et al. 2012) or the determination of the denominator in case-population studies (Moore et al. 2013). Many studies are on-going.

Overall, more than 150 publications refer to SNDS or SNIIRAM. More may exist that did not use these identifiers.

1.9 Administrative Information

- Organisation responsible for maintaining the database
  CNAM (National health insurance system)—Health Data Hub.
- Funding
  Public funding by health insurance system.
- Contact details (administrative, scientific, and technical contact)
  Contact any of several research units using the database;
  Institut National des données de santé
  19, rue Arthur Croquette
  94220 Charenton-le-Pont
  Tél: 01 45 18 43 90
  Fax: 01 45 18 43 99
- URL of website
  https://www.health-data-hub.fr/
  https://www.indsante.fr/fr/deposer-une-demande.

2 Practical Experience with the Database

The database has proven to be suitable for drug utilisation studies, drug safety studies, comparative effectiveness studies, and market access studies. Studies on long-term effects are limited to the data years that are currently available (15 years in some cases). Longer term data will be made available in time.

Studies based on SNDS data can be of any of the standard pharmacoepidemiological designs based on exposures or events: cross-sectional studies, cohort studies, nested case–control studies, self-controlled case studies, and case-population studies.

The SNDS database is currently being used in several international projects in cooperation with OHDSI, EHDEN, and other networks in Europe and worldwide.

Different research teams have developed different tools to manage and analyse the data.

The main challenge in using the database lies in the size and complexity of the database. Some extractions can be very large and consequently require significant computing power, as well as data-managing resources.

References

Basson M, Mezzarobba M, Weill A et al (2016) Severe intestinal malabsorption associated with olmesartan: a French nationwide observational cohort study. Gut 65(10):1664–1669. https://doi.org/10.1136/gutjnl-2015-309690

Bernard MA, Benichou J, Blin P et al (2012) Use of health insurance claim patterns to identify patients using nonsteroidal anti-inflammatory drugs for rheumatoid arthritis. Pharmacoepidemiol Drug Saf 21(6):573–583. https://doi.org/10.1002/pds.3221

Bezin J, Girodet PO, Rambelomanana S et al (2015) Choice of ICD-10 codes for the identification of acute coronary syndrome in the French hospitalization database. Fundam Clin Pharmacol 29(6):586–591. https://doi.org/10.1111/fcp.12143

Bezin J, Duong M, Lassalle R et al (2017) The national healthcare system claims databases in France, SNIIRAM and EGB: Powerful tools for pharmacoepidemiology. Pharmacoepidemiol Drug Saf 26(8):954–962. https://doi.org/10.1002/pds.4233

Blin P, Lassalle R, Dureau-Pournin C et al (2012) Insulin glargine and risk of cancer: a cohort study in the French National Healthcare Insurance Database. Diabetologia 55(3):644–653. https://doi.org/10.1007/s00125-011-2429-5

Blin P, Dureau-Pournin C, Foubert-Samier A et al (2015) Parkinson's disease incidence and prevalence assessment in France using the national healthcare insurance database. Eur J Neurol 22(3):464–471. https://doi.org/10.1111/ene.12592

Duong M, Salvo F, Pariente A et al. (2014) Usage patterns of 'over-the-counter' vs. prescription-strength nonsteroidal anti-inflammatory drugs in France. Br J Clin Pharmacol 77 (5):887–895. https://doi.org/10.1111/bcp.12239

Fagot JP, Blotiere PO, Ricordeau P et al (2013) Does insulin glargine increase the risk of cancer compared with other basal insulins? A French nationwide cohort study based on national administrative databases. Diabetes Care 36(2):294–301. https://doi.org/10.2337/dc12-0506

Gilleron V, Gasnier-Duparc N, Hebbrecht G (2018) Certification des comptes: Une incitation à la traçabilité des processus de contrôle. Revue Hospitaliere de France 582:42–46

Health Data Hub (2020) https://www.health-data-hub.fr/. Accessed 2 Feb 2020

Maura G, Blotiere PO, Bouillon K et al (2015) Comparison of the short-term risk of bleeding and arterial thromboembolic events in nonvalvular atrial fibrillation patients newly treated with dabigatran or rivaroxaban versus vitamin K antagonists: a French nationwide propensity-matched cohort study. Circulation 132(13):1252–1260. https://doi.org/10.1161/CIRCULATIONAHA.115.015710

Moore N, Gulmez SE, Larrey D et al (2013) Choice of the denominator in case population studies: event rates for registration for liver transplantation after exposure to NSAIDs in the SALT study in France. Pharmacoepidemiol Drug Saf 22(2):160–167. https://doi.org/10.1002/pds.3371

Moulis G, Lapeyre-Mestre M, Palmaro A et al (2015) French health insurance databases: what interest for medical research? Rev Med Interne 36(6):411–417. https://doi.org/10.1016/j.revmed.2014.11.009

Neumann A, Weill A, Ricordeau P et al (2012) Pioglitazone and risk of bladder cancer among diabetic patients in France: a population-based cohort study. Diabetologia 55(7):1953–1962. https://doi.org/10.1007/s00125-012-2538-9

Neumann A, Maura G, Weill A et al (2014) Comparative effectiveness of rosuvastatin versus simvastatin in primary prevention among new users: a cohort study in the French national health insurance database. Pharmacoepidemiol Drug Saf 23(3):240–250. https://doi.org/10.1002/pds.3544

Plateforme des Données de Santé (2020) Accéder aux données de santé. https://www.indsante.fr/fr/deposer-une-demande. Accessed 2 Feb 2020

Quantin C, Bouzelat H, Dusserre L (1996) Irreversible encryption method by generation of polynomials. Med Inform (Lond) 21(2):113–121. https://doi.org/10.3109/14639239608995013

Quantin C, Bouzelat H, Dusserre L (1997) A computerized record hash coding and linkage procedure to warrant epidemiological follow-up data security. Stud Health Technol Inform 43(Pt A):339–342

Quantin C, Bouzelat H, Allaert FA et al (1998a) Automatic record hash coding and linkage for epidemiological follow-up data confidentiality. Methods Inf Med 37(3):271–277

Quantin C, Bouzelat H, Allaert FA et al (1998b) How to ensure data security of an epidemiological follow-up: quality assessment of an anonymous record linkage procedure. Int J Med Inform 49(1):117–122. https://doi.org/10.1016/s1386-5056(98)00019-7

Thurin N, Blin P, Rouyer M et al (2018) Identifying patients with metastatic castration-resistant prostate cancers (mCRPC) in the SNDS database: Camerra Study. Pharmacoepidemiol Drug Saf 27:71–72

Thurin N, Rouyer M, Gross-Goupil M et al (2019) Validation of a complex algorithm for the diagnosis of metastatic castration-resistant prostate cancer within a claims database. Pharmacoepidemiol Drug Saf 28:165–165

Tuppin P, de Roquefeuil L, Weill A et al (2010) French national health insurance information system and the permanent beneficiaries sample. Rev Epidemiol Sante Publique 58(4):286–290. https://doi.org/10.1016/j.respe.2010.04.005

Weill A, Paita M, Tuppin P et al (2010) Benfluorex and valvular heart disease: a cohort study of a million people with diabetes mellitus. Pharmacoepidemiol Drug Saf 19(12):1256–1262. https://doi.org/10.1002/pds.2044

Agenzia Regionale di Sanità della Toscana (ARS)

Rosa Gini

Abstract Italy has a *universal*, single-payer healthcare system funded by the general taxation: the national government provides regional governments with funding, which they must dedicate to ensure that their resident population has access to a nationally-defined list of services. Starting in the mid-nineties, regional governments were requested to electronically record services provided to their population and to transmit the information to the national government.

1 Database Description

1.1 Introduction

Agenzia regionale di sanità della Toscana (ARS) is an agency of the Tuscany Region in Italy and acts as a technical and scientific consultant both to the regional government and to the Regional Council of Tuscany.

1.2 Database Characteristics

Italy has a *universal*, single-payer healthcare system funded by the general taxation: the national government provides regional governments with funding, which they must dedicate to ensure that their resident population has access to a nationally-defined list of services. Starting in the mid-nineties, regional governments were requested to electronically record services provided to their population and to transmit the information to the national government. The list of services whose recording is compulsory has grown steadily. The information is recorded by the local

R. Gini (✉)
Agenzia regional di sanità della Toscana—ARS, Via Pietro Dazzi 1, Florence, Italy
e-mail: rosa.gini@ars.toscana.it

© Springer Nature Switzerland AG 2021   141
M. Sturkenboom and T. Schink (eds.), *Databases for Pharmacoepidemiological Research*, Springer Series on Epidemiology and Public Health,
https://doi.org/10.1007/978-3-030-51455-6_11

healthcare providers and transmitted in a standard electronic format to the region, which in turn transmits it to the national government (Trifiro et al. 2019).

The core data that ARS has access to are the healthcare administrative databases of the population of the Italian region of Tuscany, which amounts to around 3.6 million inhabitants. The Tuscany Region transmits a copy of its healthcare administrative databases to ARS, which is entitled by regional law to use it for its institutional purposes, upon permission of a board representing the Regional Council.

As is the case in every Italian region, the reason for entering the database is the registration with a primary care physician, which may happen upon immigration or upon birth; the reason for exiting the database is emigration or death.

Upon permission by a regional ethical review board, ARS may also access and link with its core data the cancer registry, the congenital anomaly registry and the rare disease registry, all collected on the whole Tuscan population. On occasion, ARS may request to retrieve information from medical records and/or laboratory results of specific subpopulations and link it to its core data.

All the data transferred to ARS is pseudonymized with a regional identifier.

Data collection of the most important tables has been available since 2003. The database is updated every 2–3 months, and the lag time is about 2–3 weeks, but data is incomplete for 4–5 months.

1.3   Available Data

The administrative databases contain tables that are described in the next paragraphs.

Registry of inhabitants

Right to healthcare is granted to all persons who are legal inhabitants of Tuscany. In order to access healthcare, inhabitants (or their parents in case of children) must request a primary care physician, which is a general practitioner for adults or a pediatrician for children. The registry of inhabitants records the date of birth, date of registration, date of exit (if persons transfer out of Tuscany), date of death, identifier of the primary care physician, citizenship, and address. The registry is longitudinal.

Hospital discharge records

Hospital discharge records are created when a person is discharged after hospital admission, which may last one or multiple days. A record includes the date of admission, principal discharge diagnosis (which is the diagnosis which justifies the cost allocated to the admission), up to five secondary and ancillary diagnoses, up to six diagnostic and surgical/medical procedures during the hospital stay, discharge date, and status at discharge (including death). Diagnoses and procedures are coded using an Italian modification of the ICD9-CM coding system. Records from recent years also contain the education level and diagnoses may be labeled as 'present on admission'.

If the record refers to a birth, the code of the hospital discharge record of the mother is included.

Specialist visits, diagnostic tests

The decision to include drugs in the national drug formulary, i.e., deciding which drugs will be covered by the National Healthcare System, falls within the remit of the Italian Medicines Agency (*Agenzia Italiana del Farmaco*, AIFA). In general, all "life-saving" and chronic medications are refundable, i.e., approximately 70% of all marketed drugs in Italy.

Three data sources record dispensations of drugs reimbursed by the healthcare system:

- dispensings in community pharmacies
- dispensings in hospital pharmacies for outpatient use
- dispensings in hospital pharmacies for inpatient use.

The third data source (drugs for inpatient use) is the only administrative source lacking the patient identifier: The identifier of the ward where the patient is admitted is the only information recorded, and the identity of the patient may only be obtained by probabilistic record linkage.

All three sources record the amount of product dispensed, and the product which is labeled by the Italian code for marketing authorization, as released by AIFA. This in turn can be linked to brand name, ATC, number of defined daily doses (DDD) dispensed, and number and strength of posologic units (if applicable). The batch number is also available.

Outpatient activity

Inhabitants have the right to access a number of outpatient healthcare services: specialist visits, diagnostic tests, rehabilitation procedures, and therapeutic procedures. This list of services is updated regularly by the national government and coded with a national coding system. Tuscany may add additional services coded in the regional coding system, or record an additional, more detailed regional code. It must be noted that specialist visits are recorded but diagnoses are not; and utilization of tests is recorded but results are not.

Services are recorded with date (in case of recurring services, start date, end date, and number of episodes of care) and place of service.

Exemptions

Inhabitants are requested to contribute financially to some of their healthcare at the point of service. Exemption from this requirement is granted to children younger than six and to the elderly (unless they are wealthy). Moreover, exemption is granted for specific healthcare services to patients who have a diagnosis that requires recurring use of those services.

The records of exemptions from copayment contain the date of exemption and the ICD-9-CM code of the disease.

Emergency admission

Upon admission to an emergency service, the following information is recorded: date, anamnesis, diagnoses, procedures, and possible admission to hospital. Anamnesis is provided in free text, diagnoses and procedures in ICD-9-CM.

Other administrative databases

Other administrative databases collect mental healthcare, services in residential, semi-residential, and home settings, and rehabilitation services.

Non-administrative databases

Besides administrative databases, ARS also receives a copy of other registries.

In the case of births or still births (i.e., number of weeks of gestation higher than 22) information is recorded on the place of birth, on socio-economic characteristics of the parents, on the pregnancy (e.g., gestational age, body mass index before pregnancy, smoke status during pregnancy), on the delivery, on characteristics of the newborn (e.g., weight), and possibly on congenital anomalies or the cause of death.

Other registries are: the spontaneous abortions and induced terminations registry, the death registry, the vaccine registry (also recorded with batch number), and the pathology registry, which are collected on the whole Tuscan population.

1.4 Strengths and Limitations

A major strength of the ARS database is its size, comprehensiveness of a large Italian region and long follow-up time.

Record linkage and its quality

The potential of the ARS database lies in the possibility of linking within and across data tables. With the exception of inpatient drug use, record linkage is deterministic. The quality of record linkage is determined by the quality of recording of the personal identifier. When conducting descriptive and analytic studies, study subjects should be restricted to those recorded in the inhabitant registry, because those are the only ones whose care is systematically recorded in the ARS database. After 2010, the registry of inhabitants compares well with the sex- and age-specific counts released by the

National Institute of Statistics. Moreover, person identifiers (whose pseudonymization is received by ARS) are increasingly compiled automatically. However, a small amount of loss to record linkage needs to be taken into account.

Completeness

A strength of administrative databases is their internal completeness, due to legal and funding motivations. However, external completeness needs to be discussed, since access to private healthcare is common in Italy to shorten time to access to healthcare.

Private hospitalization can be considered residual in Tuscany.

Medicinal products which are not reimbursed are not recorded, but even reimbursed drugs may often be purchased over-the-counter (OTC) if they are cheap or if the copayment is comparable to the price. According to AIFA estimates, in Italy in 2017, 1708.2 DDDs per 1000 inhabitants were dispensed. Of those, 66.2% were reimbursed by the National Healthcare System, while 33.8% were purchased by patients OTC.

As for outpatient activities, according to the National Institute of Statistics, in 2012/2013, around 40% of specialist visits (excluding primary and dental care), 23% of specialist diagnostic tests, and 13% of blood tests were paid privately by patients.

Healthcare and events which are not recorded

Primary care visits are not recorded, since primary care physicians are paid based on the number of persons they assist. As already mentioned, therapies administered during inpatient care are not recorded, nor are diagnoses issued by specialists or results of diagnostic tests recorded.

1.5 Validation

Validation of samples of records from hospitalizations, access to emergency care, or specialist visits is possible via access to medical records. Emergency care and pathology registers also have free text records which can be used for validation purposes.

1.6 Governance and Ethical Issues

According to regional law, ARS can execute studies on its database, provided the control board of the Regional Council approves the activity.

Enrichment with external sources, such as validation or access to laboratory result, needs to be approved by the Ethical Review Board of the corresponding hospitals.

1.7 Administrative Information

ARS is a public institution whose budget is provided by the Regional Government
of Tuscany.

Contact details

Organization/affiliation: Agenzia regionale di sanità della Toscana—ARS via
Pietro Dazzi 1, Florence, Italy

Website: www.ars.toscana.it

Reference

Trifiro G, Gini R, Barone-Adesi F et al (2019) The role of European healthcare databases for
   post-marketing drug effectiveness, safety and value evaluation: where does Italy stand? Drug Saf
   42(3):347–363. https://doi.org/10.1007/s40264-018-0732-5

Caserta Record Linkage Database

Gianluca Trifirò, Valentina Ientile, Janet Sultana, and Michele Tari

Abstract The Italian publicly funded National Health Service (NHS) provides universal health care, mainly free of charge, to all NHS beneficiaries, that is, the whole Italian population. The NHS has three levels of management. At the national level, the health ministry is responsible for upholding citizens' rights to health care and its main aim is to define the so-called essential levels of health care, i.e., the services that the NHS must supply free of charge after payment of a registration and maintenance fee.

1 Database Description

1.1 Introduction

The Italian publicly funded National Health Service (NHS) provides universal health care, mainly free of charge, to all NHS beneficiaries, that is, the whole Italian population. The NHS has three levels of management. At the national level, the health ministry is responsible for upholding citizens' rights to health care and its main aim is to define the so-called essential levels of health care, i.e., the services that the NHS must supply free of charge after payment of a registration and maintenance fee. The Ministry transfers the responsibilities of health care governance to the single regions, giving the regions a strong independence in the service management. Each

G. Trifirò (✉)
Department of Diagnostics and Public Health, University of Verona, Verona, Italy
e-mail: gianluca.trifiro@unime.it

V. Ientile · J. Sultana
Department of Biomedical and Dental Sciences and Morpho-functional Imaging, University of Messina, Messina, Italy

M. Tari
Local Health Unit of Caserta, Caserta, Italy

© Springer Nature Switzerland AG 2021
M. Sturkenboom and T. Schink (eds.), *Databases for Pharmacoepidemiological Research*, Springer Series on Epidemiology and Public Health,
https://doi.org/10.1007/978-3-030-51455-6_12

region is then divided into Local Health Units (LHUs), which have a direct role in the management of health care services in their respective areas within the region.

The Caserta record linkage database contains individual claims databases with information on health care services covered by the NHS. All claims databases from the Caserta LHU can be linked to each other through anonymized unique patient identifiers. The most widely used claims databases include drug dispensing databases and hospital discharge diagnosis databases. The degree of patient coverage over the catchment area is very high, since practically all persons living in Caserta, as in all Italian cities, are NHS beneficiaries.

Information in the Caserta record linkage database was recorded as early as 2000 and reached its maximum completeness and consistency starting in 2009. In the following years, several disease (such as chronic obstructive pulmonary disease, hypertension, diabetes mellitus) and health care service (low protein diet products) registers were launched in the catchment area, further increasing the volume of available health care data. In addition, a new system based on electronic prescriptions for drugs prescribed by specialists was introduced in 2015. The value of these electronic prescriptions is that they contain information on the dosing regimen as well as on the indication of use of the dispensed drugs, which is not available in pharmacy claims. The claims database can be linked to other useful data sources, such as electronic medical record databases including prescriptions with associated indication of use sent by general practitioners (GPs). The GP prescription database was set up by the Caserta LHU in 2000 with the initial aim of facilitating clinical auditing of GPs practicing in the Caserta area concerning the management of the most frequent acute and chronic diseases. Data was collected until 2015 and various attempts to restart it have not yet succeeded. This GP database is the only one in Italy which allows the systematic linkage of GP prescription data to claims data on a patient level. The Caserta linkage database has been used extensively for research over the past decade, including studies on drug utilization (Oteri et al. 2010; Ingrasciotta et al. 2014; Trifirò et al. 2007; Sultana et al. 2015), drug safety (Ingrasciotta et al. 2015), risk minimization measures (Viola et al. 2016) and disease epidemiology (Trifirò et al. 2014). The Caserta linkage database has also been used to conduct studies within a network of databases in the context of schizophrenia research (Sultana et al. 2019) and more widely, to conduct studies on the use and safety of biologic drugs (Ingrasciotta et al. 2019; Belleudi et al. 2019; Marciano et al. 2018).

1.2   Software for Data Collection

In addition to traditional claims databases, information on prescriptions mainly issued by specialists is collected through Sani.A.R.P., a health information system used in the Campania Region. Sani.A.R.P. was launched by the Caserta LHU in 2002 with the aim of managing prescriptions more efficiently by using an online platform. Since 2013, Sani.A.R.P. has been considered an essential part of the Regional Health Information System and many prescribing and dispensing pathways are progressively monitored and managed using this platform. Sani.A.R.P. collects data concerning electronic prescriptions in a community setting with over 6000 prescribers. It allows real-time monitoring of health care delivery in partner pharmacies and integrates patient-level data on health care from diagnosis onwards. The use of Sani.A.R.P. has also reduced medication errors by linking prescriptions to the regional health system and the regional formulary, thus verifying its temporal validity. Sani.A.R.P. is ethically transparent, as it is mandatory to collect informed consent from patients who are directly registered on the portal. Since patients explicitly give their consent to share their clinical information, prescribers are able to access the patient's drug history.

1.3   Data Sources

As previously mentioned, the Caserta linkage database consists of several components which can be linked to each other via anonymized unique patient identifiers: claims databases, disease registries and a general practicioner (GP) prescription database. The Caserta linkage claims database currently contains demographic and clinical information on 1,159,385 persons residing in the Caserta catchment area from 2009 to 2019. Of these, 985,275 were active as of 31 December 2019. For a subset of 654,378 (66.4%) subjects, GP prescriptions with associated indication of use can be linked to the claims databases at the patient level. The general characteristics of the underlying population are shown in Table 1. The average follow-up time of persons registered in the database is about 8.0 years for the whole population and 5.4 years for the GP subset. The shorter average follow-up for the GP subset is due to the necessity of using a dedicated algorithm to identify valid observation periods based on the availability of data for a specific GP. Data collection stopped in 2014.

1.3.1   Claims Databases

Since most of the health care costs in Italy are covered by the NHS, electronic data are collected for administrative purposes from pharmacies, hospitals, laboratories, and outpatient specialist centres in the context of primary, secondary, and tertiary care. NHS claims data are collected for patients from birth until death. Claims databases in Italy are very similar within each Italian region and within each city. They have been described in great detail elsewhere (Trifirò et al. 2019). Caserta claims data conform to this description.

There is a specific claims database from the Caserta LHU for each branch of health care service provided. These databases can be linked to GPs' prescriptions at the patient level through anonymized unique patient identifiers. Due to the fact that data are anonymized, it is not possible to re-contact persons in the database for the collection of additional data. However, it is possible to identify the GPs caring for specific patients, to contact the GPs, and to ask them for further information. This

Table 1 General characteristics underlying population for the Caserta record linkage database (2009–2019) and for the sub-population identified directly from the GP prescription database (2000–2015)

	Overall Caserta LHU residents N = 1,159,385 (%)	GP prescription database N = 654,378 (%)
Sex		
Male	573,435 (49.5)	318,572 (48.7)
Female	585,950 (50.5)	335,806 (51.3)
Mean age ± SD	35.5 ± 23.2	39.5 ± 20.5[a]
Age classes (years)		
<45	755,756 (65.2)	398,645 (60.9)
45–64	253,014 (21.8)	166,134 (25.4)
65–80	117,073 (10.1)	73,253 (11.2)
>80	33,542 (2.9)	16,346 (2.5)
Mean follow-up (years)	8.0 ± 3.0	5.4 ± 2.0
Cumulative person-years	9,338,503	3,511,084

[a]GPs in Italy only have patients who are 14 years or older; younger patients are visited by family pediatricians. *Abbreviations* GP—general practitioners; LHU—local health unit; SD—standard deviation

can be useful when validating diagnoses identified through algorithms. Usually, the claims databases are updated every six months and the lag time for new data to be available is about one year. The individual claims databases are outlined below.

- *Demographic registry*: These data consist of an updated list of inhabitants who are registered with a GP practicing in the Caserta LHU catchment area. This registry contains information about age, gender, date of registration in the regional health care system, and where applicable, date of death or deregistration of the persons cared by GP. There is no information on the cause of death.
- *Drug dispensing database*: This database contains data on outpatient drug dispensing which occurs via direct distribution through public or private pharmacies. The database contains data concerning only the dispensing of drugs which are reimbursed by the Italian National Health System (NHS) for persons registered with the Caserta LHU. Drug dispensing data contain information on the drug name, number of prescribed packages, the national drug code, and cost of the packages. The national drug code (*Autorizzazione Immissione in Commercio*) is assigned to each medication when it is approved to be marketed in Italy. It is specific to the active pharmaceutical product, the strength, route of administration, and marketing authorization holder. This means that through this code, all drugs identified in the database can be described in detail. Drug information in the database is also coded using the Anatomic and Therapeutic Chemical (ATC) classification code. From 2015, approximately 70% of all pharmacy claims for drugs covered by the NHS collected from community pharmacies had the indication of use registered through the International Classification of Diseases, 9th

edition, with clinical modifications (ICD-9-CM) code. Over-the-counter drugs are not reimbursed in Italy. For this reason, prescriptions for these drugs cannot be captured in the Caserta claims linkage database. Drugs which are reimbursed by the NHS but which are not bought through the NHS are also not captured. Information on the duration of a pharmacy claim is deduced based on the assumption that the doses prescribed are in line with the 'defined daily dose' as outlined by the World Health Organization.

- *Therapeutic plans database*: This database contains information on expensive drugs which can only be prescribed by qualified specialists. Specifically, the generic name of the drug prescribed, the date of dispensing, the indication of use, and the dosing regimen including daily dosage and duration are captured.
- *Hospital discharge database*: This database contains information from hospital discharge records for persons living in the Caserta LHU catchment area. Each hospital discharge record contains the admission and discharge date, the primary diagnosis (i.e., the main cause of hospitalization) as well as up to five secondary diagnoses and performed hospital procedures with associated costs. Diagnoses are coded using ICD-9-CM codes. Data concerning discharge diagnoses from hospitals within as well as outside (around 5–10% of all hospitalizations) Caserta LHU are captured. In the latter case, persons living inside the LHU Caserta catchment area have been treated in hospitals outside of this area, which leads to approximately one year extra lag time for data collection.
- *Emergency department admissions database*: This data concerns the reasons for admission to emergency departments of the hospitals in Caserta LHU, coded using ICD-9 CM codes. Date of admission and discharge are also available.
- *Referrals for outpatient diagnostic tests and specialist's visits database*: This database contains the referrals for both outpatient radiologic and laboratory diagnostic tests which are performed in public health care centres and are reimbursed by the NHS. In addition, special ambulatory procedures (e.g., dental extraction) and specialist visits are also registered. The procedure or examination costs based on the regional formulary are reported. Data are coded using a regional diagnostic test coding system and are available for all residents in the catchment area of the Caserta LHU. The date of a procedure or examination as well as the name of the laboratory where the tests were carried out are also available. The results of these tests are available for approximately 20% of the catchment population covered in the whole claims database.
- *Laboratory tests values database*: Around 20% of the laboratory tests for people residing in Caserta are performed in public health care clinics using a common software facilitating centralization of the results of these tests, which are captured in a dedicated database.
- *Database of co-payment exempt patients*: This database contains coded information about specific diseases (often chronic and/or debilitating diseases such as diabetes and Parkinson's disease, respectively) or socioeconomic factors that render a subject eligible for exemption from health care co-pay, i.e., from the contribution fees for a particular service. For patients with an exemption code, the date of start and, if applicable, end of exemption are available.

1.3.2 Frailty Registry

For all persons who are ≥65 years, yearly comprehensive geriatric evaluation forms have to be electronically filled by their GP (Guerriero et al. 2015). Currently, for about 80% of elderly persons in the catchment area, there is at least one evaluation form. The available information concerns drug prescriptions, co-morbidities, and functional status. The functional status is a rich source of geriatric data as it contains the results of specific evaluation scales on accommodation, activities of daily living, mobility, nursing needs, social conditions, mental conditions, ability to speak and hear, seeing ability, physical activity, urinary and intestinal continence, as well as smoking status, alcohol consumption, and weight and body mass index. The evaluation of the forms is carried out by the GPs once a year with the obligation to record the information.

1.3.3 Clinical and Disease Registries

From 2015, the Caserta LHU has launched several disease- and therapy-specific registries to evaluate the appropriate use of health care resources and to monitor health care expenditure. Currently, registries for diabetic patients, hypertensive patients, coeliac disease patients, patients undergoing dialysis, and those with chronic kidney disease on a low protein diet are available. These databases contain data which can be linked to pharmacy claims and to clinical values of specific tests. For example, it is possible to identify the blood pressure values, low density cholesterol level values, glycated hemoglobin, and body mass index, etc. In 2018, there were 63,275 patients in the diabetes registry (5% of persons in the Caserta claims database) and 213,599 persons with hypertension in the hypertension registry (18.4% of persons in the Caserta claims database).

1.3.4 GP Prescription Database

GPs act as gatekeepers in the Italian national health care system for patients aged 14 years or older, issuing drug prescriptions and referring patients to specialists for examinations, hospitalizations (except for those via emergency department), and diagnostic tests. GPs who contribute to the GP database and record prescription data during their daily clinical practice use dedicated software and send anonymized data on prescriptions and indications of use to a coordinating centre on a monthly basis. All data are checked for completeness and stored in a central server. The GP prescription database covers about 60% of the inhabitants of the Caserta catchment area, as not all GPs practicing in the same area transfer data periodically to the central database. A comparison of the population identified from the claims database and from the GP prescription database is outlined in Table 2.

The GP prescription database contains information on drug prescriptions issued by GPs with the related indication of use coded using ICD-9-CM. Prescriptions written by specialists are also updated to the patient prescription history in the Caserta claims

Table 2 Overview of available data in the Caserta claims linkage database

Type of database	Data source	Starting from	Population covered
Claims	Demographic registry	2000	Caserta LHU population (reference) (%)
	Drug dispensing (from either private pharmacies or direct distribution from specialist center) database	2004	100
	Oncologic drug registry	2013	100
	Therapeutic plan database	2011	100
	Hospitalization and hospital procedures database	2000	100
	Emergency department admissions	2012	100
	Request for outpatient diagnostic tests and specialist visits database	2007	100
	Registry for exemption code-granted patients	2000	100
	Laboratory test values	2014	~20
	GPs' prescriptions with associated indication of use	2000	~63
Frailty database	Multidimensional geriatric assessment	2013	~80% of ≥65 years old
Disease registries	Disease-registries (e.g. diabetes mellitus, celiac disease, etc.)	2015	Disease specific

Abbreviation GP—general practitioner; LHU—local health unit

linkage database if the drugs are reimbursed by the NHS. For each prescription, the date of prescription, anonymized physician code, number of prescribed drug packages as well as the national drug code are available. As with the pharmacy claims database, the duration of the prescription is not available, but is deduced based on the assumption that the doses prescribed are in line with the 'defined daily dose' as outline by the World Health Organization.

1.4 Strengths and Limitations

The main strength of the Caserta record linkage database is its multifaceted patient data derived from both clinical and administrative data sources in a large general population with several years of follow-up. The high coverage of the population in the catchment area is another important strength of the claims database, as practically all persons living in Caserta are NHS beneficiaries and would therefore have their data captured. Since most medications available in Italy are covered by the NHS, there is also a high coverage of medications used, provided that they are purchased through the NHS. Another important strength is the availability of the information about indications of drug use. While these are available only up to 2015 from the database containing GP prescriptions, the electronic prescriptions which started being collected in 2015 have continued providing this information. The presence of yearly comprehensive geriatric evaluations, available for approximately 80% of the elderly persons living in Caserta, is another strength of the Caserta data. In general, such information is rarely recorded routinely in claims databases. Data related to frailty can be very useful if adjusted for confounding, which is usually unmeasured. The data in Caserta has expanded in recent years. For example, recently, data collection has begun for a pregnancy registry, which contains detailed information about maternal health as well as information on the delivery and infant health. This pregnancy registry allows mother-baby linkage, which is very useful for pharmacoepidemiological studies. Pregnant women can currently only be identified for data analyses using specific ICD-9-CM codes indicating pregnancy identified from the hospital discharge database and/or the GPs' prescriptions with indications. Altogether this information provides a very detailed overview of the general population, making the Caserta record linkage database a valuable tool for pharmacoepidemiological research.

The Caserta data also has some limitations. The hospital discharge database is the main manner in which explicit diagnoses are recorded in all of the Caserta claims databases. This means that persons who are not hospitalized will likely not have any other diagnoses recorded in other claims. In addition, the diagnoses from the hospital discharge claims are more likely to concern acute rather than chronic diseases. As a result, the identification of diseases in the Caserta claims data is usually done through proxies (e.g., using anti-diabetic drugs to identify diabetics) or through complex algorithms, based on patient characteristics, which are relevant to a specific disease. There are also some limitations concerning drug use capture, such as the lack of data on dosing regimen for all drugs that are dispensed without a therapeutic plan. All information on drugs that are not covered by the National Health Service (e.g., benzodiazepines) as well as drugs dispensed during hospital stays are also not captured. Another limitation is that data concerning laboratory test results, geriatric evaluations, and GP prescriptions are only available for a subset of the Caserta population that can be linked to the claims database population.

1.5   Quality Checks

There are several quality checks that are performed on the Caserta claims linkage database at different phases of data collection and analysis. The completeness of the data is checked in-house (e.g., missing records, correct and/or valid data format, duplicate records), data quantity and quality over time is compared to ensure that

it is consistent (e.g., comparing new data to past validated data) for internal validation, and external validation is conducted by bench-marking, i.e., by comparing the
demographic characteristics of the population under study, frequency of drug utilization as well as comorbidities in the single databases with other databases and/or
national estimates as provided by the Italian national statistics office. Frequencies
of recorded codes and patient numbers are calculated yearly to identify unexpected
differences in available data. An external check is also conducted using IQVIA
data for Caserta, allowing checks on drug purchasing and costs related to both reimbursed and not-reimbursed drugs purchased in pharmacies and hospitals. This type of
external check provides a reliable drug-level measure about the proportion of drug
prescriptions/dispensing that are non-reimbursed (mainly over-the-counter drugs),
and that are, for this reason, not recorded in the Caserta claims linkage database.
This validation provides an overview of the volume of dispensed drugs that cannot
be otherwise captured in the Caserta claims linkage database.

1.6 Governance and Ethical Issues

The use of Caserta claims and associated data is allowed through a specific agreement
which is signed by the Caserta Local Health Unit (data owners) and the public
institution requesting data use (e.g., University of Messina). Data contained in the
Caserta record linkage database are fully anonymized and securely transferred and
stored in a central server. All studies carried out using the Caserta record linkage
database are non-interventional, observational, retrospective studies which in Italy do
not require any approval from the Ethical Committee (only notification) or informed
consent for included subjects as long as data privacy is guaranteed. Therefore, the
Ethical Committee of the Academic Hospital G. Martino of Messina is only notified
of all studies conducted using the Caserta record linkage database. All observational
studies are carried out according to the terms of the above mentioned agreement and
with the active participation of a special team of health professionals and researchers
from Caserta LHU. Sharing data at the patient level is not allowed, while fully
anonymized aggregated data can be shared in case of multiple database studies.

1.7 Publications

Several studies were published in the area of chronic kidney disease (Ingrasciotta
et al. 2014, 2015; Trifirò et al. 2014; Sultana et al. 2015), diabetes (Trifirò et al. 2016;
Rafaniello et al. 2015), and cardiovascular diseases (Trifirò et al. 2008a; Ferrajolo
et al. 2014; Piacentini et al. 2005) using the Caserta record linkage database. Drug
utilization and/or safety studies were also conducted on central nervous system drugs
(Trifirò et al. 2007, 2008b; Alacqua et al. 2009; Oteri et al. 2010) and the effectiveness
and safety of bisphosphonates (Lapi et al. 2013; Ghirardi et al. 2014a, b). The Caserta

record linkage database was also used to assess the effect of an educational program in primary care (Arcoraci et al. 2014) and the effects of the L'Aquila earthquake on the prescribing pattern of antidepressant and antipsychotic drugs (Trifirò et al. 2013). The Caserta data have also been widely used to study biologics along with other databases in Italy (Ingrasciotta et al. 2019; Belleudi et al. 2019; Marciano et al. 2018). Today the Caserta claims linkage database Arianna is increasingly used to carry out epidemiological studies in several research fields as well as post-authorization safety studies, many of which are currently in progress.

References

Alacqua M, Trifirò G, Spina E et al (2009) Newer and older antiepileptic drug use in Southern Italy: a population-based study during the years 2003–2005. Epilepsy Res 85(1):107–113. https://doi.org/10.1016/j.eplepsyres.2009.03.002

Arcoraci V, Santoni L, Ferrara R et al (2014) Effect of an educational program in primary care: the case of lipid control in cardio-cerebrovascular prevention. Int J Immunopathol Pharmacol 27(3):351–363. https://doi.org/10.1177/039463201402700305

Belleudi V, Trotta F, Addis A et al (2019) Effectiveness and safety of switching originator and biosimilar epoetins in patients with chronic kidney disease in a large-scale italian cohort study. Drug Saf 42(12):1437–1447. https://doi.org/10.1007/s40264-019-00845-y

Ferrajolo C, Arcoraci V, Sullo MG et al (2014) Pattern of statin use in southern Italian primary care: can prescription databases be used for monitoring long-term adherence to the treatment? PLoS ONE 9(7):e102146. https://doi.org/10.1371/journal.pone.0102146

Ghirardi A, Di Bari M, Zambon A et al (2014a) Effectiveness of oral bisphosphonates for primary prevention of osteoporotic fractures: evidence from the AIFA-BEST observational study. Eur J Clin Pharmacol 70(9):1129–1137. https://doi.org/10.1007/s00228-014-1708-8

Ghirardi A, Scotti L, Vedova GD et al (2014b) Oral bisphosphonates do not increase the risk of severe upper gastrointestinal complications: a nested case-control study. BMC Gastroenterol 14:5. https://doi.org/10.1186/1471-230x-14-5

Guerriero F, Orlando V, Tari DU et al (2015) How healthy is community-dwelling elderly population? Results from Southern Italy. Transl Med UniSa 13:59–64

Ingrasciotta Y, Sultana J, Giorgianni F et al (2014) The burden of nephrotoxic drug prescriptions in patients with chronic kidney disease: a retrospective population-based study in Southern Italy. PLoS ONE 9(2):e89072. https://doi.org/10.1371/journal.pone.0089072

Ingrasciotta Y, Sultana J, Giorgianni F et al (2015) Association of individual non-steroidal anti-inflammatory drugs and chronic kidney disease: a population-based case control study. PLoS ONE 10(4):e0122899. https://doi.org/10.1371/journal.pone.0122899

Ingrasciotta Y, Belleudi V, Trotta F et al (2019) In search of predictors of switching between erythropoiesis-stimulating agents in clinical practice: a multi-regional cohort study. Biodrugs. https://doi.org/10.1007/s40259-019-00385-y

Lapi F, Cipriani F, Caputi AP et al (2013) Assessing the risk of osteonecrosis of the jaw due to bisphosphonate therapy in the secondary prevention of osteoporotic fractures. Osteoporos Int 24(2):697–705. https://doi.org/10.1007/s00198-012-2013-y

Marciano I, Ingrasciotta Y, Giorgianni F et al (2018) Pattern of use of biosimilar and originator somatropin in Italy: a population-based multiple databases study during the years 2009–2014. Front Endocrinol (Lausanne) 9:95. https://doi.org/10.3389/fendo.2018.00095

Oteri A, Trifirò G, Gagliostro MS et al (2010) Prescribing pattern of anti-epileptic drugs in an Italian setting of elderly outpatients: a population-based study during 2004–07. Br J Clin Pharmacol 70(4):514–522. https://doi.org/10.1111/j.1365-2125.2010.03619.x

Piacentini N, Trifirò G, Tari M et al (2005) Statin-macrolide interaction risk: a population-based study throughout a general practice database. Eur J Clin Pharmacol 61(8):615–620. https://doi.org/10.1007/s00228-005-0972-z

Rafaniello C, Arcoraci V, Ferrajolo C et al (2015) Trends in the prescription of antidiabetic medications from 2009 to 2012 in a general practice of Southern Italy: a population-based study. Diabetes Res Clin Pract 108(1):157–163. https://doi.org/10.1016/j.diabres.2014.12.007

Sultana J, Musazzi UM, Ingrasciotta Y et al (2015) Medication is an additional source of phosphate intake in chronic kidney disease patients. Nutr Metab Cardiovasc Dis 25(10):959–967. https://doi.org/10.1016/j.numecd.2015.06.001

Sultana J, Hurtado I, Bejarano-Quisoboni D et al (2019) Antipsychotic utilization patterns among patients with schizophrenic disorder: a cross-national analysis in four countries. Eur J Clin Pharmacol 75(7):1005–1015. https://doi.org/10.1007/s00228-019-02654-9

Trifirò G, Barbui C, Spina E et al (2007) Antidepressant drugs: prevalence, incidence and indication of use in general practice of Southern Italy during the years 2003–2004. Pharmacoepidemiol Drug Saf 16(5):552–559. https://doi.org/10.1002/pds.1303

Trifirò G, Alacqua M, Corrao S et al (2008a) Statins for the primary prevention of cardiovascular events in elderly patients: a picture from clinical practice without strong evidence from clinical trials. J Am Geriatr Soc 56(1):175–177. https://doi.org/10.1111/j.1532-5415.2007.01486.x

Trifirò G, Savica R, Morgante L et al (2008b) Prescribing pattern of anti-Parkinson drugs in Southern Italy: cross-sectional analysis in the years 2003–2005. Parkinsonism Relat Disord 14(5):420–425. https://doi.org/10.1016/j.parkreldis.2007.10.010

Trifirò G, Italiano D, Alibrandi A et al (2013) Effects of L'Aquila earthquake on the prescribing pattern of antidepressant and antipsychotic drugs. Int J Clin Pharm 35(6):1053–1062. https://doi.org/10.1007/s11096-013-9822-8

Trifirò G, Sultana J, Giorgianni F et al (2014) Chronic kidney disease requiring healthcare services: a new approach to evaluate epidemiology of renal disease. Biomed Res Int 2014:268362. https://doi.org/10.1155/2014/268362

Trifirò G, Parrino F, Pizzimenti V et al (2016) The management of diabetes mellitus in patients with chronic kidney disease: a population-based study in Southern Italy. Clin Drug Investig 36(3):203–212. https://doi.org/10.1007/s40261-015-0367-6

Trifirò G, Gini R, Barone-Adesi F et al (2019) The role of European Healthcare Databases for post-marketing drug effectiveness, safety and value evaluation: where does Italy stand? Drug Saf 42(3):347–363. https://doi.org/10.1007/s40264-018-0732-5

Viola E, Trifirò G, Ingrasciotta Y et al (2016) Adverse drug reactions associated with off-label use of ketorolac, with particular focus on elderly patients. An analysis of the Italian pharmacovigilance database and a population based study. Expert Opin Drug Saf 15(sup 2):61–67. https://doi.org/10.1080/14740338.2016.1221401

Pedianet Database

Anna Cantarutti and Carlo Gaquinto

Abstract Pedianet is an independent network of family paediatricians established in 1998 to collect information from outpatient family paediatricians in Italy for clinical and epidemiological research (e.g., pharmacovigilance studies, studies on prescribing patterns, and studies of the efficiency of health services). The Pedianet database's beginning dates back to January 2000. The Pedianet system has the advantage of collecting data at a population level as a by-product of routine activities, therefore generating a far larger quantity of data than ad hoc studies.

1 Database Description

1.1 Introduction

Pedianet is an independent network of family paediatricians established in 1998 to collect information from outpatient family paediatricians in Italy for clinical and epidemiological research (e.g., pharmacovigilance studies, studies on prescribing patterns, and studies of the efficiency of health services). The Pedianet database's beginning dates back to January 2000. The Pedianet system has the advantage of collecting data at a population level as a by-product of routine activities, therefore generating a far larger quantity of data than ad hoc studies.

In January 2007, a new law came into force in Europe, which states that for registration of new drugs it is mandatory to present a Paediatric Investigation Plan to the European Medicines Agency (EMEA). In addition, there are a number of

A. Cantarutti (✉)
Unit of Biostatistics, Epidemiology and Public Health, Department of Statistics and Quantitative Methods, University of Milano-Bicocca, Via Bicocca Rego Arcimboldi 8, Milan, Italy
e-mail: anna.cantarutti@unimib.it

C. Gaquinto
Department of Woman and Child Health, University of Padova, Via Giustiniani 3, Padova, Italy
e-mail: carlo.giaquinto@unipd.it

© Springer Nature Switzerland AG 2021   159
M. Sturkenboom and T. Schink (eds.), *Databases for Pharmacoepidemiological Research*, Springer Series on Epidemiology and Public Health,
https://doi.org/10.1007/978-3-030-51455-6_13

incentives for companies to obtain a paediatric licence for drugs that are already on the market, both under patent and "off patent". In this context, the role of Pedianet not just as a database (especially for pharmacovigilance studies) but as an organised structure in which different competencies converge is essential. This is being confirmed by the presence and participation of Pedianet in important European projects, such as TEDDY (Ceci et al. 2009), which is an EU-funded Network of Excellence (NoE), EU-ADR, EU-ADR alliance (both on pharmacovigilance), EMIF (European Medical Information Framework) and ADVANCE (Accelerated development of vaccine benefit-risk collaboration in Europe) as well as by the increasing interest European institutions, research groups, and pharmaceutical companies are showing to collaborate with Pedianet.

1.2   Database Characteristics

The Pedianet system is based on the transmission of specific data (determined by individual studies) from computerised clinical files, which the paediatricians in the network fill out during their daily professional activities. Data are anonymously collected and validated by a central server in Padua. The database is owned and maintained by the *Società Servizi Telematici* (So.Se.Te). Approximately 200 paediatricians throughout the country (3% of all Italian paediatricians) have thus far been participating in the project, regularly sending information on their activities for the Pedianet database. The coordination of the database and data analyses is carried out by a scientific committee, which includes internationally well-known paediatricians, epidemiologists, and researchers. In Italy, paediatric primary care is provided exclusively by primary care paediatricians (PCPs). Primary care includes general first-access care for children and adolescents (0–16 years), which is provided by PCPs paid through a state collective agreement. The Italian Public Health Care System requires that all children have an identified primary care provider (Corsello et al. 2016).

Data collection started in January 2000 with a 3-year test period and is still ongoing. Pedianet counts about 265,000[1] children aged between 0 and 16 years old. Children enter the database with the first visit recorded by their paediatrician and exit when reaching the age of 14 and/or changing residence and/or dying. The average follow-up time is 14 years, demographic and socioeconomic status information are recorded respectively for parents and the child. The Pedianet database is representative of the paediatric Italian population.

The data from paediatric general practitioners and family paediatricians form a unique resource, both for studying individual diseases, as well as for studying the interactions between different areas of health care and population health. The database is updated in real time.

---

[1] On December 31, 2015.

1.3 Available Data

The data include demographic information as well as information on inpatient diagnoses (48,000,001), drug prescriptions (31,500,001), anthropometric measures (16,400,001), specialist medical examinations (12,000,001), and physical examinations or lab tests (16,000,001).

Demographic data include year of birth, age, sex, region of residence, nationality, and information about the parents (e.g., nationality, smoking habits, educational level of the mother and the socioeconomic level, were recorded). In addition, the type of breastfeeding at 1, 3, 6, 9, and 12 months after birth, parity, Apgar score at 1, 5, and 10 min after birth, gestational age, birth weight, birth height, jaundice and family illnesses are recorded. Additional information on the health status of the mother may also be available but is not routinely documented. Date and cause of death of a patient are also recorded in the Pedianet database.

Information on outpatient diagnoses and symptoms includes primary and ancillary diagnoses, the date of diagnosis, and diagnostic certainty. Diagnoses are coded using the International Classification of Diseases, version 9 (ICD-9) with at least four digits. Outpatient prescriptions, treatment, including immunizations, and diagnostic procedures (laboratory tests and physical examinations) are also recorded.

Outpatient prescription information, both for reimbursed and non-reimbursed drugs, includes the date of prescription and the date of dispensation, the indication, the ATC code, the Italian MinSan code, the number of prescribed packages, and the dose prescribed.

Information about physical examinations and laboratory tests is generally documented, including the measured value, the date, and if necessary, the reason for performing the examination or test.

Patients can be re-contacted through the participating paediatrician to gather additional information. It is also possible to identify family members (brothers and sisters) within the database.

The Pedianet project team is now developing a system to link Pedianet databases with other administrative databases such as the Immunisation database or the hospitalization database. This will greatly improve the completeness of data available for research.

1.4 Strengths and Limitations

A major strength of the Pedianet database is its size. The database counts 265,000 Italian children aged from 0 to 16 years old. Information on diagnoses, prescriptions, and outcomes are quite comprehensive reflecting the field work of paediatricians. The size and the long follow-up time allow studying rare events and rare exposures.

Finally, the data are produced in clinical practice and thereby represent a unique observational experience that allows studying the dynamics of the various aspects of healthcare (including effectiveness and impact studies) as well as the state of health of the population.

The main limitations of the database include the lack of information of the family environment, an underreporting of hospitalization and immunization data, and the lack of many OTC prescriptions. This makes Pedianet not fully appropriate for studies on non-specific outcomes. However, these studies can be performed through prospective observational cohort studies which have been successfully carried out using the Pedianet network.

1.5 Validation

Validation is an important process to make Pedianet data suitable for both prospective and retrospective studies thanks to the possibility to contact paediatricians to check the validity of the information. Data validation is ensured through:

1. Checking the correspondence of data with information on the child's medical record
2. Contacting the treating doctor to ask for patient information and comparing this information with that in the Pedianet database
3. Checking for outliers
4. Ensuring that the medication prescribed to a patient is consistent with the diagnosis
5. Ensuring that the results of medical tests performed are consistent with the diagnoses.

In the near future, data will be directly transferred to the Pedianet database from the electronic health records (the so called *Fascicolo Sanitario Elettronico*, FSE), which collects all hospitalization, medical tests, and examinations done. From then, the validation of these data is no longer necessary, or will at least be faster.

1.6 Governance and Ethical Issues

The Pedianet database has been registered according to the Italian law. Data are included in the database only after written informed consent is obtained from the parents of the child. Data are collected anonymously on a central server in Padua, where it is validated and prepared for research.

Access to the database is allowed only for Pedianet researchers in the context of research projects that have been approved by both the Steering Committee and the Ethics Review Board (if required). It is not permitted to give third parties access to the data. Patient level data cannot be shared, however aggregated data may be shared with research partners, e.g., for pooled analysis.

The coordination of the projects and data analysis is carried out by a scientific committee that includes internationally well-known paediatricians, epidemiologists, and researchers.

1.7   Documents and Publications

Over 30 clinical epidemiological studies on major paediatric diseases or pharma-covigilance have been carried out or were ongoing up to 31th December, 2015. These studies have resulted in over 70 publications and conference presentations.

Relevant papers on risk quantification include Dona et al. (2016); Menniti-Ippolito et al. (2000); Sturkenboom et al. (2005). Some examples of published results of studies on the incidence of specific disease are Cantarutti et al. (2015); Pacurariu et al. (2015); Nicolosi et al. (2003); Barbato et al. (2003).

1.8   Administrative Information

The database is maintained and owned by the Società Servizi Telematici Srl. The maintenance of the database is funded through different research projects. Studies carried out to date have been financed by public bodies (European Commission, *Istituto Superiore di Sanità*, AIFA, *Consiglio Nazionale delle Ricerche, Regione Veneto, Aziende Socio Sanitarie, Istituto Zooprofilattico delle Venezie*, etc.), or private groups such as pharmaceutical companies or international research groups.

Contact Details
Organisation/affiliation: Società Servizi Telematici Srl, Via G. Medici 9/A, 35121 Padua (PD), Italy

Administartive Contact: Carlo Giaquinto
   carlo.giaquinto@unipd.it
   (+39) 049 8726723
   Website: http://www.pedianet.it/en/

References

Barbato A, Panizzolo C, Biserna L et al (2003) Asthma prevalence and drug prescription in asthmatic children. Eur Ann Allergy Clin Immunol 35(2):47–51

Cantarutti A, Dona D, Visentin F et al (2015) Epidemiology of frequently occurring skin diseases in Italian children from 2006 to 2012: a retrospective, population-based study. Pediatr Dermatol 32(5):668–678. https://doi.org/10.1111/pde.12568

Ceci A, Giaquinto C, Aboulker JP et al (2009) The task-force in Europe for drug development for the young (TEDDY) network of excellence. Paediatr Drugs 11(1):18–21. https://doi.org/10.2165/0148581-200911010-00008

Corsello G, Ferrara P, Chiamenti G et al (2016) The child health care system in Italy. J Pediatr 177s:S116–s126. https://doi.org/10.1016/j.jpeds.2016.04.048

Dona D, Mozzo E, Scamarcia A et al (2016) Community-acquired rotavirus gastroenteritis compared with adenovirus and norovirus gastroenteritis in Italian children: a pedianet study. Int J Pediatr 2016:5236243. https://doi.org/10.1155/2016/5236243

Menniti-Ippolito G, Raschetti R, Da Cas R et al (2000) Active monitoring of adverse drug reactions in children. Italian Paediatric Pharmacosurveillance Multicenter Group. Lancet 355(9215):1613–1614. https://doi.org/10.1016/s0140-6736(00)02219-4

Nicolosi A, Sturkenboom M, Mannino S et al (2003) The incidence of varicella: correction of a common error. Epidemiology 14(1):99–102. https://doi.org/10.1097/00001648-200301000-00024

Pacurariu AC, Straus SM, Trifiro G et al (2015) Useful interplay between spontaneous ADR reports and electronic healthcare records in signal detection. Drug Saf 38(12):1201–1210. https://doi.org/10.1007/s40264-015-0341-5

Sturkenboom M, Nicolosi A, Cantarutti L et al (2005) Incidence of mucocutaneous reactions in children treated with niflumic acid, other nonsteroidal antiinflammatory drugs, or nonopioid analgesics. Pediatrics 116(1):e26–e33. https://doi.org/10.1542/peds.2004-0040

BIFAP Program: A Data Resource for Pharmacoepidemiological Research in Spain

Miguel Gil, Miguel Angel Maciá, Julio Bonis, Consuelo Huerta,
Elisa Martín-Merino, Arturo Álvarez, Verónica Bryant, and Dolores
Montero on behalf of BIFAP Team

Abstract BIFAP includes information routinely collected by primary care physicians (PCPs) in their practices (real-world data). In 2018, the BIFAP database included anonymized and prospectively recorded data in the electronic medical records (EMR) of 7566 PCPs (6419 General Practitioners (GPs)/1147 pediatricians) up to the end of 2018.

BIFAP Team: Alicia Gonzalez, Carlos León, Luz León, Ana Llorente, Mar Martín.

M. Gil (✉) · M. A. Maciá · J. Bonis · C. Huerta · E. Martín-Merino · A. Álvarez · V. Bryant ·
Dolores Montero on behalf of BIFAP Team
BIFAP Program, Pharmacoepidemiology and Pharmacovigilance Medicines for Human Use
Department, Spanish Agency of Drugs and Medical Devices AEMPS, Campezo Street 1, 28022
Madrid, Spain
e-mail: mgilg@aemps.es

M. A. Maciá
e-mail: mamacia@aemps.es

C. Huerta
e-mail: chuerta@aemps.es

E. Martín-Merino
e-mail: emartinm@aemps.es

A. Álvarez
e-mail: aalvarez_externo@bifap.aemps.es

V. Bryant
e-mail: vbryant@aemps.es

Dolores Montero on behalf of BIFAP Team
e-mail: dmontero@aemps.es

© Springer Nature Switzerland AG 2021
M. Sturkenboom and T. Schink (eds.), *Databases for Pharmacoepidemiological
Research*, Springer Series on Epidemiology and Public Health,
https://doi.org/10.1007/978-3-030-51455-6_14

1 Database Description

1.1 Introduction

Spain has a National Health Service (NHS) that provides universal access to health services to the Spanish population through the Regional Healthcare Services. PCPs at NHS primary care centers have a central role. They act as gatekeepers of the system and also exchange information with other levels of care to ensure the continuity of care. Most (98.9%) of the population is registered with a PCP under the Spanish NHS (Ministerio de Sanidad Consumo y Bienestar Social 2019) and, in addition, most drug prescriptions are written at the primary care level (Bernal-Delgado et al. 2018).

BIFAP (*Base de Datos para la Investigación Farmacoepidemiológica en Atencion Primaria*) is a longitudinal population-based database of computer-based medical patient records, from PCPs belonging to the NHS, and situated in any one of the participating Autonomous Communities (Regions) throughout Spain (www.bifap.org). BIFAP is a non-profit program financed by the Spanish Agency on Medicines and Medical Devices (AEMPS), a government agency belonging to the Ministry of Health, Consumer Affairs and Social Welfare. Ten out of 17 regions of Spain collaborate in the program and participation of the regions in BIFAP is voluntary (Maciá-Martínez et al. 2020).

The main use of BIFAP is for research purposes in order to evaluate the adverse and beneficial effects of drugs and drug utilization patterns as used in the general population under real conditions of use.

1.2 Database Characteristics

BIFAP includes information routinely collected by primary care physicians (PCPs) in their practices (real-world data). In 2018, the BIFAP database included anonymized and prospectively recorded data in the electronic medical records (EMR) of 7566 PCPs (6419 General Practitioners (GPs)/1147 pediatricians) up to the end of 2018. The valid study period in BIFAP starts in 2001 when the EMRs where fully implemented throughout Spain (Salvador Rosa et al. 2002). Information before EMR implementation is available as registered by the GP.

The BIFAP database is updated yearly. The total number of patients available for studies in the 2018 database is 12 million (2.3 million pediatric patients), representing 102 million person-years of follow-up. The mean follow-up of patients in the database is 8.6 years and the number of patients with follow-ups of 5 years or longer is 8.9 million (Fig. 1).

The number of patients with up-to-date information in 2018 (active patients) is 8 million, representing 17% of the total Spanish population. This percentage increases to 57.6% if only the seven regions currently providing EMR data are considered.

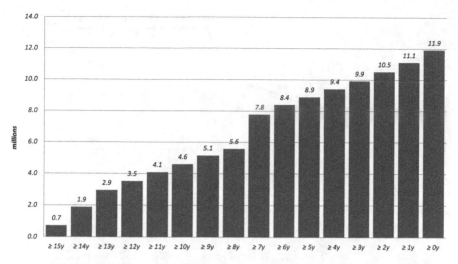

Fig. 1 Distribution of years of follow-up of patients included in BIFAP database. Y-axis: N° of patients in BIFAP (in millions). X axis: Minimum (≥) number of years (y) patients are followed in BIFAP database (for instance, 7.8 million patients have at least 7 seven years of person-time of follow-up in BIFAP)

The whole population of five Spanish regions (Aragón, Asturias, Castilla y Leon, Murcia, and Navarra) is currently covered (population-based scheme) and inclusion of the whole population of the other participants' regions is foreseen within the next two years. The yearly evolution of the number of active patients in BIFAP and the geographical distribution of patient data contributing to BIFAP within Spain are shown in Figs. 2 and 3, respectively.

1.3 Available Data in BIFAP

The PCPs' electronic medical records contain details on demographics, prescriptions, episodes of care (diagnoses/symptoms), specialist referrals, other additional health data (test results, interventions, etc.) and clinical notes registered as free text. Detailed information is included in the following subsections and summarized in Table 1.

Information in BIFAP is anonymized and no patient's personal identifiers are included in the BIFAP database. Most, but not all participating regions share the same EMR software. Consequently, there is heterogeneity in how the information is provided to BIFAP. The information is harmonized into a BIFAP common data model in order to be available for research purposes. The structure of the BIFAP common data model is displayed in Fig. 4.

Administrative/Sociodemographic information

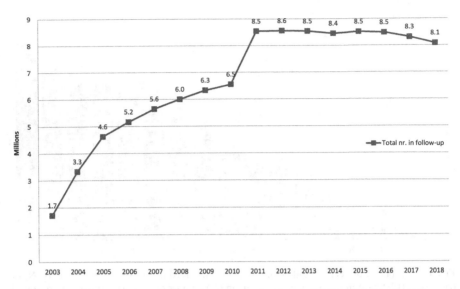

Fig. 2 Annual number of patients with active follow-up in the period 2003–2018. *Active follow-up defined as, at least, one day of follow-up in the corresponding year

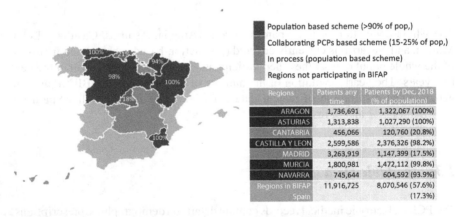

Fig. 3 Geographical distribution of patient data contributing to BIFAP in Spain

BIFAP data include information on the dates patients were registered or left a PCP's practice. Additional demographic data such as age and sex are also collected. Date of death is registered in primary care for administrative purposes whilst the cause of death is available only if registered by the PCPs. No structured information is available on the socioeconomic status and ethnicity of patients. Nevertheless, this information might be available as free text or by using related codes for an undetermined number of patients depending on the PCP's registering habits.

Health problems information (Episodes of care)

Table 1 Data available in BIFAP

Type of patient data	Data available
Administrative data	Dates when patients were registered or have left a PCP's practice, including date of death
Socio-demographic data	Age, gender
Lifestyle data/additional health data	Smoking, alcohol intake, weight, height, blood pressure
	Laboratory test results
Health problems in primary care	Diseases/symptoms leading to patient consultation (episodes of care)
Results of diagnostic procedures	Laboratory, imaging
	Recorded either in structured format or as free text
Referrals to specialists/information of other levels of care	Referrals to specialists (out-patient/in-patient) and to emergency services
	Essential data derived from referral (new diagnoses, interventions, results of specialized tests, etc.) are recorded either in structured format or as free text
Hospital discharge diagnosis	Through linkage with hospital registries; present coverage: 50% of patients included in BIFAP in the last 5 years
Interventions: medicines	Medicines prescriptions
	Dispensings (coverage in 2018: 75% of all recorded prescriptions)
	Vaccination records
Interventions: other	Recorded either in structured format or as free text
Death	Date of death included for administrative purposes
	Cause of death through linkage with Spanish Mortality Registry (expected 2021)

Currently, two coding systems with different levels of granularity coexist in BIFAP: The International Classification of Primary Care (ICPC) (WONCA International Classification Committee 1998) and the International Classification of Diseases (ICD-9) (Centers for Disease Control and Prevention 2015). The ICPC is the coding system for eight of the participant regions, and its granularity is limited as compared with ICD-9 (~1300 vs. ~13,000 codes, respectively).

In EMR software, the episode of care is coded and also labeled as incident symptom/diagnosis (DI), personal history (PH), and/or clinical problem list (CPL). Any action taken by the PCP and related to that episode (referrals, prescriptions, procedures, laboratory tests, radiology, etc.), and the additional clinical notes as free text, must be linked to the DI. The clinical notes as free text, once anonymized, can

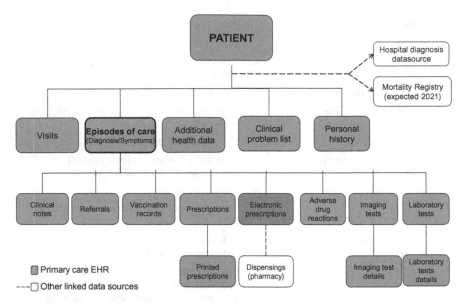

Fig. 4 Structure of the BIFAP Common Data Model

be used: To better characterize the coded entries for validation purposes; to identify diagnoses not properly coded or to obtain specific information about the diagnosis registered by the PCP (i.e., cancer stage, specific interventions, etc.).

To facilitate the identification of the episode of care, the EMR software contains an internal thesaurus where a list of descriptors of diseases, signs or symptoms is linked to the different dictionary codes. Often, these descriptors provide more detailed information than that in the corresponding code. Also, only for ICPC-based EMR software, new descriptors can be included at the local level, and the PCPs can also modify or add information to the selected episode of care descriptor. This EMR software flexibility results in a large number of different diagnosis descriptors in the BIFAP database (8.5 million).

To standardize this, BIFAP has developed its own research dictionary (ICPC-BIFAP) by adding a fourth digit to the original three-digit ICPC code of the most frequently used descriptors, increasing its granularity. In 2018, the ICPC-BIFAP dictionary included 5100 indexed terms. Concerning the regions coding with ICD-9, the diagnosis information received in BIFAP is already normalized, given the high granularity of the medical terms dictionary information and the quality control procedures performed. Thus, no further actions are performed in BIFAP. Both together, ICPC-BIFAP and ICD-9 codes cover about 88.7% of all diagnoses registered in BIFAP (221.8 million).

To ease the management of events in epidemiological studies, specific algorithms have been developed that identify valid clinical events to be included in the BIFAP catalog of events. Clinical event algorithms include related codes in both ICD-9 and ICPC-based BIFAP dictionaries. Depending on the characteristics of the event and, in order to maximize its sensibility and specificity, the algorithms might also include laboratory test results, additional health data, string text search strategies in GP clinical notes, etc.

The validity of the clinical event algorithms is addressed by reviewing a sample of cases (internal validity) and by comparing epidemiological measurements (i.e., incidence, prevalence) with the available evidence. To date, the BIFAP catalog of events includes 260 events including those most frequently used in pharmacoepidemiological studies and also others developed in the context of the studies already performed with the database.

Drug prescription information

Drug prescription information in BIFAP includes the product name, the active substance, number of prescribed packages, the intended duration, the dosage regimens, the strength and the indication for the prescription. Prescriptions are coded according to the Anatomical Therapeutic Chemical (ATC) classification system (WHO Collaborating Centre for Drug Statistics Methodology 2019).

Drug prescription information in BIFAP is based on prescription by PCPs who are responsible for most of the drug prescriptions in the Spanish NHS. Prescriptions for patients are generated directly by the computer and prescription details (drug type, dosage, etc.) are recorded digitally. Electronic drug prescription systems linked to community pharmacies are being progressively implemented in the different regions participating in BIFAP. This also facilitates the identification of dispensings by pharmacies. In 2018, 75% of the prescriptions in BIFAP were e-prescription records (OECD/European Union 2018) (see Fig. 5).

Prescribed medicines are linked to an episode of care record (describing symptoms or diagnoses) facilitating the analysis of the prescription's indication although, in some circumstances, this linkage may not reflect the indication accurately. The

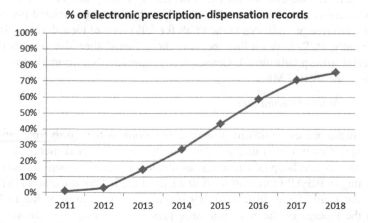

Fig. 5 Proportion of electronic prescription-dispensation records among all prescription records in BIFAP (by year)

validity of the linkage of a prescription to its indication is limited by the granularity of the medical terms dictionary, the availability of the indication as a code and the prescription habits of the PCP. So, as a sensitivity analysis, it is always recommendable to also analyze all the diagnosis information included in the clinical profile regardless of the linked code of the drug of interest.

Drugs prescribed by hospital doctors, other specialists or in the private health care setting are not registered in BIFAP in a structured way, unless the treatment is to be continued by the PCPs. Also, medications dispensed without a prescription (OTC) are not available in PCP records and thus also not in BIFAP. However, the number of drugs that can be prescribed OTC is limited in Spain.

Additional health data

EMR software allows registering other health care data such as lifestyle variables (smoking, alcohol intake, body mass index, etc.), other measurements commonly performed in the primary care setting (i.e., blood pressure, height, weight, etc.), and vaccinations.

Laboratory test results are also available as entered by the PCPs or, more frequently, by direct dump of the data into the PCPs EMR depending on the facilities available when recorded.

Information on radiology results and diagnostic procedures is available as entered by the PCPs in free text fields.

Information on other levels of care

Patients attending hospital or outpatient specialist care are usually referred by PCPs, although self-referred patients to emergency departments are also possible. The reason for the referral by the PCP is always available for administrative purposes, but the availability of results of the referral and emergency department visits in the EMRs depends on the PCPs manually entering this information, either coded or as clinical notes in free text fields. Nevertheless, hospitalized patients are frequently referred at discharge to the PCPs for follow-up of their diseases. In addition, currently, PCPs have on-line access to the patients' specialist records (outpatient specialist/hospitalizations). Consequently, specialist's information is usually available in the PCPs EMR.

Ability to link to external data

BIFAP is in the process of linking primary care records with records from other data sources, specifically coded diagnoses at hospital discharge and mortality registry information. To date, hospitalizations are available for a subset of periods and regions participating in BIFAP, representing around half of the BIFAP population in the five most recent years. Drug dispensings by pharmacies are also available in BIFAP through the linkage of the electronic drug prescription systems to the commnity pharmacies (see section drug prescription information and Fig. 5).

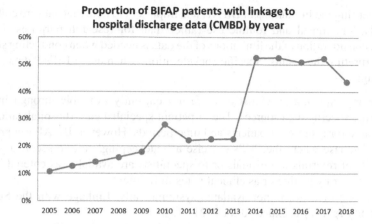

Fig. 6 Proportion of patients in BIFAP with linkage to hospitalization discharge data by year

Concerning mortality, the linkage of BIFAP primary care records with the Spanish mortality registry is expected for 2021. This will provide the cause of death as registered in the mortality registry of patients included in the BIFAP database.

1.4 Strenghts and Limitations

The main strengths of BIFAP are related to:

- Its large sample size (12 million patients) and population-based nature, covering 57.6% of the population in the seven regions providing PCPs' EMRs in BIFAP, representing the whole population in five of the participating regions.
- The longitudinal nature of the database and data availability for many years, enabling long follow-up of patients.
- The representativeness of routine clinical care and the validity and quality of the information included in the database that has been assessed in multiple validation studies.
- The availability of complete medical records from PCPs including clinical notes as free text and the linkage to other healthcare data sources like hospital registries and mortality registries.
- Complete and detailed information on characteristics of drug prescriptions and dispensings including indication, dose, and intended duration.
- The annual updates of the database facilitating accessibility and efficiency to perform pharmacoepidemiological studies without long delays.
- Support and full integration in the activities of the Agency on Medicines and Medical Devices (AEMPS). A multidisciplinary team with expertise and deep knowledge of the BIFAP database that includes senior epidemiologists, statisticians, information technologies personnel, and administrative staff.

Concerning the limitations of BIFAP, it is important to note that data are collected primarily for clinical and routine use rather than for research purposes. Consequently, consideration of the limitations of the data is needed when conducting studies and interpreting the results. Specific considerations when using BIFAP data are the following:

- Data on outpatient specialist care are not currently available through linkage with the specific data sources. The in-patient specialist care (hospitalizations) is available for a subset of patients and time periods. However, BIFAP is a primary care database where the PCPs exercise a 'gatekeeping' role to secondary care. Results of referrals to hospitals or to specialists are available as entered by the PCPs either by coding or as clinical notes in free-text.
- The cause of death is not available systematically. Linkage with the Spanish mortality registry is expected for 2021.
- Laboratory or imaging test results are not registered systematically in a structured way, being more likely to be entered if abnormal.
- Data on drugs administered or dispensed in the hospital setting or prescribed in private health care settings are not available.
- As in similar databases, treatment compliance is not recorded. Therefore, information on a prescription dispensed does not necessarily mean that the drug was actually taken.
- The linkage of a prescription to an episode of care may not properly reflect the indication of the prescription. Indication studies based exclusively in the use of linked codes are limited by the granularity of the medical terms dictionary, the availability of the indication as a code and the PCPs' prescriptions habits.

1.5   Validation

The validity of BIFAP depends on the quality and completeness of the data recorded by the PCPs. The raw data provided by participating regions undergo extensive quality control and validity checks by BIFAP database administrators for database integration purposes. Patient-level data are also assessed, with patients considered as acceptable for inclusion in the BIFAP database after several consistency and quality control checks.

Complete patients' clinical profiles as registered by the PCPs are available for research purposes. This allows performing validation studies by reviewing clinical profiles, including clinical notes as free text, in order to identify case events with a high likelihood to be true events or to establish the positive predictive value of event case detection algorithms. In addition, questionnaires might also be sent to GPs allowing researchers to verify the information captured or to obtain additional information.

Moreover, the availability of linkage of PCP records to other data sources like hospital registries, allows the cross-validation of the event of interest in both sources and eventually, the selection of the best source of information according the specific study needs.

To date, several studies including the validation of outcomes in BIFAP by clinical profile review have been performed, confirming the validity (positive and negative predictive values) of the algorithms defined to identify the clinical events in BIFAP (de Abajo et al. 2013, 2014, 2015; García-Poza et al. 2015; Gil et al. 2011, 2019b; Martín-Merino et al. 2015; Rodríguez-Martín et al. 2019a, b; Rodríguez-Miguel et al. 2019a; Saiz et al. 2017; Chacón García et al. 2010). Two of these studies (de Abajo et al. 2013, 2014) also included an additional validation via questionnaires sent to the PCPs. These two studies showed a high confirmation rate as compared to the validation performed by BIFAP researchers by reviewing clinical profiles, although the PCPs' response rate was low.

Other examples of validation of the information in BIFAP are those related to BIFAP participation in international collaborative multi-database projects in the context of the European Commission work programs (SAFEGUARD, PROTECT, ADVANCE). In this regard, the validation of seven cardiovascular, pancreatic, and cancer outcomes performed in the context of the SAFEGUARD project, which addresses the safety of oral antidiabetic drugs (Safeguard Consortium 2015), showed a high positive predictive value of the events identified by codes (range 85–97.5%) when verified by clinical profile review (including free text clinical notes) as gold standard. Also, the compliance with the vaccination schedules of HPV vaccination with 2–3 doses at patient-level has been also validated (Martín-Merino et al. 2019b).

The completeness (sensitivity) of diagnosis recording in BIFAP has also been evaluated for a number of events in benchmarking processes with other databases worldwide within the context of BIFAP international multi-database studies or other specific studies. In these studies, incidence/prevalence figures of different events are comparable to results obtained from other databases with similar characteristics (de Groot et al. 2014; Huerta et al. 2016; Requena et al. 2014) and other available evidence (i.e., literature, registries, etc.) used as gold standard (Gil et al. 2019b).

Concerning exposure information, the completeness and validity is very high given the role of PCPs as gatekeepers in the context of the Spanish NHS, and the fact that the prescription data are generated directly from the computer.

1.6   Governance and Ethical Issues

BIFAP is financed, coordinated, and administered by the Spanish Agency on Medicines and Medical Devices (AEMPS). The collaboration with the participating regions is established through a formal agreement and enables the periodic reception of anonymized electronic health care records. An Advisory Board, where representatives of these regions participate, monitors the progress of the BIFAP program.

Information in the BIFAP database neither includes patient personal identifiers nor data fields containing strong identifiers (address, name, telephone, NHS number, etc.). Before EMR data are transferred to the AEMPS, there is a process of pseudo-anonymization of personal identifiers followed by additional procedures (Article 29 Data Protection Working Party 2014) which ensure the anonymization of the data available for investigators. In addition, patients' privacy is warranted by the appropriate technical and organizational measures to minimize any potential risk of re-identification. Personal information of the PCPs and location of their practices are not available in the BIFAP database.

Access to BIFAP data follows a set of governance rules and procedures. A comprehensive governance document approved by the AEMPS in agreement with the BIFAP Advisory Board is publicly available on the BIFAP webpage. This BIFAP data access governance applies the principles of the General Data Protection Regulation (GDPR) (European Parliament 2016).

1.7 Use of BIFAP to Perform Pharmacoepidemiological Studies

The BIFAP research database is accessible to perform pharmacoepidemiological studies by independent researchers in Spain belonging to the public sector and to support the activities of the AEMPS. Independent researchers should first be accredited. Then, they have to submit a study protocol which needs to be evaluated and approved by an independent scientific committee. After that step, they have to sign a commitment document. During the implementation of the protocol data are processed and transferred following security measures adapted to the user and the characteristics of the data. The steps needed to perform a study in BIFAP are summarized in Fig. 7. The description of the projects performed with BIFAP is documented on the webpage (BIFAP 2019).

A multidisciplinary team provides support to researchers with regard to the extraction of the information for the analysis on the basis of the approved protocol specifications and the characteristics of the BIFAP database. An anonymized dataset is provided to the researchers to perform the study.

Several informatics tools have been developed for data extraction and analysis. As an example, BIFAP EXPRESS is an exploratory analysis tool based on pre-aggregated data to perform customized analyses on the BIFAP database. With BIFAP EXPRESS drug utilization indicators, population-based information at active substance level (ATC classification), and demographic characteristics (age groups/gender) are available. Several modules have been developed to date including: Prevalence drug use module and trends; indication of use and prescribed daily dose. Query results are produced in a fast and comprehensive way and can be exported supporting different formats.

The informatics tools developed to facilitate data extraction and dataset generation also include tools for the selection of potential cases of interest, incidence rate calculations and controls if needed (filter tool), the generation of covariates and exposures

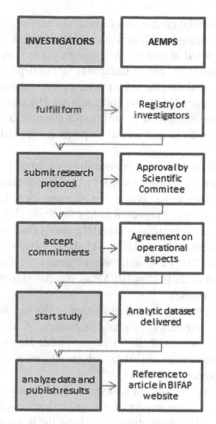

Fig. 7 Steps to perform a study in BIFAP: role of investigators and AEMPS. AEMPS: Spanish Agency of drugs and medical devices

(data creator tool), and a clinical profile viewer. Additional tools tailored to different study designs are being developed including case-control studies and comparison of incidence rates of adverse events.

1.8 Documents and Publications

To date, 69 articles have been published in peer-reviewed journals, reflecting the BIFAP contribution to the knowledge of the risks associated with drugs, either in the evaluation of potential safety signals, risk quantification or drug utilization studies (BIFAP 2019).

Relevant papers on risk quantification include the following: Those addressing the cardiovascular risk of patients exposed to several drugs including NSAIDs and non-narcotic analgesics (de Abajo et al. 2014; García-Poza et al. 2015), allopurinol (de Abajo et al. 2015; Rodríguez-Martín et al. 2019a) and calcium supplements (de

Abajo et al. 2017), colorectal cancer risk in patients exposed to NSAIDs and other drugs for pain control (Rodríguez-Miguel et al. 2019a, b), risk of typical and atypical fractures in patients exposed to oral bisphosphonates (Erviti et al. 2013a, b), risk of fractures in patients exposed to benzodiazepines or antidepressant drugs (Requena et al. 2016a; Souverein et al. 2016), risk of toxic epidermal necrolysis and Stevens-Johnson syndrome associated with benzodiazepines (Martín-Merino et al. 2015), liver injury risk in patients exposed to antibiotics (Brauer et al. 2016a; Udo et al. 2016) or risk of infections by herpes viruses in patients exposed to valproic acid (Gil et al. 2019a).

In addition, drug utilization studies are usually performed to describe the patterns and determinants of drug use. Some examples of published results are the following: Characterization of patients using standard or intensive lipid lowering therapy with statins for primary and secondary prevention (Macías Saint-Gerons et al. 2014, 2015), trend patterns of drug use in patients with Alzheimer's disease (Bonis et al. 2013), anti-osteoporotic treatments (Martín-Merino et al. 2017a) or trend patterns in benzodiazepine (Huerta et al. 2016) and antiepileptic drugs (de Groot et al. 2014) and antibiotic use (Brauer et al. 2016b) in BIFAP as compared to other seven European electronic healthcare databases.

BIFAP also contributes to obtaining estimates of the incidence or prevalence of health problems such as community acquired pneumonia (Chacón García et al. 2010; Rivero-Calle et al. 2016; Saiz et al. 2017), dementia (de Hoyos-Alonso et al. 2016), hip/femur fractures (Requena et al. 2014), colorectal cancer (Gil et al. 2019b), and acute liver injury (Ruigómez et al. 2014).

Finally, it is worth mentioning the relevant role of sources of information like BIFAP for the evaluation of the impact of risk minimization activities. For example, studies performed in the BIFAP database to evaluate the impact of risk minimization activities of calcineurin inhibitors (Oliva et al. 2012) or codein prescribing for pain in children (Hedenmalm et al. 2019).

A summary of the main areas (drug/diagnoses) of research in BIFAP, including the published articles by type of research (drug-event association studies and drug utilization) is shown in Table 2.

The full list of articles based on BIFAP data published in peer-reviewed journals is available on the website (BIFAP 2019).

Table 2 Areas of interest (drugs and diagnoses) for research in BIFAP by type of research

Drug class (ATC)	Drug-event association studies	Drug utilization studies
Drugs used in diabetes (A10B)	Cancer (bladder, pancreas, etc.) (Safeguard Consortium 2015)	Use (Safeguard Consortium 2015) (+)
	Myocardial infarction (Safeguard Consortium 2015)	
	Pancreatitis (Safeguard Consortium 2015)	
	Pneumonia (Gorricho et al. 2017)	
Calcium supplements (A12A)	Myocardial infarction (de Abajo et al. 2017; Rodríguez-Martín et al. 2019b)	
Antithrombotic agents (B01A)	Bleeding, stroke (van den Ham et al. 2019) (+)	Trends (Ibáñez et al. 2019) (+)
Low-ceiling diuretics, thiazides (C03A)	Skin cancer	
Lipid modifying agents (C10)		Indication (Macías Saint-Gerons et al. 2014, 2015)
Topical calcineurin inhibitors (D11A)		Impact of RMM (Oliva et al. 2012)
Estrogens (G03C, G03F)		Trends (Baladé Martínez et al. 2016)
Antiandrogens (G03H)	Meningioma (Gil et al. 2011)	
Antibacterials (J01)	Acute liver injury (Brauer et al. 2016a; Udo et al. 2016) (+)	Use (Brauer et al. 2016b) (+)
		Indication (urinary tract infection)[a]
Vaccines (J07)	Pertussis vaccine adverse events (Weibel et al. 2019)	Coverage (Braeye et al. 2019; Emborg et al. 2019; Martín-Merino et al. 2019a)
Antiinflammatory drugs (M01)	Myocardial infarction risk (de Abajo et al. 2014)	Indication (Sáez-Jiménez and Bonis 2015)
	Colorectal cancer (Rodríguez-Miguel et al. 2019a)	
	Gastrointestinal bleeding (de Abajo et al. 2013)	

(continued)

Table 2 (continued)

Drug class (ATC)	Drug-event association studies	Drug utilization studies
	Ischemic stroke (García-Poza et al. 2015)	
Antigout drugs (M04)	Myocardial infarction (de Abajo et al. 2015; Rodríguez-Martín et al. 2019a)	
Anti-osteoporotic drugs (M05B)	Fractures (Erviti et al. 2013a, b)	Trends (Leon Vazquez et al. 2015)
	Venous thromboembolism (Martín-Merino et al. 2018) (+)	Trends (Martín-Merino et al. 2017a) (+)
		Use (Martín-Merino et al. 2017b)
Opioids (N02A)		Impact of RMM (codeine) (Hedenmalm et al. 2019) (+)
		Impact of RMM (fentanyl)[a]
Antiepileptics (N03A)	Herpes virus infection (Gil et al. 2019a)	Use (de Groot et al. 2014) (+)
Antipsychotics (N05A)		Indication (dementia)[a]
Anxiolytics, hypnotics and sedatives (N05B, N05C)	Fractures (Requena et al. 2016a, b) (+)	Trends (Huerta et al. 2016) (+)
	SCAR (Martín-Merino et al. 2015)	Adherence (Martín-Pérez et al. 2019)
Antidepressants (N06A)	Fractures (Udo et al. 2016) (+)	Use (Abbing-Karahagopian et al. 2014) (+)
		Use (Macías Saint-Gerons et al. 2018)
Psychostimulants, agents used for ADHD and nootropics (N06B)	Valvular heart disease (Saiz et al. 2020)	Trends (Raman et al. 2018) (+)
Anti-dementia drugs (N06D)		Trends (Bonis et al. 2013)
Adrenergics, inhalants (R03A)	COPD exacerbations (Aguilar-Shea and Bonis 2019)	Trends (Rottenkolber et al. 2015) (+)
Overall	SCAR (Rodríguez-Martín et al. 2018)	

1.9 Administrative Information

The Spanish Agency on Medicines and Medical Devices fully funds BIFAP and is responsible for maintaining the database. Contact details are the following:

- Organization/Affiliation:

BIFAP Program
Pharmacoepidemiology and Pharmacovigilance Division
Department of Medicines of Human Use
Spanish Agency on Medicines and Medical Devices
Campezo 1 edificio 8
28022 Madrid
Spain
Email: equipo@aemps.es
Website: www.bifap.org

2 Practical Experience with the Database

Given the BIFAP characteristics, the database is a powerful tool to perform pharma-coepidemiological studies. Its large sample size and long-term follow-up (median follow-up 8 years) facilitate studies of rare adverse events and long-term effects/risk of drugs under real conditions of use. Studies performed with BIFAP include the main epidemiological designs (case-control, cohort, case-only designs, cross-sectional, etc.). A significant number of papers of studies with the BIFAP database have been published in peer-reviewed journals.

The BIFAP database is fully integrated in the AEMPS roles and activities as a useful tool to assist post-authorization regulatory decision-making and to generate scientific evidence on drug-related issues. This is realized by supporting routine phar-macovigilance, performing post-authorization observational safety studies, assessing drug use patterns of medicines, and evaluating the impact of regulatory actions.

BIFAP was launched in 2003 and has a multidisciplinary team to cover the different areas of the project with a deep knowledge of the data characteristics and long-time experience in performing studies with the database. BIFAP has actively participated in multiple international collaborative projects with other data sources worldwide in the context of the European Commission work programs. These projects mainly aimed to address safety issues, i.e., SAFEGUARD (CORDIS. EU research results 2019), improve the information available on the benefit-risk ratio of marketed vaccines (www.advance-vaccines.eu), develop, test, and disseminate methodological standards for the design, conduct, and analysis of pharmacoepi-demiological studies applicable to different safety issues and using different data sources (www.imi-protect.eu).

Several informatics tools have been developed for data extraction and analysis (see section "Use of BIFAP to perform pharmacoepidemiological studies"). These validated tools are useful for the standardization of the extraction and analytic proce-dures. In addition, the tools are really flexible and thus may be used in different scenarios tailored to the study requirements.

BIFAP shares common development areas and challenges with other data sources used for epidemiological research including: The accurate identification of health outcomes of interest (Lanes et al. 2015), the precise measurement of the treatment exposure, and methodological issues related to study designs, missing imputation, outliers treatment, etc.

BIFAP development areas related to specific characteristics of the database are the following:

- *Increasing the size and representativeness of the database*
  In this regard, BIFAP is open to new regions in Spain willing to participate.
- *Linkage with other health care data sources*
  Currently, BIFAP is a primary care database. A main interest for BIFAP is to link primary care information with other health care databases. Current linkage of PCP's registry in BIFAP includes hospital and mortality registries. Other health care data sources of interest are outpatient specialist and cancer registries.
- *Harmonization processes of information from different electronic medical records*
  There are different EMRs in the regions participating in BIFAP with different data models. Main challenges are the harmonization processes of the heterogeneous and evolving sources of information.
- *Improvement of processing of information contained in natural language found in free text of electronic patient records* (Nadkarni et al. 2011).

Acknowledgements The authors would like to acknowledge the excellent collaboration of the primary care practitioners and pediatricians, and the support of the regional authorities participating in the database (Aragón, Asturias, Canarias, Cantabria, Castilla y León, Castilla-La Mancha, La Rioja, Comunidad de Madrid, Murcia y Navarra). Also, we wish to thank the former members of the BIFAP team for their valuable contribution to the development of the project.

Funding information The 'Base de datos para la investigación Farmacoepidemiológica en Atención Primaria' (BIFAP) is fully financed by the Spanish Agency on Medicines and Medical Devices (AEMPS).

Disclaimer This document expresses the opinion of the authors of the paper, and may not be understood or quoted as being made on behalf of or reflecting the position of the AEMPS.

References

Abbing-Karahagopian V, Huerta C, Souverein PC et al (2014) Antidepressant prescribing in five European countries: application of common definitions to assess the prevalence, clinical observations, and methodological implications. Eur J Clin Pharmacol 70(7):849–857. https://doi.org/10.1007/s00228-014-1676-z

Aguilar-Shea AL, Bonis J (2019) COPD from an everyday primary care point of view. J Fam Med Prim Care 8(8):2644–2650. https://doi.org/10.4103/jfmpc.jfmpc_477_19

Article 29 Data Protection Working Party (2014) 0829/14/EN WP216 Opinion 05/2014 on Anonymisation techniques adopted on 10 April 2014. http://ec.europa.eu/justice/article-29/documentation/opinion-recommendation/files/2014/wp216_en.pdf. Accessed 12 Dec 2019

Baladé Martínez L, Montero Corominas D, Macías Saint-Gerons D (2016) Utilization of hormone replacement therapy in Spain: trends in the period 2000–2014. Med Clin (Barc) 147(7):287–292. https://doi.org/10.1016/j.medcli.2016.05.023

Bernal-Delgado E, Garcia-Armesto S, Oliva J et al (2018) Spain: health system review. Health Syst Transit 20(2):1–179

BIFAP (2019) Base de Datos para la Investigación Farmacoepidemiológica en Atencion Primaria. http://www.bifap.org/. Accessed 12 Dec 2019

Bonis JS, Hoyos MCA, Llorente AG et al (2013) Prevalencia de uso de fármacos para el tratamiento de la enfermedad de Alzheimer y su evolución temporal: un estudio descriptivo con la base de datos de atención primaria BIFAP. Alzheimer Realidades e investigación en demencia 54:20–27. https://doi.org/10.5538/1137-1242.2013.54.20

Braeye T, Bauchau V, Sturkenboom M et al (2019) Estimation of vaccination coverage from electronic healthcare records; methods performance evaluation—a contribution of the ADVANCE-project. PLoS ONE 14(9):e0222296. https://doi.org/10.1371/journal.pone.0222296

Brauer R, Douglas I, Garcia Rodriguez LA et al (2016a) Risk of acute liver injury associated with use of antibiotics. Comparative cohort and nested case-control studies using two primary care databases in Europe. Pharmacoepidemiol Drug Saf 25(s1):29–38. https://doi.org/10.1002/pds.3861

Brauer R, Ruigómez A, Downey G et al (2016b) Prevalence of antibiotic use: a comparison across various European health care data sources. Pharmacoepidemiol Drug Saf 25(s1):11–20. https://doi.org/10.1002/pds.3831

Centers for Disease Control and Prevention (2015) ICD—ICD-9-CM—international classification of diseases, Ninth Revision, clinical modification. https://www.cdc.gov/nchs/icd/icd9cm.htm. Accessed 12 Dec 2019

Chacón García A, Ruigómez A, García Rodríguez LA (2010) Incidence rate of community acquired pneumonia in a population cohort registered in BIFAP. Aten Primaria 42(11):543–549. https://doi.org/10.1016/j.aprim.2010.05.004

CORDIS. EU research results (2019) SAFEGUARD. https://cordis.europa.eu/project/id/282521/reporting. Accessed 12 Dec 2019

de Abajo FJ, Gil MJ, Bryant V et al (2013) Upper gastrointestinal bleeding associated with NSAIDs, other drugs and interactions: a nested case-control study in a new general practice database. Eur J Clin Pharmacol 69(3):691–701. https://doi.org/10.1007/s00228-012-1386-3

de Abajo FJ, Gil MJ, García Poza P et al (2014) Risk of nonfatal acute myocardial infarction associated with non-steroidal antiinflammatory drugs, non-narcotic analgesics and other drugs used in osteoarthritis: a nested case-control study. Pharmacoepidemiol Drug Saf 23(11):1128–1138. https://doi.org/10.1002/pds.3617

de Abajo FJ, Gil MJ, Rodríguez A et al (2015) Allopurinol use and risk of non-fatal acute myocardial infarction. Heart 101(9):679–685. https://doi.org/10.1136/heartjnl-2014-306670

de Abajo FJ, Rodríguez-Martín S, Rodríguez-Miguel A et al (2017) Risk of ischemic stroke associated with calcium supplements with or without vitamin D: a nested case-control study. J Am Heart Assoc 6(5):e005795. https://doi.org/10.1161/JAHA.117.005795

de Groot MCH, Schuerch M, de Vries F et al (2014) Antiepileptic drug use in seven electronic health record databases in Europe: a methodologic comparison. Epilepsia 55(5):666–673. https://doi.org/10.1111/epi.12557

de Hoyos-Alonso MC, Bonis J, Tapias-Merino E et al (2016) Estimated prevalence of dementia based on analysis of drug databases in the Region of Madrid (Spain). Neurología (Barcelona, Spain) 31(1):1–8. https://doi.org/10.1016/j.nrl.2014.08.008

Emborg H-D, Kahlert J, Braeye T et al (2019) ADVANCE system testing: can coverage of pertussis vaccination be estimated in European countries using electronic healthcare databases: An example. Vaccine. https://doi.org/10.1016/j.vaccine.2019.07.039

Erviti J, Alonso A, Gorricho J et al (2013a) Oral bisphosphonates may not decrease hip fracture risk in elderly Spanish women: a nested case-control study. BMJ Open 3(2):e002084. https://doi.org/10.1136/bmjopen-2012-002084

Erviti J, Alonso A, Oliva B et al (2013b) Oral bisphosphonates are associated with increased risk of subtrochanteric and diaphyseal fractures in elderly women: a nested case-control study. BMJ Open 3(1):e002091. https://doi.org/10.1136/bmjopen-2012-002091

European Parliament (2016) Regulation (EU) 2016/679 of the European Parliament and of the Council of 27 April 2016 on the protection of natural persons with regard to the processing of personal data and on the free movement of such data, and repealing Directive 95/46/EC (General Data Protection Regulation). https://eur-lex.europa.eu/eli/reg/2016/679/oj. Accessed 12 Dec 2019

García-Poza P, de Abajo FJ, Gil MJ et al (2015) Risk of ischemic stroke associated with non-steroidal anti-inflammatory drugs and paracetamol: a population-based case-control study. J Thromb Haemost 13(5):708–718. https://doi.org/10.1111/jth.12855

Gil M, González-González R, Vázquez-Calvo A et al (2019a) Clinical infections by Herpesviruses in patients treated with Valproic acid: a nested case-control study in the Spanish primary care database. BIFAP. J Clin Med 8(9):1442. https://doi.org/10.3390/jcm8091442

Gil M, Oliva B, Timoner J et al (2011) Risk of meningioma among users of high doses of cyproterone acetate as compared with the general population: evidence from a population-based cohort study. Br J Clin Pharmacol 72(6):965–968. https://doi.org/10.1111/j.1365-2125.2011.04031.x

Gil M, Rodríguez-Miguel A, Montoya-Catalá H et al (2019b) Validation study of colorectal cancer diagnosis in the Spanish primary care database, BIFAP. Pharmacoepidemiol Drug Saf 28(2):209–216. https://doi.org/10.1002/pds.4686

Gorricho J, Garjón J, Alonso A et al (2017) Use of oral antidiabetic agents and risk of community-acquired pneumonia: a nested case-control study. Br J Clin Pharmacol 83(9):2034–2044. https://doi.org/10.1111/bcp.13288

Hedenmalm K, Blake K, Donegan K et al (2019) A European multicentre drug utilisation study of the impact of regulatory measures on prescribing of codeine for pain in children. Pharmacoepidemiol Drug Saf 28(8):1086–1096. https://doi.org/10.1002/pds.4836

Huerta C, Abbing-Karahagopian V, Requena G et al (2016) Exposure to benzodiazepines (anxi-olytics, hypnotics and related drugs) in seven European electronic healthcare databases: a cross-national descriptive study from the PROTECT-EU Project. Pharmacoepidemiol Drug Saf 25(s1):56–65. https://doi.org/10.1002/pds.3825

Ibáñez L, Sabaté M, Vidal X et al (2019) Incidence of direct oral anticoagulant use in patients with nonvalvular atrial fibrillation and characteristics of users in 6 European countries (2008–2015): a cross-national drug utilization study. Br J Clin Pharmacol 85(11):2524–2539. https://doi.org/10.1111/bcp.14071

Lanes S, Brown JS, Haynes K et al (2015) Identifying health outcomes in healthcare databases. Pharmacoepidemiol Drug Saf 24(10):1009–1016. https://doi.org/10.1002/pds.3856

Leon Vazquez F, Bonis J, Bryant Cerezo V et al (2015) Prevencion de fractura osteoporotica en España: uso de farmacos antes y despues de una fractura de cadera. Revista de Osteoporosis y Metabolismo Mineral 7:54–62

Macías Saint-Gerons D, de la Fuente Honrubia C, González Bermejo D et al (2015) Clinical-epidemiological profile of patients initiating intensive statin therapy for the secondary prevention of vascular disease in Spain. Rev Esp Salud Publica 89(2):159–171. https://doi.org/10.4321/S1135-57272015000200005

Macías Saint-Gerons D, de la Fuente Honrubia C, Montero Corominas D et al (2014) Standard and intensive lipid-lowering therapy with statins for the primary prevention of vascular diseases: a population-based study. Eur J Clin Pharmacol 70(1):99–108. https://doi.org/10.1007/s00228-013-1586-5

Macías Saint-Gerons D, Huerta Álvarez C, García Poza P et al (2018) Trazodone utilization among the elderly in Spain. A population based study. Revista De Psiquiatria Y Salud Mental 11(4):208–215. https://doi.org/10.1016/j.rpsm.2016.11.003

Martín-Merino E, de Abajo FJ, Gil M (2015) Risk of toxic epidermal necrolysis and Stevens-Johnson syndrome associated with benzodiazepines: a population-based cohort study. Eur J Clin Pharmacol 71(6):759–766. https://doi.org/10.1007/s00228-015-1850-y

Martín-Merino E, Huerta-Álvarez C, Prieto-Alhambra D et al (2017a) Secular trends of use of anti-osteoporotic treatments in Spain: a population-based cohort study including over 1.5 million people and more than 12 years of follow-up. Bone 105:292–298. https://doi.org/10.1016/j.bone. 2017.08.031

Martín-Merino E, Huerta-Álvarez C, Prieto-Alhambra D et al (2017b) Cessation rate of anti-osteoporosis treatments and risk factors in Spanish primary care settings: a population-based cohort analysis. Arch Osteoporos 12(1):39. https://doi.org/10.1007/s11657-017-0331-6

Martín-Merino E, Llorente-García A, Corominas DM et al (2019a) The longitudinal incidence of human Papillomavirus vaccination in Spanish primary care in the first 6 years after approval. Pharmaceut Med 33(2):135–144

Martín-Merino E, Llorente-García A, Montero-Corominas D et al (2019b) The recording of human papillomavirus (HPV) vaccination in BIFAP primary care database: a validation study. Pharmacoepidemiol Drug Saf 28(2):201–208. https://doi.org/10.1002/pds.4674

Martín-Merino E, Petersen I, Hawley S et al (2018) Risk of venous thromboembolism among users of different anti-osteoporosis drugs: a population-based cohort analysis including over 200,000 participants from Spain and the UK. Osteoporos Int 29(2):467–478. https://doi.org/10.1007/s00 198-017-4308-5

Martín-Pérez M, Bryant V, Martín-Merino E et al (2019) Are patients adherent to benzodiazepine treatment? Results of a retrospective cohort study in primary care in Spain. Pharmacoepidemiol Drug Saf 28(s2):453. https://doi.org/10.1002/pds.4864

Ministerio de Sanidad Consumo y Bienestar Social (2019) Key indicators. Spanish national health system. http://inclasns.msssi.es/?lang=EN. Accessed 12 Dec 2019

Maciá-Martínez MA, Gil M, Huerta C et al (2020) Base de Datos para la Investigación Farmacoepidemiológica en Atención Primaria (BIFAP): A data resource for pharmacoepidemiology in Spain [published online ahead of print, 2020 Apr 26]. Pharmacoepidemiol Drug Saf. https://doi. org/10.1002/pds.5006

Nadkarni PM, Ohno-Machado L, Chapman WW (2011) Natural language processing: an introduction. J Am Med Inform Assoc 18(5):544–551. https://doi.org/10.1136/amiajnl-2011-000464

OECD/European Union (2018) Health at a Glance: Europe 2018. https://doi.org/10.1787/health_ glance_eur-2018-en

Oliva B, Gil M, Montero D et al. (2012) Patterns of topical Calcineurin inhibitor drug use. Impact of regulatory actions in off-label use. Pharmacoepidemiol Drug Saf 21(s3):156. https://doi.org/ 10.1002/pds

Raman SR, Man KKC, Bahmanyar S et al (2018) Trends in attention-deficit hyperactivity disorder medication use: a retrospective observational study using population-based databases. The Lancet Psychiatry 5(10):824–835. https://doi.org/10.1016/S2215-0366(18)30293-1

Requena G, Abbing-Karahagopian V, Huerta C et al (2014) Incidence rates and trends of hip/femur fractures in five European countries: comparison using e-healthcare records databases. Calcif Tissue Int 94(6):580–589. https://doi.org/10.1007/s00223-014-9850-y

Requena G, Huerta C, Gardarsdottir H et al (2016a) Hip/femur fractures associated with the use of benzodiazepines (anxiolytics, hypnotics and related drugs): a methodological approach to assess consistencies across databases from the PROTECT-EU project. Pharmacoepidemiol Drug Saf 25(s1):66–78. https://doi.org/10.1002/pds.3816

Requena G, Logie J, Martin E et al (2016b) Do case-only designs yield consistent results across design and different databases? A case study of hip fractures and benzodiazepines. Pharmacoepidemiol Drug Saf 25(s1):79–87. https://doi.org/10.1002/pds.3822

Rivero-Calle I, Pardo-Seco J, Aldaz P et al (2016) Incidence and risk factor prevalence of community-acquired pneumonia in adults in primary care in Spain (NEUMO-ES-RISK project). BMC Infect Dis 16(1):645. https://doi.org/10.1186/s12879-016-1974-4

Rodríguez-Martín S, de Abajo FJ, Gil M et al (2019a) Risk of acute myocardial infarction among new users of allopurinol according to serum urate level: a nested case-control study. J Clin Med 8(12):2150. https://doi.org/10.3390/jcm8122150

Rodríguez-Martín S, González-Bermejo D, Rodríguez-Miguel A et al (2019b) Risk of Myocardial infarction among new users of calcium supplements alone or combined with vitamin D: a population-based case-control study. Clin Pharmacol Ther. https://doi.org/10.1002/cpt.1636

Rodríguez-Martín S, Martín-Merino E, Lerma V et al (2018) Active surveillance of severe cutaneous adverse reactions: A case-population approach using a registry and a health care database. Pharmacoepidemiol Drug Saf 27(9):1042–1050. https://doi.org/10.1002/pds.4622

Rodríguez-Miguel A, García-Rodríguez LA, Gil M et al (2019a) Population-based case-control study: chemoprotection of colorectal cancer with non-aspirin nonsteroidal anti-inflammatory drugs and other drugs for pain control. Aliment Pharmacol Ther 50(3):295–305. https://doi.org/10.1111/apt.15333

Rodríguez-Miguel A, García-Rodríguez LA, Gil M et al (2019b) Clopidogrel and low-dose aspirin, alone or together, reduce risk of colorectal cancer. Clin Gastroenterol Hepatol 17(10):2024–2033.e2022. https://doi.org/10.1016/j.cgh.2018.12.012

Rottenkolber M, Voogd E, van Dijk L et al (2015) Seasonal changes in prescribing of long-acting beta-2-agonists-containing drugs. Respir Med 109(7):828–837. https://doi.org/10.1016/j.rmed.2015.01.010

Ruigómez A, Brauer R, Rodríguez LAG et al (2014) Ascertainment of acute liver injury in two European primary care databases. Eur J Clin Pharmacol 70(10):1227–1235. https://doi.org/10.1007/s00228-014-1721-y

Sáez-Jiménez R, Bonis J (2015) Estudio descriptivo sobre el uso de antiinflamatorios no esteroideos por vía intramuscular para el tratamiento de la lumbalgia aguda en las consultas de Atención Primaria en España durante 2002–2011. Rev Clin Med Fam [online] 8:103–109

Safeguard Consortium (2015) Final report summary—SAFEGUARD (Safety evaluation of adverse reactions in diabetes). https://cordis.europa.eu/docs/results/282/282521/final1-safeguard_final-publishable-summary-report.pdf. Accessed 12 Dec 2019

Saiz LC, Garjón J, Gorricho J et al (2017) Validation and incidence of community-acquired pneumonia in patients with type 2 diabetes in the BIFAP database. Epidemiol Infect 145(14):3056–3064. https://doi.org/10.1017/S0950268817001868

Saiz LC, Gil M, Alonso A et al (2020) Use of methylphenidate and risk for valvular heart disease: a case-control study nested in the BIFAP cohort. Pharmacoepidemiol Drug Saf. https://doi.org/10.1002/pds.4954

Salvador Rosa A, Moreno Pérez JC, Sonego D et al (2002) The BIFAP project: database for pharmaco-epidemiological research in primary care. Aten Primaria 30(10):655–661. https://doi.org/10.1016/s0212-6567(02)79129-4

Souverein PC, Abbing-Karahagopian V, Martin E et al (2016) Understanding inconsistency in the results from observational pharmacoepidemiological studies: the case of antidepressant use and risk of hip/femur fractures. Pharmacoepidemiol Drug Saf 25(s1):88–102. https://doi.org/10.1002/pds.3862

Udo R, Tcherny-Lessenot S, Brauer R et al (2016) The risk of acute liver injury associated with the use of antibiotics—evaluating robustness of results in the pharmacoepidemiological research on outcomes of therapeutics by a European consortium (PROTECT) project. Pharmacoepidemiol Drug Saf 25(s1):47–55. https://doi.org/10.1002/pds.3841

van den Ham H, Souverein P, Klungel O et al (2019) Risk of major bleeding associated with the use of individual direct oral anticoagulants compared to vitamin K antagonists in patients with non-valvular atrial fibrillation: a meta-analysis of results from multiple population-based cohort studies using a common protocol in Europe and Canada. Pharmacoepidemiol Drug Saf 28(s2):410–411. https://doi.org/10.1002/pds.4864

Weibel D, Dodd C, Mahaux O et al (2019) ADVANCE system testing: Can safety studies be conducted using electronic healthcare data? An example using pertussis vaccination. Vaccine. https://doi.org/10.1016/j.vaccine.2019.06.040

WHO Collaborating Centre for Drug Statistics Methodology (2019) Guidelines for ATC classification and DDD assignment 2020. Oslo, Norway

WONCA International Classification Committee (1998) ICPC-2. International classification of primary care. 2nd edn. Oxford University Press, Oxford and G. Berghof, *A data resource for Paramecia*, *alternative*, pp. ...

K. ... D ... aming Corp., reading, addition, Addison-Wesley, Math, Jan. pp. ... Addison-Wesley ... Cambridge ...
... J. ... posium on ... 1996, (value ... ...
WQM ... ... H. ... C. ... ... and an ... ... WQ. ... ... A ... method for construct ...
... ... H. ... ...

The Information System for Research in Primary Care (SIDIAP)

Talita Duarte-Salles, María Aragón, and Bonaventura Bolíbar

Abstract The Information System for Research in Primary Care (SIDIAP 2020) platform was created in 2010 by the Catalan Health Institute (ICS) and the IDIAPJGol Institute. It was designed to provide a valid and reliable database of selected information from electronic health records (EHRs) of patients registered in primary care centres for use in biomedical research. SIDIAP includes information from EHR data registered since January 1, 2006 by more than 30,000 health professionals during routine visits at 328 primary care centres pertaining to the ICS in Catalonia, a region in the North-East of Spain. SIDIAP has pseudo-anonymised records with 5.7 million people active in 2019.

1 Database Description

1.1 Introduction

Spain's National Health System scheme, which is decentralised to the autonomous regions, covers more than 98% of the population and is funded by general taxes. Primary care plays an essential role as it is the main entry point for accessing public health services, it is the most accessible and most commonly used health service which provides an integral and continuous care, and it is responsible for long-term prescriptions and specialist and hospital referrals. Primary care services are delivered through primary care centres, the basic unit of provision. These centres are composed of general practitioners (GPs), paediatricians, dentists, nurses and social care practitioners, nursing aids and administrative staff. As part of primary care, there is a set of support services such as sexual and reproductive health or home care at the end of life. In Catalonia, the *Institut Català de la Salut* (ICS, Catalan Health Institute)

T. Duarte-Salles · M. Aragón · B. Bolíbar (✉)
Fundació Institut Universitari per la recera a l'Atenció Primària de Salut Jordi Gol I Guarins
(IDIAPJGol), Gran Via Corts Catalanes 578, 08007 Barcelona, Spain
e-mail: bbolibar@idiapjgol.org

© Springer Nature Switzerland AG 2021   189
M. Sturkenboom and T. Schink (eds.), *Databases for Pharmacoepidemiological
Research*, Springer Series on Epidemiology and Public Health,
https://doi.org/10.1007/978-3-030-51455-6_15

is the most important public primary health care provider, covering approximately 75% of the Catalan population.

The Information System for Research in Primary Care (SIDIAP 2020) platform was created in 2010 by the ICS and the IDIAPJGol Institute. It was designed to provide a valid and reliable database of selected information from electronic health records (EHRs) of patients registered in primary care centres for use in biomedical research (Bolíbar et al. 2012; García-Gil et al. 2011).

1.2   Database Characteristics

SIDIAP includes information from EHR data registered since January 1, 2006 by more than 30,000 health professionals during routine visits at 328 primary care centres pertaining to the ICS in Catalonia, a region in the North-East of Spain. It is directly linked to primary care laboratories and to the Catalan pharmacy invoice databases. It can also be linked to other data sources, such as the hospital discharge database, on a project-by-project basis. SIDIAP has pseudo-anonymised records for more than 7 million people, with 5.7 million people active in 2019.

People can enter the database when they are born or when they visit an ICS primary care centre for the first time and leave the database when they are transferred out or die. If a person is transferred out but subsequently comes back, this person's EHR will be related again to the same SIDIAP-ID, and their EHR history will be available with the start date equalling the previous one. The SIDIAP database is updated annually at each start of the year, and the mean follow-up time of the population is ten years. SIDIAP has been previously shown to be highly representative of the Catalan population in terms of age, sex, and geographic distribution (Bolíbar et al. 2012). It provides an excellent source of population-based data and reliably reproduces the actual conditions of clinical practice. The high quality of these data has been previously documented, and SIDIAP has been successfully applied to epidemiological studies of key exposures and outcomes (García-Gil et al. 2011).

The database is listed in the European Network of Centres for Pharmacoepidemiology and Pharmacovigilance (ENCePP) catalogue (ENCePP 2020). Also, it has been mapped in accordance with the Observational Medical Outcomes Partnership Common Data Model (OMOP-CDM) from the Observational Health Data Sciences and Informatics (OHDSI) community network, which will allow evidence generation using standardised open source analytic tools and promote collaborative studies with other databases worldwide (Observational Health Data Sciences and Informatics 2019).

1.3 Available Data

The SIDIAP data comprises the clinical information registered by any primary health care professional (GPs, nurses, paediatricians, gynaecologists, midwives, dentists, and social workers) in EHRs as well as external information related to the primary care visit, such as the results of laboratory tests, pharmacy dispensations, and other external data.

The available information includes:

- Demographic data: Age, date of birth (only month and year can be provided), sex, type of residency area (urban or rural), and nationality
- Mortality: Date of death
- Some socioeconomic indicators (SES):

  - The ecological MEDEA index (Domínguez-Berjón et al. 2008): The MEDEA index is assigned in quintiles through the census tract to each individual in the database.
  - The pharmaceutical copayment level related to the income level and work condition of the person (Generalitat de Catalunya 2015).
  - Since 2014, social class based on occupation has also been available for those individuals who have taken sick leave at least once.

- Disease diagnoses registered by primary healthcare professionals during a visit using the International Classification of Diseases, Tenth Revision, Clinical Modification (ICD-10-CM) codification system
- Medication (prescription and dispensation): The SIDIAP includes all the drugs prescribed in a primary health care centre (with posology and frequency of taking available) as well as the drugs purchased at the pharmacy counters per month (number of drug packages dispensed). For each drug, the defined daily dose (DDD) recommended by the WHO, the strength, the number of units per package, and the administration route are also available. Drugs purchased over-the-counter or administered in hospitals are not included. Drug information is available from the Anatomical Therapeutic Chemical (ATC7) Classification System
- Laboratory test requests by primary health care professionals and their results (e.g., cell count, serology, biochemistry, etc.)
- Physical examination results and routine measurements (e.g., blood pressure, weight, height, body mass index, spirometry results, test scores, measurements related to child growth, etc.)
- Referral to other specialists by primary health care professionals including the cause of referral (ICD-10-CM code to be validated by the specialist)
- Sick leave periods: Time and cause (ICD-10-CM code)
- Requested procedures in primary care (e.g., immunizations, diagnostic imaging or different scales and tests used in primary care)
- Primary care visits (date, type of professional, and place of visit—in the centre, at patient's home or telematic visit)

- Lifestyle information: Smoking status and alcohol consumption habits
- Pregnancies and related information: Date of last period, estimated date of delivery, type of childbirth, closing circumstance of the pregnancy, gestational age, etc.
- Vaccination (including the antigen and the number of administered doses)
- Adverse drug reactions to an ATC7 drug code
- Family linkage: A large number of longitudinal health records of both parents and their children (only those born since 2006) are successfully linked in SIDIAP by the ICS through the social security number.

Access to free text data is possible for a reduced sample of patients when needed information is not already available in structured variables; for example, symptoms or cause of death. In order to analyse free text data, this information has to be anonymised beforehand.

SIDIAP also may gather additional information from patients through questionnaires to health professionals which can be administered through the ICS.

Furthermore, on a project-by-project basis, SIDIAP can be linked to other sources of clinical information thanks to the collaboration with the PADRIS programme of the Department of Health (AQUAS 2020). Thus, it is possible to have access to hospital admission data and other sources such as mental health hospitals.

1.4 Strengths and Limitations

The main strengths of SIDIAP are its large size and the high population representativeness by age, sex, and region (Bolíbar et al. 2012), including approximately 75% of the population living in Catalonia, as well as the type and amount of information available including demographic and lifestyle-related variables such as nationality, socioeconomic status, body mass index, smoking or alcohol exposures. Also, the assessment of drug exposure is assumed to be quite complete in SIDIAP since information on both prescription and dispensation is available.

Another strength of SIDIAP is the direct collaboration with the health provider (ICS) which allows the improvement of the EHR system for data collection and therefore also the improvement of the quality of the registered information. Thanks to this close collaboration SIDIAP has also been able to link with external data sources, to link mother- and father-child EHR data, and to obtain additional data from the population through questionnaires to GPs.

As shown below, the high external validity of the register of a wide number of outcomes has been demonstrated. Also, SIDIAP has been mapped in accordance with the OMOP-CDM, which facilitates and promotes multi-database studies and helps with data management and data analyses (Observational Health Data Sciences and Informatics 2019).

As this is a primary care database, information on specialist prescribing, drug dispensing in hospital setting, drugs purchased over the counter, and actual drug intake is missing. Furthermore, major attention has to be paid to underreporting, missing data, misclassification and confounding, the general limitations of real-world databases.

1.5 Validation

Different validation processes have been carried out in order to determine the quality and potential use of its information.

1.5.1 Internal Validation

Quality checks to identify duplicate patient IDs are performed centrally at each SIDIAP database update, which is done annually. As the original data are distributed in different servers by regions, stratifications of variables by geographical zone and years are performed in order to check if a concept is registered using the same codes or if data homogenisation is needed. Heat maps and other visual representations for the registration of the information by week of the year are checked during each database update in order to quickly detect any possible problems in the original ETL procedure. SIDIAP also checks logical values for measurements. In the biochemistry data case, consistency for tests taken in different laboratories is assessed, and unit conversion is undertaken when needed.

In addition, a specific quality control is performed for each requested project before data is delivered to research teams. In this step, all the data selected for the project are checked, including the calculation of counts, percentiles, maximums and minimums, incidences and prevalences. A quality check report is shared with researchers before data delivery to ensure an early detection of any inconsistencies in the data extraction.

1.5.2 External Validation

The external validation of the record of several outcomes that have been previously accessed in SIDIAP included:

- Twenty-five types of incident cancer cases were validated in SIDIAP using the population-based cancer registries of Girona and Tarragona as the gold standard. The sensitivity (76% for overall cancer), the positive predictive values (PPV; 61% for overall cancer), and the time difference between the date of diagnosis entered in SIDIAP versus that in the cancer registries (≤3 months of difference for most cancers between the two sources) were calculated for overall and site-specific cancers (Recalde et al. 2019).

- Alzheimer's disease and dementia diagnoses in primary care was validated using additional information provided by GPs through an online survey, and the Girona Dementia Registry. PPVs for Alzheimer's disease ranged from 72.3 to 89.8%, and sensitivities from 71.4 to 83.3%, depending on the gold standard used (Ponjoan et al. 2019a). The overall PPV of dementia diagnoses was estimated as 91.0% (Ponjoan et al. 2019b).
- Cardiovascular risk factors, including systolic and diastolic blood pressure, glucose, total cholesterol, triglycerides, HDL-C, LDL-C, weight, and height, as well as recorded diagnoses of diabetes, hypertension, hypercholesterolemia, smoking, and obesity were validated against data from a cohort study in the region of Girona in Catalonia. The prevalence of these cardiovascular risk factors and their association with the incidence of vascular disease observed in SIDIAP were consistent with those observed in a longitudinal epidemiological population-based study in which a standardised methodology was used to obtain the information (Ramos et al. 2012).
- Musculoskeletal Disorders: Rheumatoid arthritis prevalence (4.2/1000 in 2012) and incidence (0.20/1000 person-years) observed in SIDIAP were similar to those of other Southern European regions. Also, 73.9% of cases that had a rheumatoid factor measurement were seropositive (≥ 10 IU/mL) (Fina-Aviles et al. 2014). Ankylosing spondylitis was validated against HLA B27 laboratory test results; 62.4% of all people with a diagnosis registered in primary care also had a positive result in this test (Muñoz-Ortego et al. 2014). Finally, fractures registered in SIDIAP were validated by comparing data to hospital admission and patient-reported fracture records. In the comparison between SIDIAP and hospital discharge data, sensitivity was 60.1% and PPV was 70.8% In the comparison with the patient-reported fracture records, corresponding sensitivity and PPVs were, respectively: 56.1% and 82.1% for wrist/forearm; 66.7% and 92.3% for hip; and 50%, and 37.5% for clinical spine fractures (Pagès-Castellà et al. 2012).

1.6 Governance and Ethical Issues

IDIAPJGol is the institution in charge of the management of SIDIAP. There is a Steering Committee comprised by the ICS and the IDIAPJGol that establishes the strategic plan and evaluates the general performance of the database and its services.

SIDIAP can only provide patient level data to public research organisations or to projects required by a regulatory agency such as the European Medicines Agency (EMA). All projects have to be approved by a Scientific Committee and an Ethical Committee. Data have to be used exclusively for the approved protocol and giving data access to third parties is not allowed. Patient IDs are pseudonymised by the ICS for data protection reasons. Therefore, informed consent from patients is not required. Furthermore, in each project, different methods for de-identification, specifically generalisation and deletion, can be applied in some cases (e.g., rare events, sensitive personal information).

1.7   Documents and Publications

Since 2010, the SIDIAP data have been used in 262 research projects which have generated 153 scientific publications in high-impact journals. The full list of all conducted projects and publications can be found on the SIDIAP website (SIDIAP 2020).

The main areas of research that have been investigated in SIDIAP are cardiovascular diseases, diabetes, musculoskeletal disorders, respiratory problems, cancer, and different pharmacoepidemiology studies. Furthermore, different types of studies have been carried out and papers have already been published:

1. Health management (resources and costs in the management of different diseases)
   Example: A population-based study analysing the costs of poor glycaemic control in type 2 diabetes mellitus (Mata-Cases et al. 2020)
2. Epidemiology

   2.1. Incidence and prevalence of different diseases
        Example: A retrospective cohort study about the incidence and risk factors of clinically diagnosed knee, hip, and hand osteoarthritis (Prieto-Alhambra et al. 2013)
   2.2. Risk and prognostic factors
        Example: A matched retrospective cohort studying the risk and predictors of cirrhosis and hepatocellular carcinoma in adults with diagnosed NAFLD (Alexander et al. 2019)
   2.3 Associations between different factors and diseases
        Example: A retrospective cohort studying the association between chronic immune-mediated inflammatory diseases and cardiovascular risk (Baena-Díez et al. 2018).

3. Geographical distribution and environmental factors
   Example: A self-controlled case series study about the association between sudden changes in ambient temperature and cardiovascular hospitalisations (Ponjoan et al. 2017)
4. Evaluation of health care interventions and health policies
   Example: A clinical trial evaluating a new decision tool for improving the adequacy of anticoagulant therapy (Dalmau et al. 2018)
5. Pharmacoepidemiology
   Different types of pharmacoepidemiological studies can be done with SIDIAP, some of the studies carried out were drug utilization studies (DUS) and post-authorisation safety studies (PASS) required by the European Medicines Agency and other regulatory agencies.

   5.1 DUS with different medicines and diseases
        Example: A retrospective cohort study with the use of Apixaban (Ainhoa et al. 2018)

5.2 PASS with different medicines and diseases
    Example: A cohort and nested case-control study about acute liver injury
    and the use of Agomelatine and other antidepressants (Pladevall-Vila et al.
    2019)

5.3 Prescription evaluation and adequacy
    Example: A retrospective cohort study of the therapeutic inertia in type 2
    diabetes mellitus (Mata-Cases et al. 2018)

5.4 Effectiveness of medicines
    Example: A retrospective cohort study with the use of statins for primary
    prevention of cardiovascular events and mortality in old persons (Ramos
    et al. 2018).

1.8 Administrative Information

The database is maintained by IDIAPJGol and funded by own resources.

Contact details

Organization/affiliation: Fundació Institut Universitari per a la recerca a
l'Atenció Primària de Salut Jordi Gol i Gurina (IDIAPJGol)
    Gran Via de les Corts Catalanes, 587, 08007 Àtic
    Barcelona, Spain.

Administrative Contact: Anna Moleras
    e-mail: sidiap@idiapjgol.info
    phone: +34 93 482 46 94
    Scientific and technical contacts: Bonaventura Bolibar
    e-mail: bbolibar@idiapjgol.org
    phone: +34 93 482 46 94

Website: https://www.sidiap.org/

References

Ainhoa G, Cortés J, Giner-Soriano M et al (2018) Characteristics of apixaban-treated patients, evaluation of the dose prescribed, and the persistence of treatment: a cohort study in Catalonia. J Cardiovasc Pharmacol Ther 23:494–501. https://doi.org/10.1177/1074248418778544

Alexander M, Loomis A, Lei J et al (2019) Risks and clinical predictors of cirrhosis and hepatocellular carcinoma diagnoses in adults with diagnosed NAFLD: real-world study of 18 million patients in four European cohorts. BMC Med 17:95. https://doi.org/10.1186/s12916-019-1321-x

AQUAS (2020) Programa d'analítica de dades per a la recerca i la innovació en salut. http://aquas.gencat.cat/ca/ambits/analitica-dades/padris/. Accessed 20 Feb 2020

Baena-Díez JM, Garcia-Gil M, Comas-Cufí M et al (2018) Association between chronic immune-mediated inflammatory diseases and cardiovascular risk. Heart 104(2):119–126. https://doi.org/10.1136/heartjnl-2017-311279

Bolíbar B, Fina Avilés F, Morros R et al (2012) Base de datos SIDIAP: la historia clínica informatizada de Atención Primaria como fuente de información para la investigación epidemiológica. Med Clin (Barc) 138(14):617–621. https://doi.org/10.1016/j.medcli.2012.01.020

Dalmau R, Gonçalves A, Forcadell E et al (2018) A new clinical decision support tool for improving the adequacy of anticoagulant therapy and reducing the incidence of stroke in nonvalvular atrial fibrillation: a randomized clinical trial in primary care. Medicine 97:e9578. https://doi.org/10.1097/MD.0000000000009578

Domínguez-Berjón MF, Borrell C, Cano-Serral G et al (2008) Constructing a deprivation index based on census data in large Spanish cities (the MEDEA project). Gac Sanit 22(3):179–187. https://doi.org/10.1157/13123961

ENCePP (2020) European Network of Centres for Pharmacoepidemiology and Pharmacovigilance. http://www.encepp.eu/encepp/viewResource.htm?id=4646. Accessed 19 Feb 2020

Fina-Aviles F, Medina M, Méndez L et al (2014) The descriptive epidemiology of rheumatoid arthritis in Catalonia: a retrospective study using routinely collected data. Clin Rheumatol 35. https://doi.org/10.1007/s10067-014-2801-1

García-Gil MDM, Hermosilla E, Prieto-Alhambra D et al (2011) Construction and validation of a scoring system for the selection of high-quality data in a Spanish population primary care database (SIDIAP). Inform Prim Care 19(3):135–145. https://doi.org/10.14236/jhi.v19i3.806

Generalitat de Catalunya (2015) Consell Assessor per a la Sostenibilitat i el Progrés del Sistema Sanitari. Medicaments i Productes Sanitaris. https://catsalut.gencat.cat/ca/serveis-sanitaris/atencio-farmaceutica/financament-public-medicaments/. Accessed 18 Feb 2020

Mata-Cases M, Franch-Nadal J, Real J et al (2018) Therapeutic inertia in patients treated with two or more antidiabetics in primary care: factors predicting intensification of treatment. Diabetes Obes Metab 20(1):103–112. https://doi.org/10.1111/dom.13045

Mata-Cases M, Rodríguez-Sánchez B, Mauricio D et al (2020) The association between poor glycemic control and health care costs in people with diabetes: a population-based study. Diabetes Care: dc190573. https://doi.org/10.2337/dc19-0573

Muñoz-Ortego J, Vestergaard P, Rubio JB et al (2014) Ankylosing spondylitis is associated with an increased risk of vertebral and nonvertebral clinical fractures: a population-based cohort study. J Bone Miner Res 29(8):1770–1776. https://doi.org/10.1002/jbmr.2217

Observational Health Data Sciences and Informatics (2019) The book of OHDSI-observational health data sciences and informatics. OHDSI, San Bernardino, CA

Pagès-Castellà A, Carbonell C, Avilés F et al (2012) Burden of osteoporotic fractures in primary health care in Catalonia (Spain): a population-based study. BMC Musculoskelet Disord 13:79. https://doi.org/10.1186/1471-2474-13-79

Pladevall-Vila M, Pottegård A, Schink T et al (2019) Risk of acute liver injury in agomelatine and other antidepressant users in four European countries: a cohort and nested case–control study using automated health data sources. CNS Drugs 33. https://doi.org/10.1007/s40263-019-00611-9

Ponjoan A, Blanch J, Alves-Cabratosa L et al (2017) Effects of extreme temperatures on cardiovascular emergency hospitalizations in a Mediterranean region: a self-controlled case series study. Environ Health 16(1):32. https://doi.org/10.1186/s12940-017-0238-0

Ponjoan A, Garre-Olmo J, Blanch J et al (2019a) How well can electronic health records from primary care identify Alzheimer's disease cases? Clin Epidemiol 11:509–518. https://doi.org/10.2147/CLEP.S206770

Ponjoan A, Garre-Olmo J, Blanch J et al (2019b) Epidemiology of dementia: prevalence and incidence estimates using validated electronic health records from primary care. Clin Epidemiol 11:217–228. https://doi.org/10.2147/CLEP.S186590

Prieto-Alhambra D, Judge A, Javaid M et al (2013) Incidence and risk factors for clinically diagnosed knee, hip and hand osteoarthritis: influences of age, gender and osteoarthritis affecting other joints. Ann Rheum Dis 73. https://doi.org/10.1136/annrheumdis-2013-203355

Ramos R, Balló E, Marrugat J et al (2012) Validez del Sistema de Información para el Desarrollo de la Investigación en Atención Primaria (SIDIAP) en el estudio de enfermedades vasculares: estudio EMMA. Rev Esp Cardiol 65(1):29–37. https://doi.org/10.1016/j.recesp.2011.07.017

Ramos R, Comas-Cufí M, Martí-Lluch R et al (2018) Statins for primary prevention of cardiovascular events and mortality in old and very old adults with and without type 2 diabetes: retrospective cohort study. BMJ 362:k3359. https://doi.org/10.1136/bmj.k3359

Recalde M, Manzano-Salgado C, Díaz Y et al (2019) Validation of cancer diagnoses in electronic health records: results from the information system for research in primary care (SIDIAP) In Northeast Spain. Clin Epidemiol 11:1015–1024. https://doi.org/10.2147/CLEP.S225568

SIDIAP (2020) Sistema d'Informació per al desenvolupament de la Investigació en Atenció Primària. https://www.sidiap.org/. Accessed 19 Feb 2020

Estonian Health Insurance Fund (EHIF) Database

Helis Puksand and Sirly Lätt

Abstract The Estonian Health Insurance Fund (EHIF) database is an administrative database containing claims data from Estonian healthcare providers and is financed by the Estonian Health Insurance Fund. It covers information on each medical contact, as well as on prescription medicines, medical devices and benefits for incapacity to work. Since the remuneration of the costs of treatments and prescription medicines is based on the data, the main purpose of the database is to finance healthcare and to monitor contracts.

1 Type of Database: Introduction

The Estonian Health Insurance Fund (EHIF) database is an administrative database containing claims data from Estonian healthcare providers and is financed by the Estonian Health Insurance Fund. It covers information on each medical contact, as well as on prescription medicines, medical devices and benefits for incapacity to work. Since the remuneration of the costs of treatments and prescription medicines is based on the data, the main purpose of the database is to finance healthcare and to monitor contracts.

1.1 Database Characteristics

Information on medical contacts (physician visit, hospital stay, etc.), including all diagnostic tests and treatment provided, is based on claims data retrieved from all healthcare providers that have signed a contract with EHIF and that offer healthcare financed by EHIF, i.e., almost all Estonian healthcare providers. The Estonian health care system is mainly publicly funded through solidarity-based mandatory health

H. Puksand · S. Lätt (✉)
Estonian Health Insurance Fund, Lastekodu 48, Tallinn 10144, Estonia
e-mail: sirly.latt@haigekassa.ee

© Springer Nature Switzerland AG 2021
M. Sturkenboom and T. Schink (eds.), *Databases for Pharmacoepidemiological Research*, Springer Series on Epidemiology and Public Health,
https://doi.org/10.1007/978-3-030-51455-6_16

199

insurance contributions in the form of an earmarked social payroll tax. Due to that fact, the health insurance system covers about 95% of the Estonian population (around 1.3 million people). (Lai et al. 2013) In addition to the data of insured people, the database also contains some information sent by contractual partners of EHIF regarding services provided to uninsured people, for example, in case of emergencies. The database contains information from 2004 onwards.

Information on medical contacts (or 'treatment episodes') is registered by medical staff in an electronic system. This data is validated by a controlling system and enters the EHIF database a day after insertion. Medical staff has to document treatment data regularly (preferably daily), because it forms the basis for remuneration of the costs of the services provided. Most of the information (invoices) has to be inserted by the tenth of the following month, but corrections and some invoices can be inserted later, too.

In addition to medical contacts, the database also contains data on prescription medicines and medical devices like orthoses, glucose strips, etc. The database does not contain information about over the counter medicines. The prescription data is entered electronically in a prescription database, which is separate from the treatment database. Doctors, pharmacists and patients can all insert and view their information in the database. The information is visible in the prescription database right away, however, it enters the EHIF database usually a day after insertion. The prescription database is managed by EHIF. A similar system exists for medical devices. The Estonian Health Insurance Fund compensates part (0, 50, 75, 90 or 100%) of the costs of prescription medicines. The respective amount will be deducted in the pharmacy, so that a person can buy medicines at the reduced price.

The data concerning incapacity to work comes from four types of incapacity sheets—incapacity due to sickness, maternity, adoption or care allowance. A doctor documents the information from the incapacity sheets in an electronic system. The information is then transmitted to the employer, who enters additional data about the company and the salary. All information enters the EHIF database after it has been validated by a controlling system.

1.2   Available Data

The EHIF database includes information on hospitalizations, outpatient visits, primary care information, outpatient drug prescriptions, and incapacity to work of all insured and uninsured people. Data includes core patient data—person's ID number, name, date of birth, date of death, sex, and address. Furthermore, information on medical contacts includes information about the healthcare provider, doctor, type of healthcare, main and co-diagnoses, date of admission, date of discharge, regular procedures, surgical procedures, date of procedures, and amount of procedures. In outpatient care, the date of admission and the date of discharge are mostly the same, but they can also be different, e.g., in case a person has to repeat the visit or has to come back for a check-up on another day. For inpatient care, the Diagnosis Related Groups (DRGs) are also included.

Data about prescription drugs and medical devices contain the same information about the patient, doctor, and healthcare provider as the treatment episode data. In addition, there is information about the dispensing pharmacy, the diagnoses, the discount rate, the date when the medicine was prescribed, and also the date of issuing and dispensing. Furthermore, the active substance code, the level of content, and the total dispensed amount of the medicine, the prescribed dosage, the number of packages, the price of the medicine, the paid price, and the discount price are also included. If a doctor prescribes the medicine using a certain trade name, thus prohibiting substituting the medicine with a product from a different manufacturer that uses the same active substance, a medical reason for this limitation is also documented.

Data about the incapacity to work contains also information about the patient, doctor, and healthcare provider. In addition, information about the company where the patient works and his or her salary is included. Furthermore, the data contains the start and end date of the incapacity to work, the reason why the person is incapable to work, and the type of incapacity. Since 2015, diagnostic codes have to be documented also on the incapacity sheet.

Diagnoses are coded using the International Classification of Diseases, version 10 (ICD-10). For each treatment episode, there has to be one main diagnosis which can be supplemented by up to ten co-diagnoses. Prescription and incapacity to work data contain only one diagnosis. The active substance code of medicine is coded using the Anatomical Therapeutic Chemical (ATC) Classification System. For surgical procedures, the NOMESCO Classification of Surgical Procedures is applied.

The database does not include information about vaccinations that cannot be coded with ICD-10. It also does not include information about laboratory results and physical examination results. In Estonia, there is a different database for doctors, which includes all the information about laboratory and physical examination results. EHIF does not manage this database. However, the EHIF database does contain information about the dates and frequencies of procedures and laboratory tests.

EHIF data contains hardly any information about lifestyle. It is possible to see whether a person is insured, which for adults usually means that the person has a job. Obesity and alcohol abuse can be coded as a diagnosis.

EHIF data is automatically connected to the Business Register, which contains information about healthcare providers, such as address, register number, etc. Patient's contact data (i.e., address, telephone number, etc.) comes from the Population Registry. Information about a person's insurance status comes automatically from the Employment Registry. Other data sources could be linked to the EHIF database through the person's ID numbers if the Estonian Data Protection Inspection allows it.

1.3   Strengths and Limitations

The EHIF database has many strengths, with the main strength being the significant amount of information it contains. The data is updated regularly and data is accessible very quickly. The data is inserted electronically and the database is automatically updated, which makes it fast and easy to use for both doctors and EHIF. The primary strength of the prescription database may be that it contains information from the medical staff in addition to the information from the pharmacies. The database also contains information about prescriptions that were never actually filled. Furthermore, it is possible to examine differences in the data by comparing information documented by doctors to that documented by pharmacies.

The main limitation of the EHIF database is the validity of the data. Accuracy can only be guaranteed up to a certain level. For example, documented indications (diagnosis codes) may occasionally be incorrect. Since diagnosis codes are not a basis for financing, doctors are not sufficiently motivated to document them correctly. There is, however, a system in place to make sure that the majority of data inserted is correct and constant improvements are being made by adding additional automatic checks and analyzing the submitted data.

1.4   Validation

Data is validated on two levels. Firstly, when the data is inserted by the medical staff, automatic checks are performed to verify whether the data format is right and whether the information is coded correctly. Later, after the data has been inserted into the database, economists check the data periodically. Some things that form the basis for remuneration, such as the dates of the invoices, are checked every month, while other data is checked more occasionally. If data is incorrect, medical staff has to make corrections or the bill will be credited.

1.5   Governance and Ethical Issues

Access to the claims data is granted only to certain employees of the Estonian Health Insurance Fund. It is not permitted to give third parties access to the database or to identifiable data. Some of the aggregated data is published on the website of EHIF and although everyone can make a request for additional aggregated data, every request is assessed separately to avoid the possibility of identification of individuals. Every data request must be well grounded.

If a large amount of patient level data is requested, EHIF concludes a data exchange contract, determining that the data will not be accessible to third parties. In order to prevent the identification of individuals in the data, the person's ID number must be pseudonymized as a rule. If the requested data contains rare conditions or might be identifiable EHIF insists on approval from the Estonian Data Protection Inspection. All data requests must be approved by the legal department and the data protection department of EHIF.

No areas of research are excluded. The only reasons why EHIF might decline the provision of data are: (i) the request is not well grounded or (ii) the data is too identifiable and the inquirer does not have approval from Estonian Data Protection Inspection.

1.6   Administrative Information

The Estonian Health Insurance Fund is responsible for maintaining the databases. The database maintenance is funded from the EHIF budget and does not have any extra funding.

Contact Details

Organization/affiliation: Estonian Health Insurance Fund
   Lembitu 10, 10114 Tallinn, Estonia

Administrative Contact: email: info@haigekassa.ee
   tel: +372 6208 430

Website: https://www.haigekassa.ee/en

Reference

Lai T, Habicht T, Kahur K et al (2013) Estonia: health system review. Health Syst Transit 15(6):1–196

Icelandic Medicines Registry (IMR)

Larus S. Gudmundsson, Olafur B. Einarsson, and Magnus Johannsson

Abstract The Icelandic Medicines Registry (IMR) is a prescription database containing all prescriptions filled in pharmacies for individuals living in Iceland who are covered by the Icelandic social insurance system. The IMR was set up for the Directorate of Health to evaluate national use of prescription medicines, to monitor drug prescribing, and to promote rational use of drugs.

1 Database Description

1.1 Introduction

The Icelandic Medicines Registry (IMR) is a prescription database containing all prescriptions filled in pharmacies for individuals living in Iceland who are covered by the Icelandic social insurance system. The IMR was set up for the Directorate of Health to evaluate national use of prescription medicines, to monitor drug prescribing, and to promote rational use of drugs.

L. S. Gudmundsson (✉)
Faculty of Pharmaceutical Sciences, University of Iceland, Hagi Hofsvallagata 53, 107 Reykjavik, Iceland
e-mail: larussg@hi.is

O. B. Einarsson
Supervision and Quality of Healthcare, The Directorate of Health, Katrinartuni 2, 105 Reykjavik, Iceland

M. Johannsson
Department of Pharmacology and Toxicology, University of Iceland, Hagi Hofsvallagata 53, 107 Reykjavik, Iceland

© Springer Nature Switzerland AG 2021
M. Sturkenboom and T. Schink (eds.), *Databases for Pharmacoepidemiological Research*, Springer Series on Epidemiology and Public Health,
https://doi.org/10.1007/978-3-030-51455-6_17

1.2 Database Characteristics

The IMR covers drug prescribing information from general practitioners and specialists with license in Iceland. It also covers prescriptions filled in pharmacies. The IMR does not include medication dispensed in hospitals. Everyone who has been a legal resident in Iceland for six months automatically becomes a member of the Icelandic social insurance system, regardless of nationality. This applies unless intergovernmental treaties say otherwise. Laws on building a prescription database were passed in parliament (Althingi) in 2003. The IMR was operational in 2005 and it contains prescription information from January 2002 with full coverage from 2003. For the data years 2002–2010, the database contains information on dugs dispensed in general practice and not on those dispensed in institutions (e.g., hospices and retirement homes) and hospitals. Over this period, the IMR is estimated (from sales data) to cover about 80% of all prescription medication dispensed in Iceland. As of 2011, IMR also includes medication dispensed in institutions, thus covering about 90% of all prescription medication dispensed in Iceland. Since 2002 to date, about 99% of the Icelandic population, irrespective of residence, has been insured. From 2003 to 2014, the median person follow-up time was 10.03 years, IQR 6.18 years.

The database was maintained by the Social Insurance Administration (*Tryggingastofnun rikisins*) until 2014, since then it has been maintained by the Directorate of Health. In 2015, the IMR became a real-time database. The national prescription databases in Denmark, Finland, Iceland (IMR), Norway, and Sweden have been compared and are considered similar in their data structure and population coverage (Furu et al. 2010). In 2014, the number of people with one or more medication dispensed in a pharmacy in Iceland was 247,670 representing 76.0% of the total population (326,000) and in 2019, this number was 264,125 or 75.2% of the population (356,991).

1.3 Data Description

The IMR has information on sex, birth year, age, and residence of each individual. The information on each prescription in the database includes the de-identified social security ID (*kennitala*) of the patient, the name of the prescriber, the date of issue, the date when the drug was dispensed, the Nordic Article number, the ATC code of the drug, the total amount dispensed in Defined Daily Doses (DDDs) and the prescribed dose, form, package, and number of units. Since 2015, also a text providing information on the dosing of the medication is included in the database. The IMR does not include data on diagnoses, operations, hospitalizations, lifestyle information or socioeconomic status. Results of laboratory tests and physical examinations are not included. De-identified social security ID allows for linkage to other databases for research purposes, applications for such linkage must be approved by the National Bioethics Committee and by the Data Protection Authorities. Examples of such

Table 1 National registers that can be linked to the IMR using personal ID

Registry	Responsibility	Data processing	From year	Items registered including
Icelandic Cancer Registry	DH[a]	ICS[a]	1955	Cancer diagnosis
Icelandic Infectious Disease Registry	HSCDC[a]	HSCDC	1997	Infectious diseases
Icelandic Vaccination Registry	HSCDC	HSCDC	2002	Vaccinations
Icelandic Accident Registry	DH	DH	2002	Accidents
Icelandic Hospital Discharge Registry	DH	DH	1999	In hospital diagnoses
Causes of Death Registry	DH	DH	1996	ICD coded cause of death
Icelandic Birth Registry	DH	NUHI	1982	Pregnancy, delivery, birth defects
Icelandic Registry of Contact with Primary Health Care	DH	DH	2004	Diagnosis in primary health care

[a]DH—The Directorate of Health; ICS—Icelandic Cancer Society; HSCDC—Health Security and Communicable Disease Control; NUHI—National University Hospital of Iceland (*Landspitali Haskolasjukrahus*)
Table modified with permission (Johannsson and Haraldsdottir 2012)

linkage are date of death, link to family members, history of accidents, and history of pregnancy for women. Other databases that can be linked to the IMR can be seen in Table 1. It is not possible to re-contact patients in order to gather additional information.

1.4 Strengths and Limitations

A major strength of the IMR database is its coverage of over 90% of all prescriptions and representativeness. In 2014, the total number of dispenses in the database were over 3.5 million and in 2019, the number was over 4.4 million. Non-response is not an issue due to the administrative nature of the data. Except for hospital inpatient and over-the-counter (OTC) therapy, which are not included in IMR, ascertainment of drug exposure is assumed to be quite complete. Due to the nature of administrative claims data, not all variables of interest can be assessed in the desired detail. This applies, for example, to diagnosis, indication for medication administered, and comorbid conditions. Additionally, an incomplete assessment must be assumed for OTC medication. Data on drugs administered during hospitalization are not available.

It is recorded if a prescription was actually picked-up from the pharmacy. Information on adherence, that is, how much of the dispensed medication is actually used by the patients is not available.

1.5 Validation

For validation purposes, the prescriptions dispensed in Iceland that have been documented in the IMR were compared to information from the Icelandic Medicines Agency on all medications imported and domestically produced that were sold to pharmacies in Iceland. Around 1500 drug items (using Nordic Article Numbers) were compared for the years 2007, 2008, 2012, and 2013 (Table 2). Dispensed medication in pharmacies in DDDs was compared with medication sold to pharmacies in DDDs as a ratio where 100% is considered full concordance. The concordance for the 25th and the 75th percentiles of the ratios was between 91 and 97% and the concordance between the medians was between 77 and 101%. The concordance was better for the years 2012–2013 compared to 2007–2008 since the medians ranged from 91 to 97% for the years 2007–2008 but 97–98% for the years 2012–2013 (Table 2).

For a more detailed comparison, three groups of drugs were selected that are primarily dispensed in general pharmacies (less in hospitals) and that tend to be used regularly by patients. The medians for the ratios between the amount of drugs in DDDs dispensed in pharmacies and the amount of drugs in DDDs sold to pharmacies ranged from 91 to 102%. More detailed information about this study, such as the included ATC groups, can be retrieved from the study report (Aradottir et al. 2015).

Table 2 Dispensed drugs (in DDDs) according to the IMR as a ratio of sales (in DDDs) according to Icelandic Medicines Agency, all drugs that were sold in magnitude greater than 200 DDDs/year in 2007–2008 and 2012–2013

Year	2007	2008	2012	2013
Prev. of Nordic Article N.[a]	*1563*	*1660*	*1615*	*1676*
Percentile				
10th (%)	54	57	69	64
25th (%)	77	82[b]	88	86
Median, 50th (%)	91	96	97	97
75th (%)	98	102[b]	102	101
90th (%)	109	136	120	115

[a]Prevalence of Nordic Article Numbers of drug in table for each year
[b]Interpretation of table. If we look at the year 2012 there were 1615 Nordic Article Numbers for drugs sold in amount greater than 200 DDDs/year. We take the ratio for each of these Nordic Article Numbers, of drugs dispensed in pharmacies in DDDs, according to the Icelandic Medicines Registry database (IMR) divided by drugs sold to pharmacies according to the Icelandic Medicines Agency, and we sort the ratios according to magnitude. Then we can see that the 25th percentile for the ratios is 88% and the 75th percentile is 102%

1.6 Governance

IMR is financed by the government and coordinated by The Directorate of Health. The IMR research database is accessible to perform pharmacoepidemiological studies by independent researchers. Independent researchers must submit a study protocol which needs to be evaluated and approved by the National Bioethics Committee and The Data Protection Authority. An anonymized dataset is provided to the researchers to perform the study.

1.7 Related Publications

To date, a number of articles have been published in peer-reviewed journals reflecting IMR's contribution to drug utilization studies and to pharmacoepidemiological studies, that is, knowledge of the potential risks and/or benefits associated with drug use. There are a couple of reviews available, one covering pharmacoepidemiological research in Iceland, the IMR, and other databases available for pharmacoepidemiological and clinical epidemiological research (Johannsson and Haraldsdottir 2012). There are also reviews on pharmacoepidemiological research in the Nordic countries (Wettermark et al. 2013; Furu et al. 2010).

There are examples of drug utilization studies covering Iceland using the IMR, for example, on psychotropic drug use in children (Zoega et al. 2009), ADHD drugs in adults (Geirs et al. 2014), and use of proton-pump inhibitors among adults (Halfdanarson et al. 2018).

There are studies covering the Nordic countries, using the IMR and corresponding databases in the other Nordic countries, for example, on use of Attention-Deficit/Hyperactivity Disorder (ADHD) drugs (Furu et al. 2017; Karlstad et al. 2016; Zoega et al. 2011). There is also an example of an international study covering use of antipsychotic drugs in 16 countries (Halfdanarson et al. 2017).

There are also pharmacoepidemiological studies, for example, on drug use, pregnancy and birth-related outcomes, use of selective serotonin reuptake inhibitors (SSRI) and serotonin and nor-adrenaline reuptake inhibitors (SNRI), and antidepressants during pregnancy (Zoega et al. 2015). SSRI use and risk of pulmonary hypertension in newborns (Kieler et al. 2012), use of (SSRIs), venlafaxine and birth defects (Furu et al. 2015), SSRI use during pregnancy and risk of stillbirth and infant mortality (Stephansson et al. 2013), use of antidepressants and association with elective termination of pregnancy, and methylphenidate and amphetamine use in pregnancy (Kieler et al. 2015) and risk of congenital malformations (Huybrechts et al. 2018).

Other examples include use of opioids, sedatives, and proton-pump inhibitors (PPIs) and risk of fractures (Thorsdottir et al. 2017), PPI use and risk of cancer (Halfdanarson et al. 2019a), use of PPIs and mortality among patients with prostate cancer (Halfdanarson et al. 2019b), and association between prescription of hypnotics/anxiolytics and mortality in multimorbid and non-multimorbid patients in primary care (Linnet et al. 2019). One of the first studies published based on data from the IMR showed an increased risk of cardiovascular events following the use of Rofecoxib, mainly among young adults (Gudbjornsson et al. 2010). This study led to safer treatment for patients suffering from arthritis.

1.8 Administrative Information

The government funds the IMR and the Directorate of Health is responsible for maintaining the database. Contact details are the following:

- Organization/Affiliation:

  The Directorate of Health in Iceland
  Email: landlaeknir@landlaeknir.is
  Website: landlaeknir.is

References

Aradottir AB, Gudmundsson LS, Jonsdottir LS et al (2015) Icelandic Medicines Registry—role and operation 2005–2014. Directorate of Health, Reykjavik, Iceland

Furu K, Karlstad O, Zoega H et al (2017) Utilization of stimulants and atomoxetine for attention-deficit/hyperactivity disorder among 5.4 million children using population-based longitudinal data. Basic Clin Pharmacol Toxicol 120(4):373–379. https://doi.org/10.1111/bcpt.12724

Furu K, Kieler H, Haglund B et al (2015) Selective serotonin reuptake inhibitors and venlafaxine in early pregnancy and risk of birth defects: population based cohort study and sibling design. BMJ 350:h1798. https://doi.org/10.1136/bmj.h1798

Furu K, Wettermark B, Andersen M et al (2010) The Nordic countries as a cohort for pharmacoepi-demiological research. Basic Clin Pharmacol Toxicol 106(2):86–94. https://doi.org/10.1111/j.1742-7843.2009.00494.x

Geirs DP, Pottegard A, Halldorsson M et al (2014) A nationwide study of attention-deficit/hyperactivity disorder drug use among adults in Iceland 2003–2012. Basic Clin Pharmacol Toxicol 115(5):417–422. https://doi.org/10.1111/bcpt.12243

Gudbjornsson B, Thorsteinsson SB, Sigvaldason H et al (2010) Rofecoxib, but not celecoxib, increases the risk of thromboembolic cardiovascular events in young adults-a nationwide registry-based study. Eur J Clin Pharmacol 66(6):619–625. https://doi.org/10.1007/s00228-010-0789-2

Halfdanarson O, Zoega H, Aagaard L et al (2017) International trends in antipsychotic use: a study in 16 countries, 2005–2014. Eur Neuropsychopharmacol 27(10):1064–1076. https://doi.org/10.1016/j.euroneuro.2017.07.001

Halfdanarson OO, Fall K, Ogmundsdottir MH et al (2019a) Proton pump inhibitor use and risk of breast cancer, prostate cancer, and malignant melanoma: an Icelandic population-based case-control study. Pharmacoepidemiol Drug Saf 28(4):471–478. https://doi.org/10.1002/pds.4702

Halfdanarson OO, Pottegard A, Bjornsson ES et al (2018) Proton-pump inhibitors among adults: a nationwide drug-utilization study. Therap Adv Gastroenterol 11:1756284818777943. https://doi.org/10.1177/1756284818777943

Halfdanarson OO, Pottegard A, Lund SH et al (2019b) Use of proton pump inhibitors and mortality among Icelandic patients with prostate cancer. Basic Clin Pharmacol Toxicol. https://doi.org/10.1111/bcpt.13379

Huybrechts KF, Broms G, Christensen LB et al (2018) Association between methylphenidate and amphetamine use in pregnancy and risk of congenital malformations: a cohort study from the international pregnancy safety study consortium. JAMA Psychiatry 75(2):167–175. https://doi.org/10.1001/jamapsychiatry.2017.3644

Johannsson M, Haraldsdottir S (2012) Research in pharmacoepidemiology in Iceland. Laeknabladid 98(4):217–222

Karlstad O, Zoega H, Furu K et al (2016) Use of drugs for ADHD among adults-a multinational study among 15.8 million adults in the Nordic countries. Eur J Clin Pharmacol 72(12):1507–1514. https://doi.org/10.1007/s00228-016-2125-y

Kieler H, Artama M, Engeland A et al (2012) Selective serotonin reuptake inhibitors during pregnancy and risk of persistent pulmonary hypertension in the newborn: population based cohort study from the five Nordic countries. BMJ 344:d8012. https://doi.org/10.1136/bmj.d8012

Kieler H, Malm H, Artama M et al (2015) Use of antidepressants and association with elective termination of pregnancy: population based case-control study. BJOG 122(12):1618–1624. https://doi.org/10.1111/1471-0528.13164

Linnet K, Sigurdsson JA, Tomasdottir MO et al (2019) Association between prescription of hypnotics/anxiolytics and mortality in multimorbid and non-multimorbid patients: a longitudinal cohort study in primary care. BMJ Open 9(12):e033545. https://doi.org/10.1136/bmjopen-2019-033545

Stephansson O, Kieler H, Haglund B et al (2013) Selective serotonin reuptake inhibitors during pregnancy and risk of stillbirth and infant mortality. JAMA 309(1):48–54. https://doi.org/10.1001/jama.2012.153812

Thorsdottir G, Benedikz E, Thorgeirsdottir SA et al (2017) Do opioids, sedatives and proton-pump inhibitors increase the risk of fractures? Laeknabladid 103(5):231–235. https://doi.org/10.17992/lbl.2017.05.136

Wettermark B, Zoega H, Furu K et al (2013) The Nordic prescription databases as a resource for pharmacoepidemiological research–a literature review. Pharmacoepidemiol Drug Saf 22(7):691–699. https://doi.org/10.1002/pds.3457

Zoega H, Baldursson G, Hrafnkelsson B et al (2009) Psychotropic drug use among Icelandic children: a nationwide population-based study. J Child Adolesc Psychopharmacol 19(6):757–764. https://doi.org/10.1089/cap.2009.0003

Zoega H, Furu K, Halldorsson M et al (2011) Use of ADHD drugs in the Nordic countries: a population-based comparison study. Acta Psychiatr Scand 123(5):360–367. https://doi.org/10.1111/j.1600-0447.2010.01607.x

Zoega H, Kieler H, Norgaard M et al (2015) Use of SSRI and SNRI antidepressants during pregnancy: a population-based study from Denmark, Iceland, Norway and Sweden. PLoS One 10(12):e0144474. https://doi.org/10.1371/journal.pone.0144474

Databases in North America

The Régie de l'assurance maladie du Québec (RAMQ) Databases

Machelle Wilchesky and Samy Suissa

1 Database Description

1.1 Introduction

In Quebec, administrative data are collected for the purposes of health system management and provider payment. Individuals are eligible for health care coverage once they have established residence and have registered with the *Régie de l'assurance maladie du Québec* (RAMQ) for a health card. Persons residing outside of Québec for more than 183 days,[1] and non Canadian students with the exception of those covered under a social security agreement.[2] In 2018–2019, a total of 8 million persons residing in all regions of the province (95% of the population) were covered

M. Wilchesky (✉)
Department of Family Medicine and Division of Geriatric Medicine, McGill University, Montreal, Canada
e-mail: machelle.wilchesky@mcgill.ca

M. Wilchesky · S. Suissa
Centre for Clinical Epidemiology, Lady Davis Institute–Jewish General Hospital, Montreal, Canada

M. Wilchesky
Donald Berman Maimonides Centre for Research in Aging, 5795 Avenue Caldwell, H4W 1W3 Montreal, Canada

S. Suissa
McGill University, Montreal, Canada

[1] https://www.ramq.gouv.qc.ca/en/citizens/absence-quebec
[2] https://www.ramq.gouv.qc.ca/en/news/2020-08-12/registration-quebec-health-insurance-plan-students-covered-under-a-social-security

© Springer Nature Switzerland AG 2021
M. Sturkenboom and T. Schink (eds.), *Databases for Pharmacoepidemiological Research*, Springer Series on Epidemiology and Public Health,
https://doi.org/10.1007/978-3-030-51455-6_18

by the RAMQ health plan, of which 3.7 million (44%) were covered by the public RAMQ drug plan.[3]

1.2 A Brief History of Health and Medication Insurance in Quebec

Canada's national health insurance program has been designed to ensure that all Canadian residents have reasonable access to medically necessary hospital and physician services on a prepaid basis (Health Canada 2016). Canadian federal and provincial governments have different responsibilities in the delivery of the program, which is composed of 13 interlocking provincial and territorial health insurance plans that share certain common features and basic standards of coverage (Health Canada 2016; Madore 2005). As such, each province administers its own public health care insurance plan and is responsible for health care delivery to constituents within that province (Madore 2005). Most Canadians have access to insurance coverage for prescription medicines through public and/or private insurance plans, with federal, provincial, and territorial governments offering varying levels of coverage (Health Canada 2018). Established in 1969, the RAMQ is the government agency which administers the public health and public prescription drug insurance plans in the Province of Quebec.

Prior to 1996, the RAMQ plan provided medication coverage insurance to both the elderly (age 65 and older) and to social assistance (welfare) recipients. New legislation was then enacted to enhance the equity of access to prescription drugs by providing drug insurance for all Quebecers, including approximately 1.2 million who were previously uninsured (Martin 1996). The compulsory insurance plan (not a public drug benefit program) was implemented in two stages (Morgan 1998). In August 1996, a deductible and a 25% co-insurance charge on medication were instituted for the elderly and those on social assistance who had previously received free medications.

As of January 1, 1997, the RAMQ plan has provided medication insurance coverage for persons who were not eligible for basic coverage for prescription drugs through either group insurance or employee benefit plans ('private plans'). At this time, individuals eligible for a private plan were also mandated to join that plan and to provide coverage for their spouses and children (Régie de l'assurance maladie du Québec 2020a; Morgan et al. 2017).

---

[3]https://www.ramq.gouv.qc.ca/sites/default/files/documents/rappann1819.pdf, Accessed on November 20, 2020

1.3 Database Characteristics

Computerised administrative health databases capture health care information pertaining to fee-for-service medical claims, hospital and pharmacy records in Quebec. The two governing bodies charged with managing these data are the RAMQ and the Ministry of Health and Social Services (*Ministère de la Santé et des services sociaux*, MSSS). RAMQ manages four databases that include (1) files on demographic data, (2) drug insurance information, (3) pharmaceutical service data, and (4) fee-for-service physician billing information.[4] The MSSS manages six databases: (1) the *Maintenance et exploitation des données pour l'étude de la clientèle hospitalière* (MED-ÉCHO), which maintains files on hospital stay information; (2) the *Système d'information du Registre des traumatismes du Québec* (SIRTQ), which maintains files on trauma care; (3) the *Banque de données communes des urgences* (BDCU), which includes information on services use pertaining to episodes of care provided in emergency departments; (4) the *Système d'information sur la clientèle et les services des CLSC* (I-CLSC), (5) *Performance hospitalière (APR-DRG)* where APR-DRG groupings, resource intensity weights and other management indicators are available for in-patient and day surgeries in the acute care setting; and (6) *Registre des événements démographiques* which provides demographic event information including births, stillbirths, and deaths (See Footnote 4).

Although data are recorded in multiple files covering different domains of health care, each of these files contains a unique patient identifier that permits the linkage of these data files.

Participants of the medication insurance program are defined as individuals registered for the RAMQ plan who have filled a prescribed medication at least once during the financial period in question.[5] During the 2018–2019 fiscal year, for instance, participants of the medication insurance program included 310,758 individuals receiving social assistance, 1,361,840 individuals 65 years and older, and 1,193,561 adherents [other persons not eligible for either employee benefit plans or group insurance (private plans)].[6] Considering the age of theses participants, 235,382 were children aged 18 or younger, 1,268,937 were adults aged 18–64, and 1,361,840 were adults aged 65 and older, corresponding to medication insurance plan coverage of 15%, 24%, and 86% of the overall Quebec population within these age groups, respectively (Statistics Canada and l'Institut de la statistique du Québec 2019).

---

[4]https://www.stat.gouv.qc.ca/recherche/#/donnees/administratives/sante

[5]https://www.ramq.gouv.qc.ca/sites/default/files/documents/rappann1819.pdf, page 51, footnote 42

[6]https://www.ramq.gouv.qc.ca/sites/default/files/documents/rappann1819.pdf, page 52

1.4   Available Data

1.4.1   Available Data in the RAMQ Databases

Demographic data: The Medicare beneficiary file (*Fichier des bénéficiaires*) contains demographic information pertaining to approximately 95% of Quebec residents covered by the RAMQ plan in 2018–2019. Demographic variables include age, sex, health region and local community service center (CLSC) territory of the insured, three-digit postal code, and date and cause of death where applicable.

Drug insurance plan eligibility data: This file contains information identifying the sub-program under which the person had received coverage (adherent, social assistance, or aged 65 and over) and the start and end dates of eligibility.[7]

Prescription drug data: The RAMQ medication insurance plan covers over 7,000 medications listed on the province's formulary (*liste de medicaments)* (Régie de l'assurance maladie du Québec 2020b) which is published periodically by RAMQ. It is the most generous of the Canadian drug plans, listing a total of 33.4% of all medicines approved by Health Canada between 2008 and 2017 as compared with an average 25.6% in the drug plans in other provinces (Labrie 2019). In certain circumstances, medications not formally listed on the formulary are covered under the plan. These "exceptional medications", which are published in a separate section of the formulary, require a physician to send RAMQ a payment authorisation request and, once authorised, to include a designated code on the prescription in order for these drugs to be automatically insured.

The RAMQ drug files contain data pertaining to all filled outpatient prescriptions prescribed by a Quebec-licensed health professional to RAMQ plan participants filled at community pharmacies. Information available for each dispensed prescription includes: The dispensing date, the drug identification number (DIN), the American Hospital Formulary Service (AHFS) drug class and drug generic name/common denomination (denocom) codes, the dosage form (e.g., tablet, capsule, topical cream or inhaler), the strength, quantity and units of the drug dispensed, and the duration of treatment.[8] In addition, the database includes codes that indicate whether the prescription is new or a renewal, whether the pharmacist dispensed the exact drug as written or an equivalent medication, the drug cost and deductible contribution of the insured, the specialty of the prescribing health professional, and whether or not the prescribing health professional is registered with RAMQ and practising in Quebec (Gouvernement du Québec 2019b). The data contained within the prescription claims database has been shown to be both valid and comprehensive (Tamblyn et al. 1995).

Physician claims data: The physician claims database contains data pertaining to all physician claims for outpatient medical services remunerated on a fee-for-service basis. Fee-for-service billing represented 82% of the costs of medical services

---

[7]https://www.stat.gouv.qc.ca/recherche/#/donnees/administratives/sante/banque/1/1

[8]https://www.stat.gouv.qc.ca/recherche/#/donnees/administratives/sante/banque/1/2

rendered in the province in 2018.[9] Data elements available include the date of service, a diagnosis coded in the International Classification of Diseases (ICD) 9th Revision format, a RAMQ fee-for-service code, the location of service delivery (e.g., inpatient, emergency, clinic), and both an anonymous identifier and the medical specialty of the treating and referring physician, if applicable (See Footnote 9). Only one diagnosis code is registered by the billing physician on his request for payment, and this diagnosis is neither mandatory in order to justify the billed services nor is it validated. Validation of the RAMQ medical services claims data, however, has found diagnosis codes to be highly specific but variable in terms of their sensitivity for many conditions (Wilchesky et al. 2004).

1.4.2 Available Data in the MSSS Databases

Hospital inpatient data: The MED-ÉCHO database contains data pertaining to all discharges from Quebec hospitals providing general and specialised care. These data, compiled by hospitals and available since April 1, 1987, include acute care (physical and mental) and day surgery and contain information pertaining to hospital stays, diagnoses, procedures, services, tumors, and intensive care (Gouvernement du Québec 1987). In addition, the database also records the gestational age for planned abortions, miscarriages, and deliveries (Santos et al. 2011).

Available variables include dates of admission, discharge and length of stay, discharge type, type of admission (day surgery vs. inpatient stay), type of establishment and a de-identified establishment code, destination establishment type for patients who are transferred to another institution, and type of death (pre- or postoperative, maternal, neonatal, other). One primary and up to an additional 15 diagnoses are reported (in either ICD-9 or ICD-10-CA format for discharges taking place after April 1, 2006) as well as a diagnostic characteristic code (i.e., indicating whether a diagnosis was a complication or infection) and up to 15 procedure codes with corresponding procedure dates (Gouvernement du Québec 1987).[10] Data pertaining to the hospital department, specialty code of the associated service provider, intensive care unit code, number of days and number of episodes of admission to an ICU, and number of days a patient was admitted to a given non-ICU service is also available. Recorded hospital discharge information has been shown to be both comprehensive and valid (Levy et al. 1995; Lambert et al. 2012; Mayo et al. 1993).

The BDM-SIRTQ database contains information pertaining to admissions to the 61 designated trauma centers in Quebec. Data recorded include the date and time of the event, cause of trauma (e.g., motor vehicle accident, fall, stabbing), the location where the trauma took place (e.g., home, school, industrial area, farm) as well as the means of transport to access the trauma centre (Gouvernement du Québec 2019c; Direction générale des affaires universitaires 2009). Inclusion criteria into the registry

---

[9]https://www.stat.gouv.qc.ca/recherche/#/donnees/administratives/sante/banque/5

[10]https://www.stat.gouv.qc.ca/recherche/#/donnees/administratives/sante/banque/3

before April 1, 2010 required one or more of the following: Death as a result of injury, admission with a hospital stay of three days or more, direct admission to an intensive care unit, or inter-hospital transfer. For traumatic events after March 31, 2010, all admitted or enrolled deaths and all admitted cases were included. Trauma registry data are available from April 1998 until the last complete fiscal year (Gouvernement du Québec 2019c).

The BDCU database includes information on services use pertaining to episodes of care provided in emergency departments from April 1, 2014. It includes variables such as the date, hour, minute, and second of the start (i.e., time of registration in the emergency department at reception or by triage), and end of a treatment episode, triage code, autonomy level of the patient after triage, reason for the ER visit, primary diagnosis made by the ER physician, major diagnosis category, whether the patient was admitted to either an intensive care ward or an isolation room as well as information about transfers, death/autopsy, whether or not the patient is followed by a primary care physician. This database is also used to draw a portrait of the emergency clientele and to monitor the use of stretchers within the emergency. As such, variables pertaining to the duration of several key transitional care benchmarks such as the wait time (in minutes) before the admission request, the request for admission to the hospital center, the first triage, and the time before the patient occupied a stretcher are available for study (Gouvernement du Québec 2019a).

The I-CLSC database captures health services use within Quebec's local community service centres or *centres local de services communautaires*. This information is available from April 1, 2000, but only data from April 1, 2012 may be linked with the other databases. Variables include the date of the episode, the type of service rendered (e.g., medical, psychosocial, home care, nutrition, occupational therapy, vaccination, perinatal), reasons for any interventions rendered, and information pertaining to both the users and the providers of these services (Gouvernement du Québec 2019d).

Demographic events: In addition to the administrative health data described above, the *Fichier des évènements démographiques du Québec* contains the vital statistics data pertaining to births and deaths, including perinatal death. Information pertaining to date of death, a medical code corresponding to the underlying cause of death as well as the location (e.g., home or institution code) where the death took place is available. The *numéro d'assurance maladie* (NAM) is obtained from death certificates and is available for individuals who have died. As of the year 2000, both the initial cause of death and secondary causes of death are available (in ICD-10 format). The file also provides demographic variables on the mother, father, and baby as well as birth weight and gestational age for live births and stillbirths (Bérard et al. 2007b).[11]

---

[11] https://www.stat.gouv.qc.ca/recherche/#/donnees/administratives/sante/banque/7

1.4.3 Possibilities of Data Linkage

The RAMQ, MED-ÉCHO, and ISQ computerised databases can be linked via the health insurance number, or NAM, which is a unique identifier assigned to all legal residents of Quebec. For the purposes of research, the NAM variable is de-identified (anonymised) for each study before dissemination. Although the ISQ data does not include the NAM for individuals who are alive, mother-child linkage has been achieved using the name, surname, and date of birth of both the mother and the child (Bérard et al. 2007a). In addition, linkage to other databases such as the *Société de l'assurance automobile du Québec* (SAAQ) database has been possible, which has provided the opportunity to assess the association between exposure to various medications and the risk of motor vehicle crashes (Hemmelgarn et al. 1997; Delaney et al. 2006b; Orriols et al. 2013; Fournier et al. 2015).

1.4.4 Timeliness of Data Access

Drug data becomes available for dissemination approximately one year after they are sent to RAMQ (for example, researchers requesting data in 2009 were only able to obtain drug data for 2008 and earlier) (Rawson 2009). Physician service and hospitalisation data, however, tend to become available approximately two years after they are received by RAMQ (Rawson 2009). Delays have been an issue for researchers when acquiring Quebec data. In 2014, RAMQ indicated that one should expect a turn-around of between six to nine months following submission of a request excluding the government's *Commission d'accès à l'information* (CAI) approval process (Rawson 2009), which is required when requesting RAMQ or other health care linkable data. However, anecdotal evidence from local users suggested that linking databases historically led to delays of up to 12 months or longer although this has improved in recent years.

In 2019, the Quebec government mandated the ISQ to implement a simplified process for accessing research data in order to reduce data processing times. Since spring 2019, all requests for RAMQ and MSSS data must be made online via the "ISQ Research Data Access Point".[12] Using this new system, only one access request is necessary, regardless of the department or body holding this data, and application for authorisation from the CAI is included in the process (See Sect. 1.7).

1.4.5 Socioeconomic Status

While no specific variable for socioeconomic status or education level exists in these data per se, researchers have been successful in applying algorithms matching the three-digit postal code variable available in the RAMQ database with census data on relevant indicators (e.g., education, employment, average income, marital status) to

---

[12]https://www.stat.gouv.qc.ca/recherche/#/a-propos/guichet-acces-donnees

produce validated ecologic measures of material and social deprivation (Pampalon and Raymond 2000).

1.4.6 Variables Not Available

Information pertaining to use of over-the-counter medications, results from laboratory, imaging, or other tests, information obtained via physical examination, family medical history, and lifestyle variables such as exercise, diet, and alcohol and tobacco use are unavailable for study.

1.5 Strengths and Limitations

With 3.5 million people—representing 43% of all Quebec citizens—covered by the medication insurance program, a major strength of the RAMQ databases is the size and comprehensiveness, which results in the ability to capture important health information and events. Each database file includes a unique patient identifier that can be used to link database files and create longitudinal histories of health care and medication use. The availability of diagnostic information within all hospital and most medical visits to Quebec physicians represents an important opportunity to capture clinical outcomes for health-related research, to assemble cohorts for epidemiological study, and to engage in population-based surveillance.

One limitation of the data is the fact that the prescriptions database captures data pertaining only to outpatient prescriptions, such that longitudinal histories of medication use will have missing data during periods of hospitalisation (or other institutionalisation). When a period of time during follow-up (for a cohort study) or prior to the index date (for a case-control study) exists during which a subject cannot be recognised as being exposed, that period of time is called "immeasurable" which gives rise to the possibility of "immeasurable time bias" (Suissa 2008). When using these data to define exposure history, it is therefore necessary for researchers to employ methods and procedures to carefully account for periods where medication use is unknown (Wilchesky et al. 2012). An additional limitation of the data stems from the nature of the insurance plan in that the Quebec medications database has been found to over-represent individuals of lower socioeconomic status (Bérard and Lacasse 2009).

Other limitations of the data are inherent to the use of administrative databases in general. They do not, for example, capture over-the-counter medications or samples obtained from physicians, and, given that prescription claims data only record drugs which have been dispensed (and not taken), drug exposure can be misclassified. Studies estimating medication adherence using prescription refill data, however, have found prescription claims data to be relatively valid (Grymonpre et al. 1998; Lau et al. 1997). As is the case with other administrative data, the RAMQ databases also lack information on many potentially important confounding factors, including lifestyle information (smoking, exercise, diet), alcohol and/or illicit drug use, environmental exposures, information pertaining to work occupation, and family history of various medical conditions.

A limitation of the outpatient diagnosis data lies in the fact that only one diagnosis code is requested from physicians by RAMQ for billing, and therefore only one diagnosis is available per visit recorded in the fee-for-service physician claims database. In 2005, the prevalence of multi-morbidity among Quebec adults seen by family physicians was found to be high, with nearly 50% of patients presenting with five or more chronic conditions (Fortin et al. 2005). In 2011, the Canadian Institute for Health Information reported that seniors with three or more reported chronic conditions accounted for 40% of health care use and used an average of six prescription medications regularly (twice as many medications as seniors with only one chronic condition) (Canadian Institute for Health Information 2011). In Quebec, the diagnosis recorded on a fee-for-service physician claim is not linked to remuneration. Given both the high prevalence of multi-morbidity and the fact that acute or episodic conditions are often the underlying reason for a given patient visit, the diagnoses recorded in these administrative data represent a choice of one among possibly several diagnoses which has been made by that billing physician. It is, therefore, not all that surprising that studies which have validated RAMQ diagnoses have found them to be highly specific but much lower in sensitivity.

1.6 Validation

1.6.1 Internal Validation

A number of measures of control and verification, including inspection visits and pharmacy prescription requests made by letter to pharmacists, have been implemented by RAMQ to ensure that services have been rendered and invoiced appropriately (Régie de l'assurance maladie du Québec 2019).

1.6.2 External Validation

The RAMQ databases have been used extensively for research purposes, and information pertaining to the validity of the data contained therein has been published in a number of studies. In a 1995 study by Tamblyn et al., in which data from a regionally stratified random sample of 65,349 Quebec elderly in 1990 were used, the prescriptions claims database was found to be both comprehensive and accurate (Tamblyn et al. 1995). Data pertaining to essential variables such as drug, quantity, date dispensed, duration, and patient identifier were found to be complete with less than 0.5% missing or out of range (Tamblyn et al. 1995). Furthermore, when database information was compared with information abstracted from the clinical files of a subsample of 306 elderly patients who had attended an internal medicine clinic, 89%

had perfect matches for medication and prescribing physician, and 69.1% and 72.1% had perfect matches for quantity prescribed and prescription duration, respectively (Tamblyn et al. 1995).

The validity of diagnoses recorded within the RAMQ physician claims data has been assessed in a number of studies that have also used clinical chart information as a gold standard for comparison. In a 2001 study by Wilchesky et al., the diagnostic information abstracted from the medical charts of 14,980 patients for 14 conditions associated with drug disease contraindication were found to be highly specific but varied substantially with respect to sensitivity (Wilchesky et al. 2004). When medical claims information from both primary care and specialist physicians were combined, most diagnoses had a specificity of 95% or higher, with specificity for hypertension, Chronic Obstructive Pulmonary Disease (COPD), and glaucoma being lower at 82%, 88%, and 94%, respectively. The sensitivity of the diagnoses, however, ranged from 76% for glaucoma to 1% for postural hypotension. The same study also assessed validity of the set of diagnoses associated with the 17 conditions used to calculate the Charlson Comorbidity Index (Charlson et al. 1987; Romano et al. 1993; Deyo et al. 1992) and again found the data to be highly specific but variable in terms of sensitivity (Wilchesky et al. 2004). Similarly, Cadieux et al. assessed the accuracy of RAMQ physician billing claims for identifying episodes of acute respiratory infection in primary care and found the data to have high specificity and high positive and negative predictive value (PPV and NPV). However, sensitivity for diagnoses was below 50% (Cadieux and Tamblyn 2008). Tamblyn et al. found that using both diagnostic and procedure codes in combination provided a sensitive measure of injury occurrence in the elderly (in particular when a time window of −3 to +14 days of the recorded injury date was used), but sensitivity varied by the type of injury and by the presence of injury-specific billable procedures (Tamblyn et al. 2000). A 2017 study by Oskoui et al. reported the sensitivity and specificity of RAMQ data for cerebral palsy were 65.5% and 99.9%, respectively and that sensitivity was higher in children from rural regions, born preterm, with spastic quadriparesis, and with higher levels of motor impairment (Oskoui et al. 2017).

Finally, two recent studies have assessed the suitability of the RAMQ physician claims data for the purpose of syndromic surveillance. The first, by Chan et al., found that diagnoses in children for influenza-like illness provided an earlier signal of flu epidemic than records of visits to emergency departments (Chan et al. 2011). The second, by Cadieux et al., assessed the potential ability for these data to identify five specific syndromes (fever, gastrointestinal, neurological, rash, and respiratory, including influenza-like illness) in community health care settings and found that the diagnostic codes had low sensitivity, moderate to high PPV, and near-perfect specificity and NPV (Cadieux et al. 2011).

Assessments of validity pertaining to the other linkable databases are also available, and these studies have found the information contained within these databases to be accurate. A study by Lambert et al., conducted in a fairly large contemporary cohort of cardiac patients hospitalised in a representative sample of Quebec hospitals, found that discharge data were reliably coded and compared favourably with medical record review to predict mortality (Lambert et al. 2012). Conditions evaluated included those contained in the Charlson Comorbidity Index in addition to several other important predictors of mortality for either acute myocardial infarction (AMI), coronary angioplasty or coronary artery bypass graft. These were found to be highly specific, with high positive and negative predictive values and demonstrated sensitivities ranging from 55% for previous AMI to 94% for "diabetes without complications" (Lambert et al. 2012). In another study that assessed the accuracy of hospital discharge coding for stroke from five acute-care hospitals in Montreal where chart review was conducted by a neurologist, the primary discharge ICD-9 codes for "subarachnoid hemorrhage" and "intracerebral hemorrhage" were found to have a PPV of 100%, with overall PPV for the entire set of stroke diagnoses being between 74 and 80% (Mayo et al. 1993; Andrade et al. 2012). Finally, in a study that evaluated the validity of pregnancy-related variables recorded in Quebec administrative databases, a comparison between the ISQ demographics database file and medical charts for categorical maternal and infant characteristics found variables such as "previous pregnancy", "previous live birth(s)", and sex of the baby had near perfect sensitivity, specificity, and predictive values ranging from 92 to 99% (Vilain et al. 2008).

1.7 Governance and Ethical Issues

As mentioned in Sect. 1.4.5, researchers interested in accessing RAMQ data must now submit a request via the ISQ Research Data Access Point. Researchers outside Quebec must collaborate with a Quebec researcher who will assume responsibility for use and handling of the data. There are 12 steps in this new process (Institut de la statistique Québec 2019), the first being creating a user account followed by preparing and submitting the data request. In the second step, the ISQ assesses the completeness and feasibility of the request. If complete, the ISQ will then assess its capacity to select cohorts and link data from the various files and will verify the availability of all the variables requested for the selected research period. At this point, it is possible that the ISQ may initiate discussions with the researchers in order to clarify their needs. At the end of this step, a summary cost assessment is provided in order to confirm financial capacity to carry out the project.

The third step involves application to the *Commission d'accès à l'information* (CAI), if applicable. The ISQ will forward the final version of the data request from step two to the CAI along with all supporting documents, including the assessment report, and researchers are informed of the date these documents are sent. The CAI may request additional information from the researchers during this time. The CAI will then issue its decision and communicate it to all parties involved, namely the researcher, the data holders, and the ISQ. Upon receipt of a favourable decision by the CAI, step four involves the dissemination of the assessment report prepared by the ISQ and the documentation provided by the researcher to each data holder targeted by the access request to ask for their authorisation. Data holders (e.g., RAMQ, MSSS) must communicate their decision to the researchers within ten business days once they have received all the necessary information. Once all the necessary authorisations have been granted, step five involves a final review of the project to identify the work to be done and the preparation of contractual commitments and costs. If the researcher agrees to these terms, the commitments are signed, and the ISQ will begin working on the project.

The final steps involve preparation of and obtaining access to the research file, monitoring of the request and management of the research project until its completion, and eventual destruction of the data (Institut de la statistique Québec 2019).

1.8 Documents and Publications

The RAMQ databases have been extensively used in pharmacoepidemiological studies for a wide variety of conditions including (but not limited to): Pregnancy outcomes (Bérard et al. 2019), Alzheimer's disease (Billioti de Gage et al. 2014), cardiac arrhythmia (Essebag et al. 2003; Wilchesky et al. 2012), myocardial infarction (Bally et al. 2017, 2018), cataracts (Garbe et al. 1998), cerebrovascular disease (Perreault et al. 2009), chronic obstructive pulmonary disease (Ernst et al. 2007; Wilchesky et al. 2012), clostridium difficile (Dial et al. 2004), diabetes (Suissa et al. 2010), epilepsy (LeLorier et al. 2008), glaucoma (Garbe et al. 1997a, b), inflammatory bowel disease (Brassard et al. 2014), pneumonia (Filion et al. 2014), prostate disease (Delaney et al. 2006a), depression (Lunghi et al. 2017), and rheumatoid arthritis (Dixon et al. 2011; Bernatsky et al. 2008; Bernatsky and Ehrmann Feldman 2008).

1.9 Administrative Information

Régie de l'assurance maladie du Québec
Direction de l'analyse et de la gestion de l'information
Email: statistiques@ramq.gouv.qc.ca
http://www.ramq.gouv.qc.ca/fr/donnees-et-statistiques/donnees-sur-dem ande/chercheurs/Pages/chercheur-affilie-a-une-universite.aspx

References

Andrade SE, Harrold LR, Tjia J et al (2012) A systematic review of validated methods for identifying cerebrovascular accident or transient ischemic attack using administrative data. Pharmacoepidemiol Drug Saf 21(S1):100–128

Bally M, Dendukuri N, Rich B et al (2017) Risk of acute myocardial infarction with NSAIDs in real world use: bayesian meta-analysis of individual patient data. BMJ 357:j1909

Bally M, Beauchamp ME, Abrahamowicz M et al (2018) Risk of acute myocardial infarction with real-world NSAID s depends on dose and timing of exposure. Pharmacoepidemiol Drug Saf 27(1):69–77

Bérard A, Lacasse A (2009) Validity of perinatal pharmacoepidemiologic studies using data from the RAMQ administrative database. Can J Clin Pharmacol 16(2):e360–e369

Bérard A, Azoulay L, Koren G et al (2007a) Isotretinoin, pregnancies, abortions and birth defects: a population-based perspective. Br J Clin Pharmacol 63(2):196–205

Bérard A, Ramos E, Rey E et al (2007b) First trimester exposure to paroxetine and risk of cardiac malformations in infants: the importance of dosage. Birth Defects Res B Dev Reprod Toxicol 80(1):18–27. https://doi.org/10.1002/bdrb.20099

Bérard A, Sheehy O, Zhao J-P et al (2019) Associations between low-and high-dose oral fluconazole and pregnancy outcomes: 3 nested case-control studies. CMAJ 191(7):E179–E187

Bernatsky S, Ehrmann Feldman D (2008) Discontinuation of methotrexate therapy in older patients with newly diagnosed rheumatoid arthritis: analysis of administrative health databases in Québec, Canada. Drugs Aging 25(10):879–884

Bernatsky S, Clarke A, Suissa S (2008) Lung cancer after exposure to disease modifying antirheumatic drugs. Lung Cancer 59(2):266–269. https://doi.org/10.1016/j.lungcan.2007.06.013

Billioti de Gage S, Moride Y, Ducruet T et al (2014) Benzodiazepine use and risk of Alzheimer's disease: case-control study. BMJ 349:g5205

Brassard P, Bitton A, Suissa A et al (2014) Oral corticosteroids and the risk of serious infections in patients with elderly-onset inflammatory bowel diseases. Am J Gastroenterol 109 (11):1795–1802; quiz 1803. https://doi.org/10.1038/ajg.2014.313

Cadieux G, Tamblyn R (2008) Accuracy of physician billing claims for identifying acute respiratory infections in primary care. Health Serv Res 43(6):2223–2238. https://doi.org/10.1111/j.1475-6773.2008.00873.x

Cadieux G, Buckeridge DL, Jacques A et al (2011) Accuracy of syndrome definitions based on diagnoses in physician claims. BMC Public Health 11:17. https://doi.org/10.1186/1471-2458-11-17

Canadian Institute for Health Information (2011) Seniors and the health care system: what is the impact of multiple chronic conditions? https://secure.cihi.ca/free_products/air-chronic_disease_aib_en.pdf

Chan EH, Tamblyn R, Charland KM et al (2011) Outpatient physician billing data for age and setting specific syndromic surveillance of influenza-like illnesses. J Biomed Inform 44(2):221–228

Charlson ME, Pompei P, Ales KL et al (1987) A new method of classifying prognostic comorbidity in longitudinal studies: development and validation. J Chron Dis 40(5):373–383

Delaney JAC, Lévesque LE, Etminan M et al (2006a) Furosemide use and hospitalization for benign prostatic hyperplasia. Can J Clin Pharmacol 13(1):e75–e80

Delaney JAC, Opatrny L, Suissa S (2006b) Warfarin use and the risk of motor vehicle crash in older drivers. Br J Clin Pharmacol 61(2):229–232. https://doi.org/10.1111/j.1365-2125.2005.02548.x

Deyo RA, Cherkin DC, Ciol MA (1992) Adapting a clinical comorbidity index for use with ICD-9-CM administrative databases. J Clin Epidemiol 45(6):613–619

Dial S, Alrasadi K, Manoukian C et al (2004) Risk of Clostridium difficile diarrhea among hospital inpatients prescribed proton pump inhibitors: cohort and case-control studies. CMAJ 171(1):33–38

Direction générale des affaires universitaires, médicales, infirmières et pharmaceutiques (2009) Cadre Normatif Système D'information Du Registre Des Traumatismes Du Québec

(SIRTQ). Gouvernement du Québec. https://publications.msss.gouv.qc.ca/msss/fichiers/2019/ 19_CN-SIRTQ.pdf. Accessed 5 Feb 2020

Dixon WG, Kezouh A, Bernatsky S et al (2011) The influence of systemic glucocorticoid therapy upon the risk of non-serious infection in older patients with rheumatoid arthritis: a nested case–control study. Ann Rheum Dis 70(6):956–960. https://doi.org/10.1136/ard.2010.144741

Ernst P, Gonzalez AV, Brassard P et al (2007) Inhaled corticosteroid use in chronic obstructive pulmonary disease and the risk of hospitalization for Pneumonia. Am J Respir Crit Care Med 176(2):162–166. https://doi.org/10.1164/rccm.200611-1630OC

Essebag V, Hadjis T, Platt RW et al (2003) Amiodarone and the risk of bradyarrhythmia requiring permanent pacemaker in elderly patients with atrial fibrillation and prior myocardial infarction. J Am Coll Cardiol 41(2):249–254

Filion KB, Chateau D, Targownik LE et al (2014) Proton pump inhibitors and the risk of hospi-talisation for community-acquired pneumonia: replicated cohort studies with meta-analysis. Gut 63(4):552–558

Fortin M, Bravo G, Hudon C et al (2005) Prevalence of multimorbidity among adults seen in family practice. Ann Fam Med 3(3):223–228. https://doi.org/10.1370/afm.272

Fournier J-P, Wilchesky M, Patenaude V et al (2015) Concurrent use of benzodiazepines and antidepressants and the risk of motor vehicle accident in older drivers: a nested case-control study. Neurol Ther 4(1):39–51. https://doi.org/10.1007/s40120-015-0026-0

Garbe E, LeLorier J, Boivin JF et al (1997a) Inhaled and nasal glucocorticoids and the risks of ocular hypertension or open-angle glaucoma. JAMA 277(9):722–727

Garbe E, LeLorier J, Boivin JF et al (1997b) Risk of ocular hypertension or open-angle glaucoma in elderly patients on oral glucocorticoids. Lancet 350(9083):979–982. https://doi.org/10.1016/ s0140-6736(97)03392-8

Garbe E, Suissa S, LeLorier J (1998) Association of inhaled corticosteroid use with cataract extraction in elderly patients.[Erratum appears in JAMA 1998 Dec 2;280(21):1830]. JAMA 280 (6):539–543

Gouvernement du Québec (1987) Cadre Normatif du Système MED-ÉCHO (Maintenance et exploitation des données pour l'étude de la clientèle hospitalière). Révision: Avril 2019. https:// publications.msss.gouv.qc.ca/msss/fichiers/2000/00-601.pdf. Accessed 2 Feb 2020

Gouvernement du Québec (2019a) Banque de données communes des urgences (BDCU). https:// www.stat.gouv.qc.ca/recherche/#/donnees/administratives/sante/banque/6/34. Accessed 28 Jan 2020

Gouvernement du Québec (2019b) Fichier des services pharmaceutiques couverts par la RAMQ. https://www.stat.gouv.qc.ca/recherche/#/donnees/administratives/sante/banque/1/2. Accessed 6 Jan 2020

Gouvernement du Québec (2019c) Système d'information du registre des traumatismes du Québec (SIRTQ). https://www.stat.gouv.qc.ca/recherche/#/donnees/administratives/sante/ban que/5. Accessed 28 Jan 2020

Gouvernement du Québec (2019d) Système d'information sur la clientèle et les services des CSSS - mission CLSC (I-CLSC). https://www.stat.gouv.qc.ca/recherche/#/donnees/administrati ves/sante/banque/4/12. Accessed 28 Jan 2020

Grymonpre RE, Didur CD, Montgomery PR et al (1998) Pill count, self-report, and pharmacy claims data to measure medication adherence in the elderly. Ann Pharmacother 32(7–8):749–754

Health Canada (2016) Canada's health care system. http://www.hc-sc.gc.ca/hcs-sss/medi-assur/ index-eng.php. Accessed 25 Jan 2020

Health Canada (2018) Prescription drug insurance coverage. http://www.hc-sc.gc.ca/hcs-sss/pha rma/acces/index-eng.php. Accessed 25 Jan 2020

Hemmelgarn B, Suissa S, Huang A et al (1997) Benzodiazepine use and the risk of motor vehicle crash in the elderly. JAMA 278(1):27–31

Institut de la statistique Québec (2019) Research Data Access Point. https://www.stat.gouv.qc.ca/ recherche/documents/GuichetdAcces_Demarche_Web_an.pdf. Accessed 29 Jan 2020

Labrie Y (2019) Lessons from the Quebec Universal Prescription Drug Insurance Program. https://www.fraserinstitute.org/studies/lessons-from-the-quebec-universal-prescription-drug-ins urance-program. Accessed 12 Feb 2020

Lambert L, Blais C, Hamel D et al (2012) Evaluation of care and surveillance of cardiovascular disease: can we trust medico-administrative hospital data? Can J Cardiol 28(2):162–168

Lau HS, de Boer A, Beuning KS et al (1997) Validation of pharmacy records in drug exposure assessment. J Clin Epidemiol 50(5):619–625

LeLorier J, Duh MS, Paradis PE et al (2008) Clinical consequences of generic substitution of lamotrigine for patients with epilepsy. Neurology 70(22 Pt 2):2179–2186

Levy AR, Mayo NE, Grimard G (1995) Rates of transcervical and pertrochanteric hip fractures in the province of Quebec, Canada, 1981–1992. Am J Epidemiol 142(4):428–436

Lunghi C, Moisan J, Grégoire J-P et al (2017) The association between depression and medication nonpersistence in new users of antidiabetic drugs. Value Health 20(6):728–735

Madore O (2005) The Canada health act: overview and options. Library of Parliament, Parliamentary Information and Research Service, Ottawa

Martin M (1996) Quebec employs user-pay philosophy in launching drug-insurance plan. CMAJ 155(11):1604

Mayo N, Danys I, Carlton J et al (1993) Accuracy of hospital discharge coding for stroke. Can J Cardiol 9:121D–121D

Morgan S (1998) Quebec's drug insurance plan: a prescription for Canada? Health Policy Research Unit, Centre for Health Services and Policy Research, University of British Columbia. https://open.library.ubc.ca/cIRcle/collections/facultyresearchandpublications/52383/items/1.0048455. Accessed 14 Jan 2020

Morgan SG, Gagnon M-A, Charbonneau M et al (2017) Evaluating the effects of Quebec's private–public drug insurance system. CMAJ 189(40):E1259–E1263

Orriols L, Wilchesky M, Lagarde E et al (2013) Prescription of antidepressants and the risk of road traffic crash in the elderly: a case-crossover study. Br J Clin Pharmacol 76(5):810–815. https://doi.org/10.1111/bcp.12090

Oskoui M, Ng P, Dorais M et al (2017) Accuracy of administrative claims data for cerebral palsy diagnosis: a retrospective cohort study. CMAJ open 5(3):E570

Pampalon R, Raymond G (2000) A deprivation index for health and welfare planning in Quebec. Chronic Dis Can 21(3):104–113

Perreault S, Ellia L, Dragomir A et al (2009) Effect of statin adherence on cerebrovascular disease in primary prevention. Am J Med 122(7):647–655

Rawson NSB (2009) Access to linked administrative healthcare utilization data for pharmacoepidemiology and pharmacoeconomics research in Canada: anti-viral drugs as an example. Pharmacoepidemiol Drug Saf 18(11):1072–1079. https://doi.org/10.1002/pds.1822

Régie de l'assurance maladie du Québec (2020a) Prescription drug insurance: Eligibility for prescription drug insurance. http://www.ramq.gouv.qc.ca/en/citizens/prescription-drug-insura nce/Pages/eligibility.aspx. Accessed 29 Jan 2020

Régie de l'assurance maladie du Québec (2020b) Publications: Liste des médicaments. http://www.ramq.gouv.qc.ca/fr/publications/citoyens/publications-legales/Pages/liste-medicaments. aspx. Accessed 6 Feb 2020

Régie de l'assurance maladie du Québec (2019) Données et statistiques: Enquêtes, inspections et vérifications. http://www.ramq.gouv.qc.ca/fr/donnees-et-statistiques/Pages/enquetes-ins pections-et-verifications.aspx. Accessed 1 Feb 2020

Romano PS, Roos LL, Jollis JG (1993) Adapting a clinical comorbidity index for use with ICD-9-CM administrative data: differing perspectives. J Clin Epidemiol 46(10):1075–1079; discussion 1081–1090

Santos F, Sheehy O, Perreault S et al (2011) Exposure to anti-infective drugs during pregnancy and the risk of small-for-gestational-age newborns: a case–control study. BJOG 118(11):1374–1382

Statistics Canada and l'Institut de la statistique du Québec (2019) Estimations de la population (septembre 2019). Adapté par l'Institut de la statistique du Québec (ISQ). http://www.stat.

gouv.qc.ca/statistiques/population-demographie/structure/population-quebec-age-sexe.html# tri_pop=20. Accessed 2 Feb 2020

Suissa S (2008) Immeasurable time bias in observational studies of drug effects on mortality. Am J Epidemiol 168(3):329–335. https://doi.org/10.1093/aje/kwn135

Suissa S, Kezouh A, Ernst P (2010) Inhaled corticosteroids and the risks of diabetes onset and progression. Am J Med 123(11):1001–1006. https://doi.org/10.1016/j.amjmed.2010.06.019

Tamblyn R, Lavoie G, Petrella L et al (1995) The use of prescription claims databases in pharmacoepidemiological research: the accuracy and comprehensiveness of the prescription claims database in Quebec. J Clin Epidemiol 48(8):999–1009

Tamblyn R, Reid T, Mayo N et al (2000) Using medical services claims to assess injuries in the elderly: sensitivity of diagnostic and procedure codes for injury ascertainment. J Clin Epidemiol 53(2):183–194

Vilain A, Otis S, Forget A et al (2008) Agreement between administrative databases and medical charts for pregnancy-related variables among asthmatic women. Pharmacoepidemiol Drug Saf 17(4):345–353

Wilchesky M, Tamblyn RM, Huang A (2004) Validation of diagnostic codes within medical services claims. J Clin Epidemiol 57(2):131–141

Wilchesky M, Ernst P, Brophy JM et al (2012) Bronchodilator use and the risk of arrhythmia in COPD: part 2: reassessment in the larger Quebec cohort. Chest 142(2):305–311. https://doi.org/10.1378/chest.11-1597

Medicaid and Medicare

Dirk Enders, Tania Schink, and Til Stürmer

Abstract Medicaid is the largest health care program for persons with low income in the US and is jointly funded by the federal and individual state governments, while Medicare is solely funded by the federal government and provides health care for the vast majority of elderly persons. Both programs were established in 1965 and are overseen by the Centers of Medicare and Medicaid Services (CMS) of the United States Department of Health and Human Services.

1 Database Description

1.1 Introduction

Medicaid is the largest health care program for persons with low income in the US and is jointly funded by the federal and individual state governments, while Medicare is solely funded by the federal government and provides health care for the vast majority of elderly persons. Both programs were established in 1965 and are overseen by the Centers of Medicare and Medicaid Services (CMS) of the United States Department of Health and Human Services. The CMS also maintain a database with administrative data from both health care programs, which is the main source for researchers working with Medicaid or Medicare data (Leonard et al. 2017). The administrative data of Medicaid has been used to answer pharmacoepidemiological research questions since the early 1980s (Hennessy et al. 2012a). Administrative data of Medicare has increasingly been used for this purpose since the implementation of prescription drug coverage in 2006 (Hanlon and Donohue 2010).

D. Enders (✉) · T. Schink
Leibniz Institute for Prevention Research and Epidemiology—BIPS, Achterstrasse 30, 28359 Bremen, Germany

T. Stürmer
Gillings School of Global Public Health, University of North Carolina at Chapel Hill, Chapel Hill, North Carolina, USA

© Springer Nature Switzerland AG 2021　　　　　　　　　　　　　　　　　　231
M. Sturkenboom and T. Schink (eds.), *Databases for Pharmacoepidemiological Research*, Springer Series on Epidemiology and Public Health,
https://doi.org/10.1007/978-3-030-51455-6_19

1.2 Database Characteristics

Medicaid originally covered expenditures for low income pregnant women, families with children or elderly patients as well as chronically disabled patients in all federal states of the US. In 2014, the eligibility was extended to all low income patients in the course of the Patient Protection and Affordable Care Act, but extension is voluntary and varies by state. Medicare covers most patients aged 65 years and above as well as some disabled persons and patients with end-stage renal disease or amyotrophic lateral sclerosis. The Medicare program is divided into four parts. Part A is available to all Medicare enrollees and covers inpatient and hospice/nursing home care. Part B is available for an additional monthly fee and covers outpatient physician visits, services or products. Part C includes Medicare Advantage plans, which can be demanded by Part A or B enrollees and cover additional services, typically paid by an extra premium each month. However, the claims of Part C are generally not available for research through CMS. Part D was implemented in 2006 as part of the Medicare Modernization Act of 2003 and covers outpatient prescriptions. To be included in Part D, patients must enroll in stand-alone prescription drug plans or Medicare Advantage prescription drug plans, which are administered by private health insurances. As the eligibility criteria for Medicare and Medicaid overlap patients could be enrolled in both Medicare and Medicaid.

The trend of enrolled patients over time is depicted in Fig. 1. There has been a steady increase in enrolled persons over the last 50 years in both health care programs

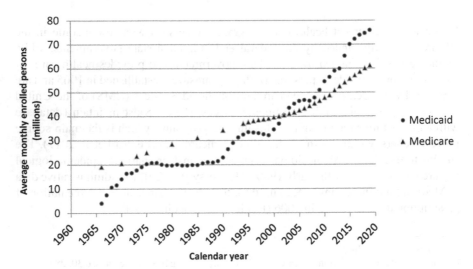

Fig. 1 Enrolled persons in Medicaid (Medicaid and CHIP Payment and Access Commission 2019) and Medicare (Centers for Medicare and Medicaid Services 2017, 2019a, b) from 1966 until 2016

with a steeper increase in enrollment for Medicaid than for Medicare (Part A or B). Table 1 shows the latest demographic characteristics. Medicaid covered 74.49 million people in 2012 and 58.48 million were enrolled in Medicare in 2017, corresponding to 23.7 and 18.0% of the US population, respectively (U.S. Census Bureau Population Division 2018). The beneficiaries of Medicaid are not representative for the US population, as children, females as well as non-white persons are over-represented due to the selective eligibility criteria of the program. For the same reason, white persons, females and seniors are overrepresented in Medicare. Over 10.6 million patients are currently enrolled in both Medicare and Medicaid (Centers for Medicare and Medicaid Services 2020).

The raw administrative data of Medicaid is processed by the CMS and made available for research purposes via research identifiable files (RIFs). For Medicaid, the administrative data needs three to four years to become available and the RIFs currently cover data from 1999 up to 2013 for all federal states and up to 2015 for some of them. The administrative data of Medicare Part A, B, and D is updated more frequently than the Medicaid data and is now available after approximately one year. Currently, the RIFs of Medicare cover the years 1999 to 2017 and 2018 data is expected to be complete at the beginning of 2020 (Part D data is available from 2006 and already includes 2018 data).

1.3 Available Data

Medicaid data is stored in five different data files, which are referred to as Medical Analytic eXtract (MAX) files by the CMS:

- The Personal Summary File contains demographic characteristics of the patients, e.g., date of birth, gender and race/ethnicity, date of death (without cause of death). It also contains information about the eligibility status (e.g., eligibility group, months of eligibility, dual eligibility to Medicare and Medicaid) and summary measures on use of the health system (e.g., number and duration of hospital stays, total number of prescribed drugs, payments).
- The Inpatient File contains all hospital stay records for enrollees using inpatient services. Included are hospital admission dates, type and begin/end of services, status at discharge and payments. Diagnoses are coded by the International Classification of Diseases, 9th Edition, Clinical Modification (ICD-9-CM and procedures by ICD-9-CM, Healthcare Common Procedure Coding System (HCPCS) level I-III or state-specific codes.
- The Other Therapy File includes claims from outpatient and inpatient physician visits (including physician specialty), as well as outpatient hospitals, clinics, home health care and hospices with respective dates. Diagnoses and procedures are coded in the same manner as in the Inpatient File. Outpatient laboratory and radiology records are also contained, but lab results are not reported.

Table 1 Demographic characteristics of the medicaid and medicare population

		Medicaid enrollees[a] (N = 74,488,564)		Medicare enrollees (Part A and/or Part B)[b] (N = 58,457,244)
Gender	Male	31,360,030 (42.10%)	Male	26,663,618 (45.61%)
	Female	43,035,479 (57.77%)	Female	31,793,626 (54.39%)
	Unknown	93,055 (0.12%)		
Age in years	<1	2,301,454 (3.09%)	Under 18	1550 (0.00%)
	1–5	11,776,704 (15.81%)	18–24	96,951 (0.17%)
	6–12	13,353,457 (17.92%)	25–34	600,268 (1.03%)
	13–14	3,316,844 (4.45%)	35–44	1,123,996 (1.92%)
	15–18	6,428,030 (8.63%)	45–54	2,258,082 (3.86%)
	19–20	2,742,867 (3.68%)	55–64	4,698,364 (8.04%)
	21–44	18,930,113 (25.41%)	65–74	28,116,983 (48.10%)
	45–64	8,832,028 (11.86%)	75–84	14,944,692 (25.57%)
	65–74	3,092,551 (4.15%)	85–94	5,879,028 (10.06%)
	75–84	2,223,220 (2.98%)	95 and older	737,330 (1.26%)
	85+	1,406,428 (1.89%)		
	Missing	84,868 (0.11%)		
Race/Ethnicity	Non-Hispanic White	30,344,114 (40.74%)	Non-Hispanic White	43,452,430 (74.33%)
	Black/African American	15,771,904 (21.17%)	Black/African American	6,110,152 (10.45%)
	Hispanic/Latino	15,147,048 (20.33%)	Hispanic	5,292,863 (9.05%)
	Asian	2,496,906 (3.35%)	Asian/Pacific Islander	1,890,556 (3.23%)
	American Indian/Alaska Native	886,563 (1.19%)	American Indian/Alaska Native	269,595 (0.46%)

(continued)

Table 1 (continued)

	Medicaid enrollees[a] (N = 74,488,564)		Medicare enrollees (Part A and/or Part B)[b] (N = 58,457,244)
Native Hawaiian/Pacific Islander	705,926 (0.95%)	Other	538,729 (0.92%)
Hispanic/Latino and one or more race	3,360,206 (4.51%)	Unknown	902,918 (1.54%)
More than one race	365,402 (0.49%)		
Not identified	5,410,495 (7.26%)		

[a]Numbers based on Medicaid Statistical Information System (MSIS) tables of 2012 (Centers for Medicare and Medicaid Services 2012). Some states didn't provide numbers for the respective year and were thus extracted from the MSIS tables of 2011 (Arizona, Colorado, District of Columbia, Florida, Hawaii, Idaho, Kansas, Louisiana, Massachusetts, Texas, Utah) and 2010 (Maine)

[b]Numbers based on CMS Chronic Conditions Data Warehouse data on total enrollment in 2017 (Centers for Medicare and Medicaid Services 2019b)

- The Prescription Drug File covers all drug claims of Medicaid, which are coded according to the National Drug Code (NDC) system. Drugs identified by other codes such as HCPCS or state-specific codes are contained in the Other Therapy file. Note that most drugs for patients which are dually eligible for Medicaid and Medicare are contained in the Medicare files. All drugs are contained with prescription date, prescription fill date, strength, quantity and duration of supply, and identification number of the prescribing physician. Non-reimbursable drugs administered at hospital and indications for drugs are not contained.
- The Long Term Care File includes claims from long-term care facilities, i.e., nursing homes, intermediate care facilities, and psychiatric facilities. The file includes admission dates to the facility, dates of services, diagnoses coded in ICD-9-CM, and discharge status of the patient.

The data of Medicare is available via numerous data files, which can be linked via unique subject identifiers:

- The Master Beneficiary Summary File contains demographic characteristics such as sex, race, region of residence, date and cause (only from 1999 to 2008) of death, monthly enrollment information for Plan C and D, and summary measures on costs and uses of services.
- The Standard Analytic Files (SAFs), also known as Medicare Claims Files, contain claims from institutional and non-institutional health care providers. Institutional data covers inpatient and outpatient data as well as claims from skilled nursing facilities, hospices, and home health agencies. Non-institutional claims cover durable medical equipment and data on physicians and free-standing facilities such as clinical laboratories. In general, diagnosis (coded in ICD-9-CM) and procedures (coded in ICD-9-CM or HCPCS) are included together with the date of service and the amount of reimbursement.
- The Medicare Provider and Analysis Review (MedPAR) Files contain inpatient hospital and/or skilled nursing facility final action claims with diagnoses and procedures (coded in ICD-9-CM) and the corresponding date of service and reimbursement amount. Contrary to the SAFs, each record represents a complete stay in a hospital or nursing facility and thus might contain multiple claims if they belong to the same stay.
- Information on prescription claims is available via the Part D Drug Event (PDE) File. This file contains one record per prescription and contains prescription date, NDC, days of supply and quantity dispensed. As in the Medicaid data, indications for drugs are missing. Further, medication administered at the hospital is covered by Plan A and is thus not contained in the PDE file. Information on prescription drug plans, pharmacies, drugs and prescribers is available in supplemental files.

Medicaid and Medicare data can be linked to each other but also to other data sources. For example, since laboratory results are absent, a study has been performed to link Medicare data of 10 eastern states data of a large national laboratory service (Hammill et al. 2015). For studies involving cancer, linkage of Medicare data with the Surveillance, Epidemiology, and End Results (SEER) program of the National

Cancer Institute is possible to obtain detailed information on cancer site, stage and histology. The Personal Summary File of Medicaid also contains state-specific case numbers identifying the Medicaid cases which each individual belongs to. Palmsten et al. (2013) used this number to identify mother-infant pairs. The authors showed that linkage is in general feasible, but the percentage of linked deliveries varies greatly by state.

1.4 Strengths and Limitations

A major strength of Medicaid and Medicare is their enormous size, which enables studies of rare events even in small subpopulations. The induced homogeneity by the eligibility criteria increases control for confounding and restriction to subpopulations might be possible, where treatment effects might be detectable in contrast to the general population. However, the non-representativeness precludes studies aiming to describe the overall US population. Further, although a small proportion of patients is included in Medicaid without gaps of enrollment (Leonard et al. 2017), membership to Medicaid is generally not stable over time precluding studies of long-term effects of most treatments (Hennessy et al. 2012b). In contrast, members of Medicare generally stay in the program once they entered such that studies with long follow-ups are possible.

As with all administrative databases, Medicaid and Medicare lack information on important confounders such as lifestyle factors (e.g. smoking, diet) or occupation. Regarding prescriptions, the databases face the common problem that over-the-counter medication is not captured. Additionally, the prescription drug plans of Medicare Part D each differ with respect to drug coverage and cost-sharing options and drug availability thus differ across plans. Prescription data in Medicaid was shown to be accurate and complete (Leonard et al. 2017), but this might not hold for low cost generics (Choudhry and Shrank 2010).

1.5 Validation

Medicaid data of each state is validated internally by the CMS (Centers for Medicare and Medicaid Services 2016) and anomalies are reported in validation tables. For both Medicare and Medicaid, reimbursement of the health care providers is determined by the recorded procedures, which are thus checked for errors and can be considered as accurate. However, a validation study comparing medical records for surgical procedures of hip fractures with Medicaid claims found some procedures coded for another purpose (Wysowski and Baum 1993).

Outpatient prescription data of Medicaid was validated in the 1980s and found to be accurate (Lessler and Harris 1984). Leonard et al. (2017) recently investigated the quality of prescription claims in Medicaid and noted that 95–99% of the prescription claims were identifiable in a commercially-available database of NDCs. Further, the absolute number of prescriptions increased steadily and consistently over time, which suggest completeness of prescription claims. Validation of prescription claims was also performed with Medicare data. Colantonio et al. (2016) e.g. validated the prescription claims of lipid lowering drugs in Medicare with self-reported drug use and observed that many beneficiaries reported drug use although no claims in Medicare exist. However, both data sources might have caused this discrepancy e.g. due to recall error in self-reports or due to missing incentives to submit claims to Medicare for reimbursement.

Leonard et al. (2017) further found that hospital data in Medicaid was underrepresented in patients aged 45 years and above due to patients with poorer health status, who are dually eligible for Medicare and Medicaid. The authors therefore advised to additionally consider Medicare data for patients 45 years and older in case hospitalization data is needed to answer the study question of interest. Further, although no gross diagnostic miscoding in the in- and outpatient claims of Medicaid occurred, the authors acknowledged that the validity of health outcomes of interest generally remains open.

The gold-standard of outcome validation represents medical record validation, which was performed in a variety of studies. Hennessy et al. (2010) e.g. reviewed codes of inpatient and emergency department encounters in Medicaid to identify sudden cardiac death and ventricular arrhythmia originating in the outpatient setting and found very good agreement with medical records. Hernandez-Trujillo et al. (2015) performed medical record validation for primary immunodeficiency disease diagnoses. They observed low positive predicted values for individual ICD-9-CM codes and propose to use additional data sources to define disease status. Different methods to retrieve medical records were summarized in a Medicare-based example study validating adverse events of special interest (Wright et al. 2017). Other methods besides medical record validation were also performed. Brouwer et al. (2015) e.g. compared an algorithm to define myocardial infarction in Medicaid HIV patients with clinical cohort data and an algorithm to identify chronic kidney disease in older Medicare adults was validated with the Reasons for Geographic and Racial Differences in Stroke (REGARDS) study (Muntner et al. 2015).

1.6 Governance and Ethical Issues

The personnel information of Medicaid or Medicare is protected under the Privacy Rule of the Health Insurance Portability and Accountability Act of 1996, which prohibits disclosure of protected health information (PHI) without written consent. Exceptions are granted for research purposes under certain conditions (Office for Civil Rights 2018). A study using PHI via research identifiable files of CMS requires a data use agreement and must be approved by the Privacy Board of CMS (Research Data Assistance Center 2020a, b). The study should assist CMS in monitoring, managing and improving the Medicaid and Medicare program and the services provided to the beneficiaries. Researchers must demonstrate experience in conducting research with files containing PHI and may only apply for the data files which are necessary to appropriately answer their study question. They further need to define a cohort in advance, since the provision costs depend on the number of patients in the cohort and the data files which are requested. However, there are some public use files containing non-identifiable data on a summary level, which can be requested without a data use agreement and without approval of the Privacy Board.

1.7 Documents and Publications

The Research Data Assistance Center (ResDaC), a contractor funded by the CMS, provides introductory workshops and webinars on Medicaid, Medicare and the corresponding data files. The ResDac website also includes a detailed description of all information included in the RIFs (https://www.resdac.org/).

Important methodological and applied example studies in pharmacoepidemiology were summarized by Hennessy et al. (2012b): Using routine data of elderly Medicaid beneficiaries of New Jersey Stürmer et al. (2005) compared conventional confounder adjustment with propensity score adjustment and adjustment using disease risk scores but found no major difference between the three methods. Schneeweiss et al. (2009) proposed an algorithm for automated confounder selection for propensity score models and evaluated its performance in three studies based on elder Medicare patients. The algorithm resulted in estimates that were all closer to the results of corresponding randomized clinical trials. Roumie et al. (2009) investigated the risk of cardiovascular events for certain non-steroidal anti-inflammatory drugs in Tennessee Medicaid enrollees and observed an increased risk for current users of rofecoxib, valdecoxib and indomethacin compared to non-users in patients without a history of cardiovascular diseases. The relation between adherence osteoporosis treatment and the risk of fractures in elderly Medicare beneficiaries was analyzed by Patrick et al. (2010), who found a consistent relation between adherence and risk reduction.

Recently conducted studies showed that Medicaid and Medicare data are still used frequently in diverse fields of epidemiological research: Leonard et al. (2018) compared new users of different antidiabetic monotherapies regarding the risk of severe hypoglycaemia in a cohort based on Medicaid beneficiaries from California, Florida, New York, Ohio and Pennsylvania and found the highest rate of serious hypoglycaemia for sulfonylureas. The prevalence of antidiabetic and antilipidemic medications in children and adolescents treated with atypical antipsychotics was estimated by Varghese et al. (2016) in Virginia Medicaid beneficiaries. The authors observed that the medication was more often prescribed in atypical antipsychotic users than in non-users. Ray et al. (2015) compared time-dependent propensity scores with conventional adjustment of time-dependent confounders and inverse-probability-of-treatment (IPT) weighted estimation of parameters in marginal structural models in a cohort of opioid users of the Medicaid population in Tennessee in the absence of confounders on the causal pathway. IPT weighted estimates were shown to be less efficient than the other two in this example. Santos et al. (2016) analyzed the use of cytomegalovirus prophylaxis in kidney transplant recipients of Medicare and found that prophylaxis use was common. In an empirical example with Medicare patients Gokhale et al. (2016) illustrated the considerable loss of power, when steps in the design study reduce sample size to minimize potential bias. Gilbertson et al. (2016) examined the influence of different time-windows for baseline confounder assessment on the mortality risk in a simulation study based on haemodialysis patients of Medicare and concluded that the timing of confounders should be taken into account for improvement of confounder control.

1.8 Administrative Information

The administrative data of Medicaid and Medicare is maintained by CMS, but ResDaC helps with data requests.

Contact details

Organization/affiliation: Research Data Assistance Center

University of Minnesota School of Public Health

Division of Health Policy and Management

420 Delaware Street SE, Mayo D355

Minneapolis, MN 55455

Administrative Contact: resdac@umn.edu

1-888-973-7322

Website: https://www.resdac.org/

References

Brouwer ES, Napravnik S, Eron JJ Jr et al (2015) Validation of medicaid claims-based diagnosis of myocardial infarction using an HIV clinical cohort. Med Care 53(6):e41–e48. https://doi.org/10.1097/MLR.0b013e318287d6fd

Centers for Medicare and Medicaid Services (2012) MSIS Tables. https://www.cms.gov/Research-Statistics-Data-and-Systems/Computer-Data-and-Systems/MedicaidDataSourcesGenInfo/MSIS-Tables.html. Accessed 1st Feb 2018

Centers for Medicare and Medicaid Services (2016) MAX validation reports. https://www.cms.gov/Research-Statistics-Data-and-Systems/Computer-Data-and-Systems/MedicaidDataSourcesGenInfo/MAX-Validation-Reports.html. Accessed 04 Jan 2018

Centers for Medicare and Medicaid Services (2017) Medicare and medicaid statistical supplement 2013 edition. https://www.cms.gov/Research-Statistics-Data-and-Systems/Statistics-Trends-and-Reports/MedicareMedicaidStatSupp/2013.html. Accessed 2 Feb 2020

Centers for Medicare and Medicaid Services (2019a) CMS fast facts. https://www.cms.gov/Research-Statistics-Data-and-Systems/Statistics-Trends-and-Reports/CMS-Fast-Facts/index.html. Accessed 2 Feb 2020

Centers for Medicare and Medicaid Services (2019b) Total medicare enrollment: part A and/or part B enrollees, by demographic characteristics, calendar year 2015. https://www.cms.gov/Research-Statistics-Data-and-Systems/Statistics-Trends-and-Reports/CMSProgramStatistics/2015/2015_Enrollment.html. Accessed 2 Feb 2020

Centers for Medicare and Medicaid Services (2020) Medicare-medicaid enrollment (MME): total medicare-medicaid enrollees by type of eligibility, calendar years 2010–2017. https://www.cms.gov/Research-Statistics-Data-and-Systems/Statistics-Trends-and-Reports/CMSProgramStatistics/2017/2017_Enrollment.html. Accessed 2 Feb 2020

Choudhry NK, Shrank WH (2010) Four-dollar generics—increased accessibility, impaired quality assurance. N Engl J Med 363(20):1885–1887. https://doi.org/10.1056/NEJMp1006189

Colantonio LD, Kent ST, Kilgore ML et al (2016) Agreement between medicare pharmacy claims, self-report, and medication inventory for assessing lipid-lowering medication use. Pharmacoepidemiol Drug Saf 25(7):827–835. https://doi.org/10.1002/pds.3970

Gilbertson DT, Bradbury BD, Wetmore JB et al (2016) Controlling confounding of treatment effects in administrative data in the presence of time-varying baseline confounders. Pharmacoepidemiol Drug Saf 25(3):269–277. https://doi.org/10.1002/pds.3922

Gokhale M, Buse JB, Pate V et al (2016) More realistic power estimation for new user, active comparator studies: an empirical example. Pharmacoepidemiol Drug Saf 25(4):462–466. https://doi.org/10.1002/pds.3872

Hammill BG, Curtis LH, Qualls LG et al (2015) Linkage of laboratory results to medicare fee-for-service claims. Med Care 53(11):974–979. https://doi.org/10.1097/mlr.0000000000000420

Hanlon JT, Donohue J (2010) Medicare part D data: a valuable tool for pharmacoepidemiology and pharmacoeconomic research. Am J Geriatric Pharmacother 8(6):483–484. https://doi.org/10.1016/S1543-5946(10)80001-7

Hennessy S, Leonard CE, Freeman CP et al (2010) Validation of diagnostic codes for outpatient-originating sudden cardiac death and ventricular arrhythmia in medicaid and medicare claims data. Pharmacoepidemiol Drug Saf 19(6):555–562. https://doi.org/10.1002/pds.1869

Hennessy S, Palumbo Freeman C, Cunningham F (2012a) US government claims databases. In: Strom BL, Kimmel SE, Hennessy S (eds) Pharmacoepidemiology, 5th edn. Wiley, Chichester, pp 209–223

Hennessy S, Palumbo Freeman C, Cunningham F (2012b) US Government claims databases. In: Strom BL, Kimmel SE, Hennessy S (eds) Pharmacoepidemiology, 5th edn. Wiley, Chichester

Hernandez-Trujillo H, Orange JS, Roy JA et al (2015) Validity of primary immunodeficiency disease diagnoses in United States medicaid data. J Clin Immunol 35(6):566–572. https://doi.org/10.1007/s10875-015-0185-x

Leonard CE, Brensinger CM, Nam Y et al (2017) The quality of medicaid and medicare data obtained from CMS and its contractors: implications for pharmacoepidemiology. BMC Health Serv Res 17(304). https://doi.org/10.1186/s12913-017-2247-7

Leonard CE, Han X, Brensinger CM et al (2018) Comparative risk of serious hypoglycemia with oral antidiabetic monotherapy: a retrospective cohort study. Pharmacoepidemiol Drug Saf 27(1):9–18. https://doi.org/10.1002/pds.4337

Lessler JT, Harris BSH (1984) Medicaid data as a source for postmarketing surveillance information: final report. Research Triangle Institute, Research Triangle Park, NC

Medicaid and CHIP Payment and Access Commission (2019) MACStats: medicaid and CHIP data book. https://www.macpac.gov/publication/macstats-medicaid-and-chip-data-book-2/. Accessed 2 Feb 2020

Muntner P, Gutierrez OM, Zhao H et al (2015) Validation study of medicare claims to identify older US adults with CKD using the reasons for geographic and racial differences in stroke (REGARDS) study. Am J Kidney Dis 65(2):249–258. https://doi.org/10.1053/j.ajkd.2014.07.012

Office for Civil Rights (2018) HIPAA privacy. https://www.hhs.gov/hipaa/for-professionals/special-topics/research/index.html. Accessed 2 Feb 2020

Palmsten K, Huybrechts KF, Mogun H et al (2013) Harnessing the medicaid analytic extract (MAX) to evaluate medications in pregnancy: design considerations. PLoS ONE 8(6):e67405. https://doi.org/10.1371/journal.pone.0067405

Patrick AR, Brookhart MA, Losina E et al (2010) The complex relation between bisphosphonate adherence and fracture reduction. J Clin Endocrinol Metab 95(7):3251–3259. https://doi.org/10.1210/jc.2009-2778

Ray WA, Liu Q, Shepherd BE (2015) Performance of time-dependent propensity scores: a pharmacoepidemiology case study. Pharmacoepidemiol Drug Saf 24(1):98–106. https://doi.org/10.1002/pds.3727

Research Data Assistance Center (2020a) Requirements for institutional review board (IRB) review and HIPAA waiver documentation for RIF DUA request submissions. https://www.resdac.org/articles/requirements-institutional-review-board-irb-review-and-hipaa-waiver-documentation-rif-dua. Accessed 2 Feb 2020

Research Data Assistance Center (2020b) Research identifiable files (RIF) requests. https://www.resdac.org/cms-data/request/research-identifiable-files. Accessed 2 Feb 2020

Roumie CL, Choma NN, Kaltenbach L et al (2009) Non-aspirin NSAIDs, Cyclooxygenase-2 Inhibitors and Risk for cardiovascular events—stroke, acute myocardial infarction, and death from coronary heart disease. Pharmacoepidemiol Drug Saf 18(11):1053–1063. https://doi.org/10.1002/pds.1820

Santos CA, Brennan DC, Saeed MJ et al (2016) Pharmacoepidemiology of cytomegalovirus prophylaxis in a large retrospective cohort of kidney transplant recipients with medicare part D coverage. Clin Transplant 30(4):435–444. https://doi.org/10.1111/ctr.12706

Schneeweiss S, Rassen JA, Glynn RJ et al (2009) High-dimensional propensity score adjustment in studies of treatment effects using health care claims data. Epidemiology 20(4):512–522. https://doi.org/10.1097/EDE.0b013e3181a663cc

Stürmer T, Schneeweiss S, Brookhart MA et al (2005) Analytic strategies to adjust confounding using exposure propensity scores and disease risk scores: nonsteroidal antiinflammatory drugs and short-term mortality in the elderly. Am J Epidemiol 161(9):891–898. https://doi.org/10.1093/aje/kwi106

U.S. Census Bureau Population Division (2018) Annual estimates of the resident population: April 1, 2010 to July 1, 2018. https://factfinder.census.gov. Accessed 2 Feb 2020

Varghese D, Kirkwood CK, Carroll NV (2016) Prevalence of antidiabetic and antilipidemic medications in children and adolescents treated with atypical antipsychotics in a virginia medicaid population. Ann Pharmacother 50(6):463–470. https://doi.org/10.1177/1060028016638861

Wright NC, Delzell ES, Smith WK et al (2017) Improving medical record retrieval for validation studies in medicare data. Pharmacoepidemiol Drug Saf 26(4):393–401. https://doi.org/10.1002/pds.4131

Wysowski DK, Baum C (1993) The validity of medicaid diagnoses of hip fracture. Am J Public Health 83(5):770

IBM MarketScan Research Databases

**Anne M. Butler, Katelin B. Nickel, Robert A. Overman,
and M. Alan Brookhart**

Abstract The IBM® MarketScan® Research Databases contain individual-level,
de-identified healthcare claims data including clinical utilization, expenditures,
insurance enrollment/plan benefit for inpatient, outpatient, prescription drug, and
carve-out services for a large population of individuals and their dependents with
employer-provided commercial insurance in the United States.

1 Database Description

1.1 Introduction

The IBM® MarketScan® Research Databases contain individual-level, de-identified
healthcare claims data including clinical utilization, expenditures, insurance enroll-
ment/plan benefit for inpatient, outpatient, prescription drug, and carve-out services
for a large population of individuals and their dependents with employer-provided
commercial insurance in the United States.

A. M. Butler (✉) · K. B. Nickel
School of Medicine, Washington University, 4523 Clayton Ave, CB 8051, St Louis, MO 63110,
USA
e-mail: anne.butler@wustl.edu

R. A. Overman
Blue Cross Blue Shield of North Carolina, Healthcare Strategy & Payment Strategic Investment,
4705 University Drive, Bldg 700, Durham, NC 27707, USA

M. A. Brookhart
Department of Population Health Sciences, Duke University, 215 Morris Street, Durham, NC
27701, USA

© Springer Nature Switzerland AG 2021   243
M. Sturkenboom and T. Schink (eds.), *Databases for Pharmacoepidemiological
Research*, Springer Series on Epidemiology and Public Health,
https://doi.org/10.1007/978-3-030-51455-6_20

1.2   Database Characteristics

In the U.S., individuals with commercial insurance (including employer- and non-group-sponsored) plans or Medicare-based plans account for approximately 55 and 20% of the population, respectively (The Henry J. Kaiser Family Foundation 2018). Two core MarketScan Databases include large samples of these populations: the IBM® MarketScan® Commercial Database and the IBM® MarketScan® Medicare Supplemental Database. Specifically, the MarketScan Commercial Database contains data from active employees, early retirees, Consolidated Omnibus Budget Reconciliation Act (COBRA) continues, and dependents insured by employer-sponsored health plans, whereas the MarketScan Medicare Supplemental Database contains data from Medicare-eligible retirees with employer-sponsored Medicare Supplemental plans. Additional data are available in the following IBM® MarketScan® Databases: Multi-State Medicaid Database, Health and Productivity Management Database, Benefit Plan Design Database, Lab Database, Health Risk Assessment Database, Dental Database, Hospital Drug Database, Weather Database, Inpatient Drug Link File, and Explorys® Claims-EMR Data Set (Hansen 2019; IBM Watson Health 2019a).

Altogether, the MarketScan Research Databases (1995–2018), constructed by IBM Watson Health, include health-related data from more than 350 unique carriers on over 200 million people residing in all 50 states and the District of Columbia (Fig. 1) (Hansen 2019). The total annual enrollee person-time increased from 26.8 million person-years in 2006 to 44.9 million person-years in 2012; 2018 contains 23.0 million person-years (Fig. 2). The annual database is typically available for purchase after an approximate two year lag time; however, early release versions of the data are also available.

1.3   Available Data

The MarketScan Commercial Database and the MarketScan Medicare Supplemental Database contain de-identified enrollee-level health data including clinical utilization, expenditures, insurance enrollment/plan benefit for inpatient and outpatient visits, and prescription drugs. Each individual in the MarketScan Databases is assigned a unique enrollee identifier, which is created by encrypting information provided by data contributors. The enrollee identifier provides links between years of data and across the MarketScan Databases. Linkage within a family, including mothers and babies, is possible in the MarketScan Commercial Database, and has become easier since 2010 when a familial id variable was first included (Panozzo et al. 2013; Cortese et al. 2015; Asfaw et al. 2012). Enrollee-level linkage to external data sources is limited; however, IBM has helped health services customers undertake unique linking projects to link the MarketScan Research Databases with external data (Hansen 2019).

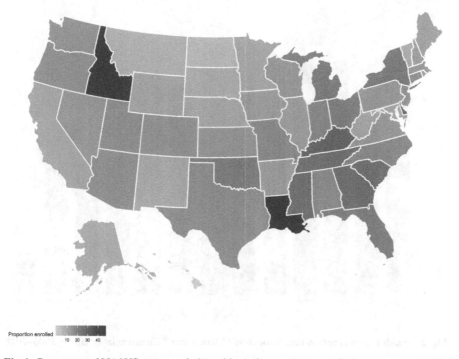

Proportion enrolled
10 20 30 40

Fig. 1 Percentage of 2016 US state population with employer or non-group insurance represented in the 2016 IBM MarketScan Commercial Database. Employer-based coverage includes those covered through a current or former employer or union, either as policyholder or as dependent. Non-group coverage includes those covered by a policy purchased directly from an insurance company, either as policyholder or as dependent. MarketScan data were person-time; results for grey states were not presented per request from IBM MarketScan (The Henry J. Kaiser Family Foundation 2018)

Both the MarketScan Commercial Database and the MarketScan Medicare Supplemental Database contain data related to demographics, medical information, health plan, financial information, drugs, and enrollment. Demographic information includes age, sex, employment status and classification, relationship to primary enrollee, state, metropolitan statistical area, and industry. Medical information includes dates of service such as admission and discharge dates for inpatient admissions, principal and secondary diagnosis codes, discharge status, major diagnostic category, principal and secondary procedure codes, diagnosis-related group (DRG), length of stay, place of service, and quantity of services. Inpatient and outpatient diagnoses are coded using the International Classification of Diseases, 9th Revision, Clinical Modification (ICD-9-CM) and ICD-10-CM codes, while procedures are coded primarily using ICD-9-CM and ICD-10-PCS procedure codes, Healthcare Common Procedural Coding System (HCPCS) procedure codes, and Current Procedural Terminology, 4th Edition (CPT-4) codes. Pregnant women can be identified by prenatal care and deliveries. Health plan information includes plan type (e.g., HMO, POS, PPO). Financial information includes several payment amounts including total,

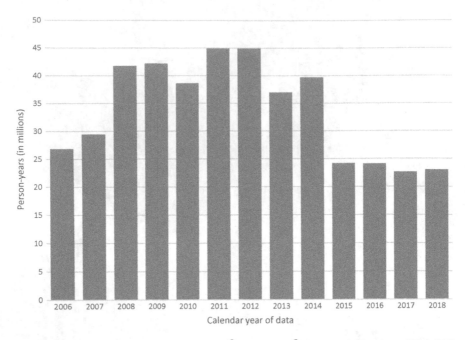

Fig. 2 Trends in annual person-time in the IBM® MarketScan® Commercial Database, 2006–2018

net, to physician, to hospital, and total admission as well as the source of the payment including patient out-of-pocket payments and employer/plan liability. Outpatient drug information includes generic product ID, average wholesale price, prescription drug payment, therapeutic class, therapeutic group, days supplied, dosage, national drug code, and refill number. Enrollment information includes dates of enrollment and disenrollment and member days. The Lab Database captures laboratory tests and results for a subset of the covered lives in both the MarketScan Commercial Database and MarketScan Medicare Supplemental Database and mainly represents lab tests ordered in office-based practice. Laboratory values are available on patients who have a test ordered and submitted to a specific large, national testing company. The laboratory test results can be linked temporally to the claims data (Brookhart et al. 2014). In the 2012 MarketScan Commercial Database, about 5% of recipients had at least one lab test result.

1.4 Strength and Limitations

The MarketScan Databases have several strengths. First, the databases offer one of the largest convenience samples in proprietary databases. Second, MarketScan data provide the ability to track enrollees and families longitudinally using the unique person-level identifier across an individual's enrollment, medical, and drug records. Thus, these data capture the full continuum of care in all reimbursed inpatient and outpatient settings: Physician office visits; hospital stays; and retail, mail order, and special pharmacies. Third, MarketScan data sources allow strong longitudinal tracking of enrollees over multiple years. Individual-level month-by-month enrollment information allows for the creation of a continuous enrollment period; however, due to what are likely administrative gaps in coverage, wherein a person is missing a month or two of enrollment data and then resumes coverage, allowances are often made to allow gaps in coverage. For example, individuals initially enrolled in 2010 have an average continuous enrollment of 2.4 years (interquartile range, 0.8–3.0 years) through 2018 (allowing a 105 day difference between the end of one month of coverage and the start of the next available month of coverage).

As a US healthcare claims database, the MarketScan data have many limitations shared by all such databases. The data generally lack clinical measures (e.g., blood pressure and body mass index), physical examination results, lifestyle factors, and patient-reported measures. However, for a selected subsample of the population, some of these measures are available in the Lab Database, the Health Risk Assessment Database, and the Explorys® Claims-EMR Data Set. The laboratory data, although representative (Brookhart et al. 2014), capture only a small fraction of the results from the laboratory tests that were ordered. The pharmacy claims capture use of outpatient prescription medications, but not over-the-counter drugs or inpatient medications. They also do not capture use of samples and the data may not capture all low-cost generic medication offered by some pharmacy chains. Claims for healthcare and medications may also be missed if enrollees are eligible for more than one insurance plan without coordination of benefits. For example, some enrollees may have Veterans Administration (VA) benefits as well as their private insurance coverage. The indication for the prescription medication is also not available. Healthcare obtained in a VA facility may not be captured in the commercial claims data. The diagnostic codes associated with hospitalizations, and particularly outpatient encounters, may not reliably identify patients with or without disease conditions due to variation in coding practices and depending on whether a comorbidity was related to a given hospitalization or outpatient visit (Brookhart et al. 2010; Nickel et al. 2016). The use of these codes and billing practices may also change over time. For example, the number of observation stays rather than direct hospital admissions has increased in patients with commercial insurance, which may lead to spurious trends in admissions and under-ascertainment of hospitalizations in studies using contemporary administrative healthcare data (Overman et al. 2014).

The MarketScan Databases also have some specific limitations beyond those shared by all US claims databases. First, the population is based on a large, non-random convenience sample from mostly large employers, which limits the generalizability of study findings. However, the MarketScan Databases provide weights which can be used to calculate more nationally representative estimates (Hansen 2019; IBM MarketScan Research Databases 2018). Second, there is little opportunity for external data linkage at the enrollee level due to data use restrictions. Third, information is not available regarding reasons for insurance disenrollment such as change of employer, switch to Medicare coverage, or death. Independent predictors of disenrollment during the calendar year (January 1 to December 30) are related to health status, including age, comorbidities, frailty, hospitalization, emergency room visits, use of durable medical equipment (DME), use of preventive care, and use of prescription medications, whereas independent predictors of year-end disenrollment (December 31) are related to health plan characteristics including insurance plan and geographic characteristics (Butler et al. 2019). Fourth, enrollees have limited enrollment durations, on average. Of enrollees beginning coverage in 2015, 18.4% had lost eligibility by six months, 31.2% by one year, and 70.7% by three years. Fifth, individuals may appear in the MarketScan Databases with different unique identifiers due to a simultaneous change in employer and insurer. Sixth, mortality information is limited to in-hospital death data obtained through the disposition at discharge, which may be inaccurate, and has not been available since 2015 (Hansen 2019). In 2015, 4.1% of patients discharged dead continued to accrue non-DME medical claims 15–365 days after death. Lastly, information is not available on race, ethnicity, or socioeconomic status; however, it is possible to approximate these variables within metropolitan statistical areas using external data sources.

1.5   Validation

MarketScan claims data undergo rigorous validation methods to ensure that claims and enrollment data are complete, accurate, and reliable. All claims have been fully paid and adjudicated (Hansen 2019). The MarketScan Databases are created as a snapshot in time and are based on a calendar-year period. For validity purposes, checks are performed for selected fields including age, sex, dates of service, zip codes, and diagnosis and procedure codes. Sanity checks are also performed on additional data to check the distribution of categorical fields. In addition, several published studies report on the use of algorithms using MarketScan data (Katz et al. 2013; Zuckerman et al. 2007; Marsico et al. 2014). Evidence suggests that trends and other patterns in biomarker levels in the MarketScan population reflect trends in nationally representative data (Brookhart et al. 2014). Validation of clinical outcomes is rare in MarketScan data due to the very limited ability to link MarketScan Databases to clinical databases.

1.6   Governance and Ethical Issues

The MarketScan Databases, which are owned by IBM Watson Health, can be licensed for research purposes. The associated license fees depend on the number of data years and the number of data products requested. Fees are discounted for academic, non-profit, and federal government funded research. Requests can be initiated at the company website: https://www.ibm.com/watson-health.

The MarketScan Databases are fully compliant with the Health Insurance Portability and Accountability Act of 1996 (HIPAA). The MarketScan Databases meet the criteria for a limited-use dataset and contain none of the data elements prohibited by HIPAA for such datasets. In addition, IBM Watson Health periodically subjects the MarketScan Databases to review by an external independent consultant to verify that the databases are fully statistically de-identified with respect to HIPAA requirements. Although meeting these requirements is optional given the current MarketScan licensing process, this additional step demonstrates the IBM Watson Health commitment to HIPAA compliance and to protecting the confidentiality of patient-level and provider-level data. All patient-level and provider-level data within the MarketScan Research Databases contain synthetic identifiers to protect the privacy of individuals and data contributors. Any public reporting of Marketscan-derived information by geography must be reviewed and approved by IBM Watson Health; this requirement comes from the data contributors. With the release of the 2017 data, additional steps have been implemented to protect the anonymity of the data contributor pool. For example, geographic areas are now masked in certain circumstances where any one data source dominates the data pool (IBM MarketScan Research Databases 2018).

1.7 Documents and Publications

The MarketScan Databases have been used in over 2000 peer-reviewed articles published in leading journals since the first article by Hillman et al. was published in the New England Journal of Medicine in 1990 (Hillman et al. 1990; IBM Watson Health 2019b). Other highly cited papers include: (a) Hu et al. Burden of migraine in the United States—Disability and economic costs (1999); (b) Naccarelli et al. Increasing prevalence of atrial fibrillation and flutter in the United States (2009); (c) Peery et al. Burden of gastrointestinal disease in the United States (2012); and (d) Crystal-Peters et al. Treating allergic rhinitis in patients with comorbid asthma: the risk of asthma-related hospitalizations and emergency department visits (2002). Research with the MarketScan Databases has made substantial contributions to the scientific literature and formulation of evidence-based healthcare guidelines in the U.S.

1.8 Administrative Information

The IBM MarketScan Research Databases are maintained and funded by IBM Watson Health.

Contact Details

Organization/affiliation: IBM Corporation
  Route 100
  Somers, NY 10589, USA

Website: https://www.ibm.com/watson-health

2 Practical Experience with the Database

The MarketScan Databases are suitable for several different types of health services studies, including comparative effectiveness research; cost effectiveness and cost offset studies; pharmacoeconomic outcomes evaluations; burden of illness analyses; surgical and pharmaceutical treatment comparisons; forecasting and modeling; assessment of best practices and benchmarking against empirical norms or clinical practice guidelines; and clinical trial planning and support (Hansen 2019).

References

Asfaw A, Pana-Cryan R, Bushnell PT (2012) Incidence and costs of family member hospitalization following injuries of workers' compensation claimants. Am J Ind Med 55(11):1028–1036. https://doi.org/10.1002/ajim.22110

Brookhart MA, Sturmer T, Glynn RJ et al (2010) Confounding control in healthcare database research: challenges and potential approaches. Med Care 48(6 Suppl):S114–S120. https://doi.org/10.1097/MLR.0b013e3181dbebe3

Brookhart MA, Todd JV, Li X et al (2014) Estimation of biomarker distributions using laboratory data collected during routine delivery of medical care. Ann Epidemiol 24(10):754–761. https://doi.org/10.1016/j.annepidem.2014.07.013

Butler AM, Todd JV, Sahrmann JM et al (2019) Informative censoring by health plan disenrollment among commercially insured adults. Pharmacoepidemiol Drug Saf 28(5):640–648. https://doi.org/10.1002/pds.4750

Cortese MM, Dahl RM, Curns AT et al (2015) Protection against gastroenteritis in US households with children who received rotavirus vaccine. J Infect Dis 211(4):558–562. https://doi.org/10.1093/infdis/jiu503

Crystal-Peters J, Neslusan C, Crown WH et al (2002) Treating allergic rhinitis in patients with comorbid asthma: the risk of asthma-related hospitalizations and emergency department visits. J Allergy Clin Immunol 109(1):57–62. https://doi.org/10.1067/mai.2002.120554

Hansen L (2019) White Paper: IBM MarketScan research databases for life sciences researchers. https://www.ibm.com/downloads/cas/0NKLE57Y

Hillman BJ, Joseph CA, Mabry MR et al (1990) Frequency and costs of diagnostic imaging in office practice–a comparison of self-referring and radiologist-referring physicians. N Engl J Med 323(23):1604–1608. https://doi.org/10.1056/nejm199012063232306

Hu XH, Markson LE, Lipton RB et al (1999) Burden of migraine in the United States: disability and economic costs. Arch Intern Med 159(8):813–818. https://doi.org/10.1001/archinte.159.8.813

IBM MarketScan Research Databases (2018) IBM MarketScan research databases user guide. IBM Watson Health, Ann Arbor, MI

IBM Watson Health (2019a) IBM explorys electronic health record (EHR) database. https://www.ibm.com/downloads/cas/6VQK0DLL. Accessed 24 Feb 2020

IBM Watson Health (2019b) IBM MarketScan research databases abbreviated bibliography. https://www.ibm.com/downloads/cas/M5K9GPXE. Accessed 20 Feb 2020

Katz AJ, Ryan PB, Racoosin JA et al (2013) Assessment of case definitions for identifying acute liver injury in large observational databases. Drug Saf 36(8):651–661. https://doi.org/10.1007/s40264-013-0060-8

Marsico M, Mehta V, Chastek B et al (2014) Estimating the incidence and prevalence of juvenile-onset recurrent respiratory papillomatosis in publicly and privately insured claims databases in the United States. Sex Transm Dis 41(5):300–305. https://doi.org/10.1097/olq.0000000000000115

Naccarelli GV, Varker H, Lin J et al (2009) Increasing prevalence of atrial fibrillation and flutter in the United States. Am J Cardiol 104(11):1534–1539. https://doi.org/10.1016/j.amjcard.2009.07.022

Nickel KB, Wallace AE, Warren DK et al (2016) Modification of claims-based measures improves identification of comorbidities in non-elderly women undergoing mastectomy for breast cancer: a retrospective cohort study. BMC Health Serv Res 16(a):388. https://doi.org/10.1186/s12913-016-1636-7

Overman RA, Freburger JK, Assimon MM et al (2014) Observation stays in administrative claims databases: underestimation of hospitalized cases. Pharmacoepidemiol Drug Saf 23(9):902–910. https://doi.org/10.1002/pds.3647

Panozzo CA, Becker-Dreps S, Pate V et al (2013) Patterns of rotavirus vaccine uptake and use in privately-insured US infants, 2006–2010. PLoS ONE 8(9):e73825. https://doi.org/10.1371/journal.pone.0073825

Peery AF, Dellon ES, Lund J et al (2012) Burden of gastrointestinal disease in the United States: 2012 update. Gastroenterology 143(5):1179–1187.e1173. https://doi.org/10.1053/j.gastro.2012.08.002

The Henry J. Kaiser Family Foundation (2018) Health insurance coverage of the total population. http://kff.org/other/state-indicator/total-population/. Accessed 18 Feb 2020

Zuckerman IH, Sato M, Hsu VD et al (2007) Validation of a method for identifying nursing home admissions using administrative claims. BMC Health Serv Res 7:202. https://doi.org/10.1186/1472-6963-7-202

Databases in Asia and Australia

The Australian Pharmaceutical Benefits Scheme (PBS) Dispensing Database

Emily A. Karanges, Melisa J. Litchfield, Leigh Mellish,
and Sallie-Anne Pearson

Abstract The Australian Pharmaceutical Benefits Scheme (PBS) database is a routinely collected, whole-of-population collection comprising data on the dispensing of medicines listed on the PBS, the Australian Government's national drug subsidy program. The database was established for administrative and payment purposes but has been used for routine monitoring, surveillance, and research for many years.

1 Database Description

1.1 Introduction

The Australian Pharmaceutical Benefits Scheme (PBS) database is a routinely collected, whole-of-population collection comprising data on the dispensing of medicines listed on the PBS, the Australian Government's national drug subsidy program. The database was established for administrative and payment purposes but has been used for routine monitoring, surveillance, and research for many years.

1.2 Setting and Database Characteristics

Australia has a publically funded universal healthcare system entitling all Australian citizens and permanent residents to a range of subsidized health services. Medicines prescribed in the community and in private hospitals are subsidized under the Commonwealth's PBS, which supports the Australian general population, or the Repatriation Pharmaceutical Benefits Scheme (RPBS) for returned servicemen and

E. A. Karanges · M. J. Litchfield · L. Mellish · S.-A. Pearson (✉)
Medicines Policy Research Unit, UNSW, Sydney, NSW 2052, Australia
e-mail: sallie.pearson@unsw.edu.au

© Springer Nature Switzerland AG 2021
M. Sturkenboom and T. Schink (eds.), *Databases for Pharmacoepidemiological Research*, Springer Series on Epidemiology and Public Health,
https://doi.org/10.1007/978-3-030-51455-6_21

women and their dependents. The database, which extends back to the early 1990s, contains whole-of-population data for Australia's 25 million residents from every State and Territory (Australian Bureau of Statistics 2019). Persons enter the database at birth and are followed until death.

The level of PBS subsidy depends on the beneficiary status of the patient. Concessional patients, including pensioners, seniors, low-income earners, expatriates, and Indigenous Australians receiving treatment for chronic illness, have a low co-payment threshold (Department of Health 2019a). Eligible veterans and their dependents are also entitled to medicines at the concessional rate and receive additional pharmaceutical items at concessional prices under the RPBS. The level of RPBS entitlement depends on the type of Repatriation Health Card held[1] (Department of Veterans' Affairs 2019b). All other patients are considered general beneficiaries and have a higher co-payment threshold. In 2019, the patient co-payment was AUD\$40.30 for general beneficiaries and AUD\$6.50 for concessional beneficiaries (Department of Health 2019b). For medicines costing more than the relevant beneficiary co-payment (i.e., over co-payment), additional costs are paid by the Commonwealth. Low-cost PBS medicines falling under the general patient co-payment (under co-payment) are not subsidized, but paid in full by the patient. Currently all PBS-listed medicines are priced above the concessional beneficiary co-payment but may be priced above or below the general beneficiary co-payment.

Prescriptions dispensed to public hospital inpatients are not PBS-subsidized; hospitals are funded by individual States and Territories and are responsible for these costs. Since 2002 the Australian Government has established individual agreements with most Australian States and Territories, enabling participating hospitals to provide discharging patients and outpatients with PBS-subsidized medicines (Department of Health 2017). At the time of writing, the state of New South Wales and the Australian Capital Territory had not signed the agreements. All private hospital inpatients are entitled to PBS-subsidized medicines.

In Australia medicines can be PBS-listed for a specific indication after approval by Australia's regulator, the Therapeutic Goods Administration. The Pharmaceutical Benefits Advisory Committee (PBAC) assesses the medicine for subsidy on the basis of efficacy, safety, and cost-effectiveness. Approved medicines are listed on the scheme as unrestricted, restricted, or authority-only medicines. The latter two categories limit the use of the medicine to certain indications, conditions, patient groups, or quantities. Where a medicine is not PBS-listed or used for a different indication, the medicine is supplied by private prescription, unsubsidized by the PBS and funded entirely by a patient or private health insurer. Once a medicine has been PBS-listed, private health insurers will not subsidize the medicine for that indication.

---

[1]Repatriation Gold Card holders (ex-prisoners of war, World War I and II veterans and mariners, and their war widows/widowers) and Orange card holders (eligible British Commonwealth and allied veterans and mariners) have full RPBS entitlements; White Card holders (other veterans and mariners) receive RPBS benefits for the treatment of specific conditions.

1.3 Available Data

When a PBS/RPBS subsidized medicine is dispensed, the administering pharmacy or hospital provides the Australian Government Services Australia (SA) with information relating to the identity of the patient, prescription dispensed, prescriber, and supplying pharmacy. The database is continually updated as the records are processed by SA. Until recently, only medicines attracting a government subsidy (over co-payment medicines) were captured in the database. As of 1 April 2012, the database was expanded to capture all under co-payment dispensings in addition to PBS and RPBS subsidized dispensings (Department of Health 2019e). Other unsubsidized medicine use including over-the-counter purchases, private prescriptions, and the majority of dispensing to public hospital inpatients is not ascertained in the dataset.

The characteristics of the dispensed medicine are described in the database using the item's Anatomical Therapeutic Chemical (ATC) code and/or PBS item code. PBS item codes provide more detail at the product level, including generic name, form, strength, administration route, quantity per unit (pack size), and approved indication (also given via streamlined authority code[2]), where relevant.

Additional data available on the prescription includes date (of prescription by the clinician, supply by the pharmacy, and/or processing of the claim by SA), script type (original or repeat), cost (to patient, government, pharmacy, and overall), brand of medicine dispensed, script category (e.g., PBS, RPBS, under co-payment), and Regulation 49[3] and Regulation 25[4] status. The prescribed dose and duration of treatment does not form part of the dispensing record. Information on the indication for prescribing is limited. Some cautious inferences can be made using the PBS item code, streamlined authority code, or through access to a separate Authority Approvals database held by SA.

Available patient information includes patient category (including general beneficiary, concessional beneficiary, etc.), age (most often supplied as month and year of birth/death), sex, and location (based on State or postcode). However, individual characteristics, such as age and sex, were not reliably collected in the PBS dataset until May 2002, and no information is available on patient ethnicity. Patient location information such as statistical area can be mapped to indices of socio-economic disadvantage. Information is also available on the prescribing doctor (including specialty and location) and the dispensing pharmacy (location).

---

[2]Authority-only prescriptions require approval from SA before prescription of the medicine is permitted. Some of these authority-only prescriptions have 'streamlined' authorization, whereby provision of an authority code by the prescriber is sufficient for the medicine to be dispensed. This is in contrast to other authority-only medicines requiring telephone or written authorization from SA. Only streamlined authority codes are provided in the PBS database; telephone or written authorisation codes are stored in a separate authority approvals database.

[3]Indicates that all repeats are supplied at the same time (previously Regulation 24).

[4]Indicates 'immediate supply necessary' prescriptions, whereby additional or early repeat supply is permitted.

A comprehensive outline of the data collection is detailed elsewhere (Mellish et al. 2015). Table 1 is an extract from this paper describing the core variables available in the PBS collection.

Medicine use can be quantified in a variety of ways in the PBS dataset, including volume of prescriptions, dispensing episodes, or costs. The strength of the medicine and quantity supplied can also be used to calculate defined daily dose (DDD) per 1000 population per day, a widely used measure of utilization allowing for standardization of drug use across countries and different forms of the drug. The DDD metric, established by the WHO Collaborating Centre for Drug Statistics Methodology, is based on the estimated mean daily dose of the drug when used for its main indication in adults (WHO Collaborating Centre for Drug Statistics Methodology 2018).

There are also opportunities for person-level linkage between the PBS/RPBS database and other routine data collections, enabling exploration of the relationships between medicines exposure and a variety of outcomes. Person-level PBS/RPBS dispensing data has been linked with Commonwealth databases such as the Medicare Benefits Scheme (MBS) collection. This database contains whole-of-population information on subsidized health care services, including visits to health care practitioners (including general practitioners, specialists, limited allied health professionals), and diagnostic and therapeutic procedures (such as pathology tests and imaging). Diagnostic information is available where MBS item numbers are diagnosis specific. MBS data include services provided to outpatients and private inpatients; however, inpatient data for public patients admitted to public hospitals is not available.

The PBS/RPBS data collection has also been linked to datasets under the custodianship of the individual Australian States and Territories, including hospital separations, emergency department presentations, cancer notifications, perinatal data, and fact and cause of death data (Colvin et al. 2009; Pratt et al. 2011; Pearson and Schaffer 2014).

Family members can be linked within the database, as they appear on the same Medicare card. However, children listed on the card may include for example stepchildren and adopted children. Children may also be listed on multiple cards (e.g., birth mother's card and step-mother's card). The only way to ensure certainty as to the relationship between family members is through birth records held by the State. These would need to be linked to the PBS dataset, a process impeded by cross-jurisdictional issues.

Maximising the value of Australia's health data has had its challenges. The federated health system, where Commonwealth or State and Territory governments are responsible for specific aspects of care, means health data collections are under the custodianship of different agencies. To undertake comprehensive health system research, data must be linked at the person level (a linkage complicated by the lack of a common patient identifier) and across jurisdictional boundaries. While Australia has a number of approved integrating authorities responsible for undertaking these large-scale, population level linkages, the ethical and governance requirements for gaining approval to link and the limited capacity of the integrating authorities have meant significant delays in data access; sometimes up to five years from initial

Table 1 Core variables present in the PBS data collection

Variable	Definition
Medicine details	
ATC code	Internationally accepted, WHO-defined codes[a] that classify medicines over five levels, starting broadly with the anatomical site of action (e.g. nervous system) and ending specifically with the chemical substance (e.g. oxycodone) (WHO Collaborating Centre for Drug Statistics Methodology 2018)
PBS item code	Pharmaceutical Benefits Scheme defined codes that provide medicine details at the product level, including generic name, form, strength, administration route, quantity per unit (pack size), and approved indication, where applicable
Medicine section	Classification according to section of the PBS Schedule (Sect. 85 or 100)
Prescription details	
Date of prescription	Date on which the prescription was written
Date of supply	Date on which the medicine was supplied/dispensed by the pharmacy or hospital
Date of processing	Date on which the claim was processed by SA
Prescription type	Describes whether the prescription is an original, repeat, deferred supply, authority, etc.
Total cost	The gross price of the prescription, including the patient contribution plus the net benefit
Patient contribution	The amount paid by the patient for the prescription
Government contribution	The benefit paid to the pharmacy by the Australian Government
Prescription category	The program under which the prescription was dispensed (e.g. PBS, RPBS, under co-payment, etc.)
Regulation 49 status	Indicates that the original supply and all repeats were dispensed at once
Streamlined authority code	Indicates the physician-declared indication or reason for prescription for *Authority required (STREAMLINED)* medicines
Patient details	
Patient identifier	A unique, scrambled patient identifier provided by the Australian Government, allowing derivation of additional patient characteristics such as age (via date of birth), sex and geographical location
Patient category	The beneficiary status of the patient (e.g. concessional, general, safety net, doctors bag, under co-payment, closing the gap); determines how much the patient contributes to their medicine cost
Patient location	The location (e.g. state, statistical area) of the patient
Measures of utilisation	
Quantity	The quantity of medicine supplied to the patient

(continued)

Table 1 (continued)

Variable	Definition
Number of dispensings/scripts	The number of prescriptions dispensed (including original and repeat)
DDD/1000 pop/day	A measure of utilisation based around the WHO Defined Daily Dose (DDD), allowing for standardisation of use across different countries and drug formulations; provides a rough estimate of the proportion of the population treated daily with the medicine of interest (WHO Collaborating Centre for Drug Statistics Methodology 2018)
Prescriber information	
Prescriber identifier	A unique, scrambled number identifying the prescribing doctor
Prescriber specialty	Identifies the specialty of the prescribing doctor (e.g. general practitioner, psychiatrist etc.)
Prescriber location	The location (e.g. state, statistical area) of the prescribing doctor
Pharmacy information	
Pharmacy identifier	A unique, scrambled number identifying the dispensing pharmacy
Pharmacy location	The location (e.g. state) of the dispensing pharmacy

Availability to researchers depends on the data extract
From: The Australian Pharmaceutical Benefits Scheme data collection: A practical guide for researchers (Mellish et al. 2015)
ATC Anatomical Therapeutic Chemical; *DDD/1000 pop/day* Defined daily dose per 1000 population per day; *SA* Services Australia; *WHO* World Health Organisation
[a]ATC codes provided in the PBS dataset may occasionally differ from those determined by WHO

ethical approval to data provision. This situation has impacted significantly on the capacity to undertake timely pharmacoepidemiology research. Moreover, the traditional approaches to ethical approvals on a project-by-project basis are inefficient and have further impeded timely output that can translate directly into clinical and policy practice.

However, Australia's health data linkage landscape has changed dramatically in recent years. The May 2017 release of the Productivity Commission (the Australian Government's independent advisory body) report on 'Data Availability and Use' (Productivity Commission 2017) promoted sweeping reform to increase access to public sector data for use between different levels of government, the private and research sectors. Australia's Department of Prime Minister and Cabinet responded formally to the Productivity Commission Report endorsing the proposed reforms and pledging AUD$65 million over the next four years to reduce the historical impediments to use and re-use of public data, including changes to existing legislation (Department of Prime Minister and Cabinet 2018). In recent years, the Australian Institute of Health and Welfare has been working with the Commonwealth and State and Territory health authorities to develop enduring linked data assets. In December 2016, the Australian Health Ministers' Advisory Council approved the National

Data Linkage Demonstration Project (NDLDP), a proof-of-concept project to determine the value of linking data from Commonwealth and State health care agencies to inform health policy and in 2019 the National Integrated Health Services Information (NIHSI) Analysis Asset (AA) was created. The NIHSI AA contains de-identified data from FY2011 onwards on admitted patient care and emergency department services, MBS and PBS data, Residential Aged Care and National Deaths Index data. This dataset is now in use by Commonwealth and State agencies, but was not available to third parties such as researchers at the time of writing.

The Department of Veterans' Affairs (DVA) RPBS dataset deserves particular mention in the context of data linkage due to its relative freedom from cross-jurisdictional restraints. The DVA oversees total healthcare for approximately 210,000 eligible veterans and their dependents across Australia (Department of Veterans' Affairs 2019a), maintaining custodianship over a variety of routine data collections including RPBS dispensing claims, medical service claims, and hospitalizations. This arrangement provides ready linkage of health data within this population. As such, the majority of studies using PBS and RPBS data linked to other datasets have employed the veteran population via person-level data held by the DVA (Pearson et al. 2015). However, the DVA cohort is elderly (average age of 74) and diminishing (Department of Veterans' Affairs 2019a), making recent efforts to extend linkage between PBS claims and other collections across Australia of vital importance.

1.4 Strengths and Limitations

As a result of its universal healthcare arrangements, Australia is one of the few countries in the world to have access to a whole-of-population dispensing database. The PBS database contains records on Australia's 25 million citizens and all PBS and RPBS listed prescriptions, amounting to more than 200 million prescriptions each year (Department of Health 2018). In 2011, the database captured approximately 75% of prescribed medicine use in Australia (Department of Health 2012). The inclusion of under co-payment medicines in the collection since April 2012 has increased the capture of prescribed medicines; for example our recent study demonstrated the PBS collection captures approximately 90% of all opioids prescribed in the Australian community (Gisev et al. 2018). The database is also highly accurate due to its administrative purpose and real-time, automated collection of claims data by pharmacies (Parkinson et al. 2011). Indeed, electronic dispensing records are considered the gold standard of prescribed medicine data information compared with patient notes and self-reported information (West et al. 1994, 1995).

However, the PBS database has several limitations.

First, the PBS database does not capture use of over-the-counter medicines; unsubsidized prescriptions dispensed privately in the community; or inpatient prescriptions in public hospitals, which are covered by hospital budgets. However, prescriptions supplied to private hospital inpatients, public hospital outpatients and discharging inpatients are captured under the Public Hospital Pharmaceutical Reforms for partic-ipating hospitals in five States and one Territory of Australia (Department of Health 2012, 2015).

Second, as previously mentioned, dispensed prescriptions were not reliably attributed to individuals until 2002, hence individual-level analyses and aggregated studies based on individual characteristics such as age and sex are possible only for more recent data. Additionally, the utilization of under co-payment medicines was not captured in the dataset until 1 April 2012 (Department of Health 2019e), resulting in under-ascertainment of low cost (often older, off-patent) medicines prior to this date. These medicines were only captured for beneficiaries with lower co-payment thresholds, such as concessional beneficiaries and DVA clients. Due to this limita-tion, many previous studies have restricted their study populations to concessional beneficiaries and DVA clients, for whom complete ascertainment of medicine use was possible (Pearson et al. 2015).

Third, the PBS database also does not ascertain the indication for which the medicine was prescribed. As mentioned above, medicines categorized as restricted and authority-only are only PBS-approved for use in certain indications. While the PBS item code and streamlined authority code provide some indication of the likely reason for use, there is no guarantee that the clinician is providing the medicine for this purpose. Further, no information on indication is available for medicines on unrestricted benefits (for which no indication is specified for PBS listing).

Fourth, despite the prescribed dose of the medicine being written on all prescriptions, these data are not recorded in a PBS dispensing claim.

Researchers should also be aware of additional features of the dataset that may impact utilization estimates, such as seasonal variations in dispensing and changes in data capture over time. The following references discuss key analytical considerations (Mellish et al. 2015; Kemp et al. 2012).

1.5 Validation

The PBS database was designed for administrative rather than research purposes. While this feature ensures the accuracy of the data, there has been little validation of the database for use in pharmacoepidemiological research. Indeed, our recent system-atic review of Australian pharmacoepidemiological research based on PBS claims demonstrates that out of 228 studies using PBS or RPBS data between 1987 and 2013, only 14 could be classified as having a methodological or validation purpose (Pearson et al. 2015). Most of these methodological studies did not validate PBS dispensing claims directly, focusing instead on validation of prescribing indicators. However, there are a range of Australian validation studies assessing the capacity to ascertain specific diagnoses and procedures in hospital data collections (Stavrou et al. 2012; Robertson et al. 2014; Goldsbury et al. 2012; Powell et al. 2001). Clearly this is important for drug safety studies.

1.6   Governance and Ethical Issues

PBS/RPBS dispensing claims are processed by the Australian Government Services Australia (previously Department of Human Services, Medicare Australia and the Health Insurance Commission) and provided to the Department of Health (DoH) and the DVA (RPBS only) for monitoring, evaluation, and health service planning. Limited aggregated (de-identified) PBS and RPBS data are publically available online through SA Services Australia 2019) or DoH (Department of Health 2019c), while more detailed, customized reports in aggregated or unit record formats can be requested from SA, DoH, or Department of Veterans' Affairs (DVA; RPBS only) to address specific research questions. Data are provided on a cost recovery basis.

The PBS dataset is also available in combination with other data in aggregated or individualized formats. The Drug Utilization Sub-Committee (DUSC) of the PBAC was established in 1989 for the assessment of medicine use and costs and to assist in decisions regarding medicine subsidy (Department of Health 2012). Until recently, DUSC maintained a database that included both the PBS/RPBS dataset and estimates of non-subsidized under co-payment and private prescriptions ascertained from an ongoing Pharmacy Guild Survey of a representative sample of approximately 370 community pharmacies. This combined dataset had the advantage of providing more complete medicine capture than the PBS database alone. Limited aggregated DUSC data can be obtained via the yearly Australian Statistics on Medicines (ASM) reports (Department of Health 2019d), available online from 1997 to 2015 (and in print from 1991 to 1996). However, the combined database ceased to exist in August 2012 when the Pharmacy Guild Survey was terminated. Although data on under co-payment medicine use are still collected (in the PBS dataset from April 2012), there is currently no comprehensive source of data on the dispensing of private prescriptions in Australia. Data received for research purposes can be released without individual patient consent. As such, various ethical and privacy issues exist, and researchers must abide by the *Privacy Act 1988* and *Health Records and Information Privacy Act 2003* with regards to the use and disclosure of data under the custodianship of the Commonwealth and the various State acts if linking to their collections. Data are provided without identifiers such as name and address details. Individuals can be tracked in the data through scrambled personal identification numbers that are assigned on a project specific basis.

1.7   Documents and Publications

The PBS claims database has been of significant value from a research perspective over the last three decades. We have recently conducted a comprehensive review of all published literature using Australia's PBS dispensing records over a 25-year period, from 1987 to 2013, identifying 228 studies using PBS data (Pearson et al. 2015). All studies in the review accessed PBS data via a waiver of individual consent; the review did not include cohort studies where patients had consented to the linkage of PBS data. These studies explored a range of research questions, primarily concerning trends in drug utilization (33%) and clinician or patient practices around medicine use (26%), including co-prescribing, potential drug interactions, medicine switching or patient adherence. Drug use and outcomes (18%), evaluations of intervention impacts (17%), and methodological issues (6%) were also examined.

The database has been used widely in both aggregated and unit-level analyses and in linked and unlinked forms. Specifically, we identified 106 analyses solely based on PBS data, approximately half of which were claim-based and half individual-level analyses. The remaining 122 studies combined PBS data with additional health data, 63 of which linked person-level dispensing claims with other routine data collections such as hospitalizations, cause of death or medical service claims. However, cross-jurisdictional issues limiting linkage of dispensing data with other health data have meant that a limited number of drug safety studies have been conducted. Recent developments in data linkage bring the promise of increased research productivity in this field.

The PBS database therefore places Australia in a powerful position to conduct pharmacoepidemiological research into the quality use of medicines. Recent years have seen the growth and development of PBS-based pharmacoepidemiological research, with a movement from descriptive drug utilization studies using aggregated data to an increasing focus on patient and clinician behavior, outcomes and interventions through individual-level analyses. Recent changes in data capture, such as the inclusion of under co-payment data in the PBS dataset from 2012, have encouraged movement away from restricted patient populations, such as concessional cohorts or DVA clients. Similarly, investments in data linkage initiatives will likely expand research opportunities, providing the means to examine as-yet understudied populations (such as children, pregnant women), medicines (such as antineoplastic (cancer) therapies), and research questions (such as outcomes).

1.8   Administrative Information

Limited Pharmaceutical Benefits Schedule statistics are publically available online in aggregated format from:

http://www.pbs.gov.au/info/browse/statistics

Requests for PBS data can be placed by contacting the Australian Government Services Australia at: statistics@servicesaustralia.gov.au.

Further information about data access is available at: https://www.servicesaustralia.gov.au/organisations/about-us/statistical-information-and-data

For information about data linkage contact:

Data Integration Services Centre (DISC) Unit

Australian Institute of Health and Welfare (AIHW)

linkage@aihw.gov.au

Australian Bureau of Statistics (ABS) Statistical Data Integration

data.integration@abs.gov.au.

References

Australian Bureau of Statistics (2019) Australian Demographic Statistics (cat. no. 3101.0): estimated resident population. https://www.abs.gov.au/ausstats/abs%40.nsf/mf/3101.0. Accessed 28 Oct 2019

Colvin L, Slack-Smith L, Stanley FJ et al (2009) Pharmacovigilance in pregnancy using population-based linked datasets. Pharmacoepidemiol Drug Saf 18(3):211–225. https://doi.org/10.1002/pds.1705

Department of Health (2012) Australian statistics on medicines 2011. http://www.pbs.gov.au/info/statistics/asm/asm-2011. Accessed 28 Oct 2019

Department of Health (2015) PBS Chemotherapy medicines review. Review of chemotherapy funding arrangements. Appendix 1: Public Hospital Pharmaceutical Reforms. http://www.health.gov.au/internet/main/publishing.nsf/Content/chemotherapy-review/$File/appendix-i.pdf. Accessed 28 Oct 2019

Department of Health (2017) PBS pharmaceuticals in hospitals review: final report. http://www.pbs.gov.au/reviews/pbs-pharmaceuticals-in-hospitals-review-files/PBS-Pharmaceuticals-in-Hospitals-Review.pdf. Accessed 28 Oct 2019

Department of Health (2018) Expenditure and prescriptions twelve months to 30 June 2018. http://www.pbs.gov.au/info/statistics/expenditure-prescriptions/expenditure-prescriptions-twelve-months-to-30-June-2018. Accessed 28 Oct 2019

Department of Health (2019a) 4. Patient charges. http://www.pbs.gov.au/info/healthpro/explanatory-notes/section1/Section_1_4_Explanatory_Notes. Accessed 28. Oct 2019

Department of Health (2019b) About the PBS—Patient co-payments. http://www.pbs.gov.au/info/about-the-pbs. Accessed 28 Oct 2019

Department of Health (2019c) PBS and RPBS Section 85 date of supply data. http://www.pbs.gov.au/info/statistics/dos-and-dop/dos-and-dop. Accessed 28 Oct 2019

Department of Health (2019d) PBS statistics. http://www.pbs.gov.au/info/browse/statistics#ASM. Accessed 28 Oct 2019

Department of Health (2019e) Report on under co-payment prescriptions 2018–19. http://www.pbs.gov.au/info/statistics/under-co-payment/ucp-data-report. Accessed 28 Oct 2019

Department of Prime Minister and Cabinet (2018) The australian government's response to the productivity commission data availability and use inquiry. https://dataavailability.pmc.gov.au/sites/default/files/govt-response-pc-dau-inquiry.pdf. Accessed 28 Oct 2019

Department of Veterans' Affairs (2019a) Treatment population statistics—quarterly report March 2019. https://www.dva.gov.au/sites/default/files/publications/datastatistical/treatmentpop/TPopMar2019.pdf. Accessed 28 Oct 2019

Department of Veterans' Affairs (2019b) Veterans' health cards. https://www.dva.gov.au/health-and-wellbeing/veterans-health-cards. Accessed 28 Oct 2019

Gisev N, Pearson SA, Karanges EA et al (2018) To what extent do data from pharmaceutical claims under-estimate opioid analgesic utilisation in Australia? Pharmacoepidemiol Drug Saf 27(5):550–555. https://doi.org/10.1002/pds.4329

Goldsbury DE, Armstrong K, Simonella L et al (2012) Using administrative health data to describe colorectal and lung cancer care in New South Wales, Australia: a validation study. BMC Health Serv Res 12:387. https://doi.org/10.1186/1472-6963-12-387

Kemp A, Paige E, Banks E (2012) Beginner's guide to using Pharmaceutical Benefits Scheme data. https://www.alswh.org.au/images/content/pdf/InfoData/linked-data/Guide_to_Using_PBS_Data_20131125.pdf. Accessed 28 Oct 2019

Mellish L, Karanges EA, Litchfield MJ et al (2015) The Australian Pharmaceutical Benefits Scheme data collection: a practical guide for researchers. BMC Res Notes 8:634. https://doi.org/10.1186/s13104-015-1616-8

Parkinson B, van Gool K, Kenny P (2011) Medicare Australia data for research: an introduction. University of Technology, Sydney. https://www.uts.edu.au/sites/default/files/2019-04/crest-factsheet-medicare-australia.pdf. Accessed 28 Oct 2019

Pearson SA, Pesa N, Langton JM et al (2015) Studies using Australia's Pharmaceutical Benefits Scheme data for pharmacoepidemiological research: a systematic review of the published literature (1987–2013). Pharmacoepidemiol Drug Saf 24(5):447–455. https://doi.org/10.1002/pds.3756

Pearson SA, Schaffer A (2014) The use and impact of cancer medicines in routine clinical care: methods and observations in a cohort of elderly Australians. BMJ Open 4(5):e004099. https://doi.org/10.1136/bmjopen-2013-004099

Powell H, Lim LL, Heller RF (2001) Accuracy of administrative data to assess comorbidity in patients with heart disease. An Australian perspective. J Clin Epidemiol 54(7):687–693. https://doi.org/10.1016/s0895-4356(00)00364-4

Pratt N, Roughead EE, Ramsay E et al (2011) Risk of hospitalization for hip fracture and pneumonia associated with antipsychotic prescribing in the elderly: a self-controlled case-series analysis in an Australian health care claims database. Drug Saf 34(7):567–575. https://doi.org/10.2165/11588470-000000000-00000

Productivity Commission (2017) Data availability and use: overview & recommendations. Report No. 82. Canberra

Robertson J, Pearson SA, Attia JR (2014) How well do NSW hospital data identify cases of heart failure? Med J Aust 200(1):25. https://doi.org/10.5694/mja13.10207

Services Australia (2019) Pharmaceutical benefits schedule statistics. https://www.servicesaustralia.gov.au/organisations/about-us/statistical-information-and-data/medicare-statistics/pharmaceutical-benefits-schedule-statistics?utm_id=9. Accessed 28 Oct 2019

Stavrou E, Pesa N, Pearson SA (2012) Hospital discharge diagnostic and procedure codes for upper gastro-intestinal cancer: how accurate are they? BMC Health Serv Res 12:331. https://doi.org/10.1186/1472-6963-12-331

West SL, Savitz DA, Koch G et al (1995) Recall accuracy for prescription medications: self-report compared with database information. Am J Epidemiol 142(10):1103–1112. https://doi.org/10.1093/oxfordjournals.aje.a117563

West SL, Strom BL, Freundlich B et al (1994) Completeness of prescription recording in outpatient medical records from a health maintenance organization. J Clin Epidemiol 47(2):165–171. https://doi.org/10.1016/0895-4356(94)90021-3

WHO Collaborating Centre for Drug Statistics Methodology (2018) Guidelines for ATC classification and DDD assignment 2019. Oslo

Japan—National Insurance Claims Database (NDB)

Daisuke Sato and Kazuhiko Ohe

Abstract The Japanese National Insurance Claims Database (NDB) is an administrative database based on claims data from Medical Insurance Claims and Specific Health Checkups and Guidance.

1 Database Description

1.1 Introduction

The Japanese National Insurance Claims Database (NDB) is an administrative database based on claims data from Medical Insurance Claims and Specific Health Checkups and Guidance.

The government enacted the Act on Assurance of Medical Care for Elderly People during the health care reform in 2008. In 2006, the Ministry of Health, Labour and Welfare (MHLW) has commenced discussions on a framework for the optimization of the healthcare expenses, which aims to evaluate the structure of the increase in healthcare expenditure (Health Insurance Bureau 2019).

The NDB was developed as a tool for investigation and analysis by MHLW in the context of the Health care reform. In addition, the NDB is used for the development of academic research in order to contribute to the implementation and evaluation of healthcare policy management.

D. Sato
Center for Next Generation of Community Health, Chiba University Hospital, Chiba University,
1-8-1 Inohana, Chuo-ku, Chiba-shi, Chiba 260-8677, Japan

K. Ohe (✉)
Department of Planning, Information and Management, The University of Tokyo Hospital, 7-3-1
Hongo, Bunkyo, Tokyo 113-8655, Japan
e-mail: kohe@hcc.h.u-tokyo.ac.jp

© Springer Nature Switzerland AG 2021
M. Sturkenboom and T. Schink (eds.), *Databases for Pharmacoepidemiological Research*, Springer Series on Epidemiology and Public Health,
https://doi.org/10.1007/978-3-030-51455-6_22

1.2 Database Characteristics

1.2.1 Sources of Data

Data contained in the NDB come from two different sources; firstly, data from all the data of Medical Insurance Claims across the country is collected on a monthly basis and secondly, data from Specific Health Checkups and Guidance (SHCG) conducted by health insurers is collected on a yearly basis. The claims data are subject to anonymous treatment by the agencies such as Health Insurance Claims Review and Reimbursement Services (HICRRS), etc., and SHCG data are subject to anonymous treatment by the insurers.

NDB data are characterized by nation-wide completeness. This means that the MHLW has collected insurance claim data of medical and dental treatments from all the medical institutions and pharmacies in Japan. Therefore the database covers nation-wide reimbursement information such as inpatient and outpatient data, prescriptions as well as SHCG data.

1.2.2 Description of Database Population

Claims data of the NDB include only the insured medical treatment data. There are uncovered treatments such as preventive treatment, cosmetic treatment, and childbirth (normal delivery).

The cumulative number of Medical Insurance Claims registered between April 2009 and January 2018 is 15.3 billion. The cumulative number of SHCG registered between the fiscal years 2009 and 2018 is 255 million. Although the NDB covers almost all medical insurance claims in Japan, as described in the next section, it covers SHCG data only from people who get the checkups at their own initiative between 40 and 74 years of age, because only this age-group is targeted by the SHGG initiative. The checkup rate among people between 40 and 74 years old is about 50%.

1.2.3 Start of Data Collection

Since 2006 the MHLW has been promoting the conversion to electronic storage of medical insurance claims, which allows medical insurance institutions to submit their claims data online and through electronic media. They have stored NDB data since the fiscal year 2009. The coverage rate of medical institutions differs from year to year because of the progress of acceptance by medical institutions. In April 2015, there were about 92 million pieces of claims data; electronic coverage reached 98.1% in total, 99.9% in medical institutions, 97.4% in medical clinics, 93.5% in dental institutions, and 99.9% in pharmacies.

Essentially, the NDB has collected the data of medical institutions in all periods and from each insurance practice. The claims data in the NDB is updated monthly with a lag time of about two months. SHCG data are updated yearly with a lag time of about one year (updated every February).

1.3 Available Data

NDB data include demographic information for patients, such as "age group", sex, insurer ID (anonymized), institution's secondary medical areas code (SMAs), and outcome ("death" or "survival").

Diagnoses (both inpatient and outpatient) are coded according to the ICD-10. In particular, in acute care, hospitals register several diagnoses distinguishing the main diagnosis from comorbidity and complications using the Japan Diagnosis Procedure Combination Code (DPC) (Sumitani et al. 2014).

The prescription claims information describes pharmaceutical names, prescription date, total dose, and number of days. NDB has prescription claims data from both outpatient and inpatient settings. They don't include data from non-reimbursable and OTC Medicines, but pharmacies on dispensed medicines.

Inpatient information on medical procedures includes date of admission, length of stay, type of medical treatment (examination, treatment, operation, surgery, medication, etc.), and the charge. Outpatient information on medical procedures includes date of visit, number of visits, type of treatment (examination, treatment, operation, surgery, medication, etc.), and payment. The coding of treatments and surgeries follow Japan's local procedure and surgical coding, which was specifically developed for insurance claiming.

The laboratory data include Japan's local codes for claiming of tests and the volume of tests executed. They do not include the result of laboratory tests. While on the other hand, the data of SHCG include date of visit, determination score (normal/abnormal), outcome scores of health guidance, and results of laboratory tests (HbA1c, LDL, HDL, etc.).

SHCG physical examination data include the results of blood pressure, body mass index (BMI), and abdominal circumference measurements.

Lifestyle information collected from an SHCG health interview sheet includes family history and lifestyle information (smoking, alcohol, exercise).

There is no data on the socioeconomic status, such as income and education level.

The NDB cannot be linked to other databases, because the data are anonymized. It is only permitted to link between claims data and SHCG data within the NDB. Family members can also not be linked.

It is not possible to access patient records for case validation or to contact patients to collect bio-samples.

1.4 Strengths and Limitations

A major strength of the NDB is its exhaustiveness or completeness of insurance claims. The NDB collects data from all insured people nationwide and covers 98.1% of the medical institutions in Japan. The insured medical treatment was based on medical practice determined by the Central Social Insurance Medical Council. It could be claimed for medical treatment in accordance with criteria for institutional structure or patients' comorbidity.

In the Japanese healthcare delivery system, insured people may visit any hospital or clinic at any time. Therefore, the NDB has claims information with the cross-medical institutions nationwide. Those data are consistent and can be used to follow patients receiving long-term care across institutions.

The NDB has several limitations. Firstly, the NDB data has no unique individual identification numbers directly derived from an individual ID such as the Social Security Number. Therefore, each individual record in the NDB only has a "hashed-value" generated from the combination of patient's name, sex, date of birth, insurer's ID, and insured number with the aim of protecting personal identification information. Theoretically hashed-value has the following characteristics.

1. It is generated as a fixed-length pseudorandom number from the source data.
2. It is extremely difficult to generate the same hash ID from different data.
3. It is impossible to reproduce the original data from a hash ID.

In the NDB, all the records have two kinds of hashed-values: the Hash-1 is generated from the combination of insurer's ID, insurer-dependent insured number, date of birth, and sex. The Hash-2 is generated from the combination of patient's full name, date of birth, and sex.

Secondly, claims do not contain exact dates, e.g., of procedures. Data is summarized as monthly information, because insurance claims are reimbursed on a monthly basis. For example, we do not know if a procedure took place before surgery or after surgery within one month.

1.5 Validation

Internal validity in claims data is verified by matching the Hash-1 and the Hash-2. Consequently, there is a possibility of mismatch because of changing owing to fluctuation of data, for example, the family name or the insurer. The rate of matching between the Hash-1 and Hash-2 is indicated to be less than 1%. The matching technique is referred to in Kubo S, Noda T, Imamura T, et al. National Database of Health Insurance Claims and Specific Health Checkups of Japan (NDB): Outline and Patient-Matching Technique. External validity is verified by comparing national health expenditures with the NDB. The component ratio of national health expenditures similarly supported the above trend, and the result of comparison with medical expenditure by diagnosis was similar.

1.6   Governance and Ethical Issues

1.6.1   Governance Structure

The owner of the NDB is the MHLW, Government of Japan. If a researcher wants to use NDB data, he or she must apply to the Expert Meeting on Provision of Medical Insurance Claims (Expert Committee) to examine the propriety of the application with applicant information, research plan, extracting item, data management, etc.
    The principal criteria are as follows.

1. The purpose of use is the development of academic research in order to contribute to the implementation and evaluation of healthcare policy management.
2. Extracting NDB data is a minimum requirement for the research. Personal information is not identified.
3. The place where NDB data will be used is a domestic area in Japan.
4. Data and the computer system shall not be connected to an external network system such as the Internet.
5. Ownership shall not be transferred to others, and information shall not be exchanged.

After examination by the Expert Committee, the MHLW submits the result to the Minister of Health, Labour and Welfare. Finally, the Minister of Health, Labour and Welfare presents a judgment on the application.

1.6.2   Ability to Share or Release Data

The MHLW provides a NDB sampling dataset, avoiding the possibility of identifying personal information. This sampling database is composed of inpatient, outpatient, Diagnosis Procedure Combination Code/Per-Diem Payment System (DPC/PDPS), and pharmacy data within a single month. The dataset is extracted from 10 and 1% of the inpatient and outpatient data, respectively. To avoid the possibility of personal identification, rare disease codes are left unidentified. Moreover, insurer and region information are deleted.
    Since April 2015, the MHLW has established an On-site Research Center where researchers having experience with the NDB data are available. The MHLW used to provide the extracted data according to proposals from each researcher. Now, the researchers can directly access the predetermined database in the On-site Research Center. The researchers can use their data files through examining the results of user analysis or extraction by Expert Committee.
    Clarifying the management responsibility, they limited data copying to only once. If a researcher used their data on multiple computers, they would have to offer the data on every computer.

The criteria of the release of study results are defined as follows by the Expert Committee.

1. The unit of patient summary may not be less than 10 patients in an SMA or a prefecture.
2. The unit of area summary may not be less than 100 patients in a municipality.
3. If it a specific institution or insurer is identified, the unit may not be less than 2.
4. The offer must specify publication in the application and submit to inspection by the Expert Committee.

1.6.3 Methods for De-Identification

The NDB does not use any personally traceable ID. The NDB uses a "hash ID" generated by patient name, sex, date of birth, and insurer number with the aim of protecting personal identifying information. The source data of the hash ID is deleted in the NDB.

Five-year age-groups are developed; those 100 years old or older are classified into one group. The region groups classify medical administration area or municipality. Cross-tabulation by the insurer in principle is not allowed (except through permission of the insurer).

Personal Identifying information such as post code, address, name and telephone number of insurers, name of doctor, insured ID, and visitor's name are eliminated from the SHCG database.

1.6.4 Ethics Committee

The NDB does not include personal identifying information. However, NDB data are subject to examination research ethics and ethical guidelines for epidemiological research. The NDB user policy stipulates data on management, terms of use, access control, period of use, data handling, release of results, Information Security Management System (ISMS), and measures against illegal use. The NDB Management Rules stipulate user access, security, written oaths, and operations.

1.7 Administrative Information

The NDB is maintained by the MHLW and funded by own resources.

Contact Details
Organization/affiliation: Office of Insurance System Advancement Promotion
   Division for Health Care and Long-term Care Integration,
   Health Insurance Bureau,
   Ministry of Health, Labour and Welfare (MHLW), Government of Japan

Administrative contact:
  email suisin@mhlw.go.jp
  Phone 03-5253-1111

Website: https://www.mhlw.go.jp/english/policy/health-medical/health-insurance/
index.html.

2   Practical Experience with the Database

2.1   Epidemiology of Psoriasis and Palmoplantar Pustulosis: A Nationwide Study Using the Japanese National Claims Database

This research indicated the national prevalence of psoriasis and palmoplantar pustu-
losis (PPP) in Japan. They determined whether psoriasis and PPP disease activity
varies by season and whether disease severity is associated with concurrent diabetes
mellitus, hyperlipidemia, and hypertension.

The limitation of this study is that psoriasis and PPP diagnosis codes have not
been validated. Therefore, the true national prevalence may be higher or lower than
that reported here. One concern is disease misclassification.

2.2   The Effectiveness of Risk Communication Regarding Drug Safety Information: A Nationwide Survey by the Japanese Public Health Insurance Claims Data

Although risk communication from the regulatory agencies and pharmaceutical
companies is very important for the proper use of approved medications, there is little
evaluative research of safety measures in Japan except our previous paper (Hanatani
et al. 2014) analyzing the hospital information database.

This study objectively evaluated the effectiveness of risk communication of
pharmaceuticals and medical devices safety information (PMDSI) directed safety
measures using the NDB.

The implementation rate of the hepatitis virus-monitoring test increased from
14% before to 18% after the warning letter announcement in March 2010 in all
methotrexate (MTX)-administered patients with rheumatoid arthritis (RA).

This research suggested that the installation of a drug information management
room (DIMR) is one of the important factors affecting risk communication.

Limitation of this study is that the NDB did not have the exact date for medical care and pharmaceutical dispensing because the claims data contain only monthly data, not daily data. Therefore, they could not determine the order of virus examination and MTX dispensing in the same month.

2.3 Regional Variations in In-Hospital Mortality, Care Processes, and Spending in Acute Ischemic Stroke Patients in Japan

This study investigated the regional variations and associations among eight outcomes and processes of care measures in each Secondary Medical Area (SMA).

The regional variations among SMAs in in-hospital mortality, spending, and tPA utilization were 3.2-, 1.7-, and 5.9-fold, respectively. Higher physician supply was significantly associated with lower in-hospital mortality and higher spending. Additionally, spending had a significantly negative correlation with regional continuity of care planning rate but a significantly positive correlation with rehabilitation rate.

This study had three limitations. Firstly, as with any analysis based on claims data, some important clinical information was not available.

Secondly, conclusion of the study concerning the associations between the physicians' workforce and the targeted measures may not be generalizable to all of Japan because this study area only included 8 of the 47 prefectures.

Thirdly, the only mortality measure that was feasible for this study approach was in-hospital mortality.

References

Hanatani T, Sai K, Tohkin M et al (2014) Evaluation of two Japanese regulatory actions using medical information databases: a 'Dear Doctor' letter to restrict Oseltamivir use in teenagers, and label change caution against co-administration of omeprazole with clopidogrel. J Clin Pharm Ther 39(4):361–367. https://doi.org/10.1111/jcpt.12153

Health Insurance Bureau. Ministry of Health Labour and Welfare (MHLW). Government of Japan (2019) An outline of the Japanese medical system. https://www.mhlw.go.jp/bunya/iryouhoken/iryouhoken01/dl/01_eng.pdf. Accessed 17 Jan 2020

Sumitani M, Yasunaga H, Uchida K et al (2014) Perioperative factors affecting the occurrence of acute complex regional pain syndrome following limb bone fracture surgery: data from the Japanese Diagnosis Procedure Combination database. Rheumatology (Oxford) 53(7):1186–1193. https://doi.org/10.1093/rheumatology/ket431

Population-Based Electronic Health Data Environment in Taiwan

K. Arnold Chan

Abstract The National Health Insurance (NHI) program in Taiwan was launched in 1995 and coverage is comprehensive and compulsory for all citizens. Since the late 1990s, NHI data has been utilized for clinical and public health research. Subsequently, additional data have become linkable to the NHI data for research purposes. This chapter describes the current status of the research environment with population-based electronic health data in Taiwan. The focus is on public domain research carried out by academic and research institutions with funding from public agencies or the private sector.

1 Database description

1.1 Introduction

The National Health Insurance (NHI) program in Taiwan was launched in 1995 and coverage is comprehensive and compulsory for all citizens. Since the late 1990s, NHI data has been utilized for clinical and public health research. Subsequently, additional data have become linkable to the NHI data for research purposes. This chapter describes the current status of the research environment with population-based electronic health data in Taiwan. The focus is on public domain research carried out by academic and research institutions with funding from public agencies or the private sector.

K. Arnold Chan (✉)
National Taiwan University Health Data Research Centre, 33 Linsen South Road, Room 526,
Taipei, Taiwan
e-mail: kachan@ntu.edu.tw

© Springer Nature Switzerland AG 2021
M. Sturkenboom and T. Schink (eds.), *Databases for Pharmacoepidemiological Research*, Springer Series on Epidemiology and Public Health,
https://doi.org/10.1007/978-3-030-51455-6_23

1.2 Database Characteristics

Four main data sources are available for epidemiology and health services research, and they are linkable through the unique national identification number for each Taiwan resident.

National Health Insurance

The NHI covers more than 99% of Taiwan residents and is administered by a government agency. Insurance coverage includes medical services (outpatient, emergency, and inpatient), pharmacy, dentistry, and eye care. Some traditional medicine services are also covered. It is population-based and coverage for infants initiates at birth. The only reasons for coverage termination are emigration to another country (less than 1% per year) or death. The Taiwan NHI started in 1995, and most investigators have been utilizing data since the late 1990s. Data are updated annually and available about 15 months after the end of the year.

Mortality statistics

Date of death and cause of death are available through vital statistics in Taiwan.

Cancer registry

The cancer registry in Taiwan started in 1979, and registry data are available for research. All cancer cases diagnosed in a hospital with 50 or more beds must be reported. In addition, data on the 15 most common cancers in Taiwan have more detailed information on treatment. Lag time before data become linkable to the other health data is about three years.

National Immunization Information System

Publicly funded and mandatory vaccinations for infants born after 1995 are recorded by the Taiwan Centers for Disease Control in this system, which include type(s) and date(s) of vaccines administered. Non-publicly funded vaccinations are also voluntarily reported by some health care providers to the same system.

1.3 Available Data

Sex and date of birth are available in the source data and are used to calculate age at specific events. More than 95% of the NHI population is ethnic Han Chinese, and the rest are aborigines (about 2.3%), non-Han Chinese spouses, and non-Han Chinese guest workers. No ethnicity data is available in NHI. The total number of citizens and non-citizens in the NHI data was approximately 24 million as of the end of 2018.

Diagnoses associated with medical services (outpatient, emergency, and inpatient) have been recorded as ICD-9 codes through the end of 2015 and as ICD-10 codes since January 1, 2016. A wide range of *medications*, including those available over-the-counter in some countries (such as low dose aspirin and certain non-steroidal anti-inflammatory drugs), are reimbursed and drug dispensing is captured in the database. A unique code is assigned to each drug formulation and dose entity, including separate codes for each generic version. The dispensing records include the amount of drug units dispensed, which, along with the dose, can be used to infer duration of drug use. Detailed drug use information during hospitalizations is also available. The World Health Organization Anatomical Therapeutic Chemical Classification System is commonly used in Taiwan, and drug libraries have been developed by research groups. Use of drugs that are not reimbursed is not captured in the database. Unique codes are assigned to surgical *procedures and examinations* (including pathology, radiology, endoscopy, laboratory, and others) for billing purposes.

Like most other health insurance claims databases in the world, no laboratory or examination results are available in NHI. Information on smoking, dietary patterns, alcohol consumption, height, and weight is also not available. Pregnancy can be inferred through codes for pre-natal examinations.

The *type* (clinics, community-based hospitals, medical centers) and *location* (within each of six regions in Taiwan defined by the insurance agency) of the medical care providers are available and have been utilized for health services research. Income levels (in strata) and broad occupation categories have been used as proxies for *socioeconomic indicators.*

Within the NHI data, a project linking mothers and newborn infants has been completed and a mother-infant(s) database is available for research. Disease-specific datasets, including that of female breast cancer, prostate cancer, hypertension, diabetes, systemic lupus erythematosus, and others have also been developed. Cohort or disease registry data can be linked with data described above. The current regulation does not yet allow obtaining written medical records from medical care providers to confirm medical events of interest or contacting individuals to administer questionnaires or obtain biological specimen.

1.4 Strengths and Limitations

The major strength of the Taiwanese electronic health data environment is the population-based nature of the NHI system. For almost the entirety of the adult population in Taiwan, almost 20 years of longitudinal health insurance claims data are available. The single payer ensures complete capture of all relevant medical events that resulted in insurance claims. For virtually all newborns after 1998 all reimbursed clinical events are captured in the NHI. Financial barriers in terms of co-payment are kept at a moderate level. Therefore, medical services and pharmaceutical coverage are available across the whole socioeconomic spectrum for Taiwan

citizens. To date, this is the largest population-based electronic health data environment for a majority Han Chinese population. In addition, patient cohorts identified
from electronic medical records systems in medical centers can be linked with the
population-based NHI and other data, resulting in cohorts with rich and relevant
clinical information and long-term follow-up.

There are three major limitations. The first is the lack of an approved process
to review medical records of those who may have experienced a medical event of
interest. So far, there is no explicit guideline on whether waiving the requirement for
individual authorization before review of full text medical records is acceptable to
the Ministry of Health and Welfare and the medical care institutions. The second is
out-of-pocket payment for certain expensive medical devices and drugs. Utilization
records of these devices or drugs are not captured in NHI. The third is the lag time
between the worldwide introduction of new drugs and devices and the availability of
those products in Taiwan. As Taiwan is not a major market, new drugs and devices
are not necessarily registered in Taiwan immediately after approval in North America
or Western Europe, and the delay may be more than one year.

1.5 Validation

The NHI data available for research has been 'cleaned,' but the detailed algorithm
and error rates with the raw claims data are not made public. Individual investigators routinely conduct additional 'cleaning' to delete apparently inconsistent data.
Investigators have conducted studies on individual disease entities, but there has been
no system level effort to conduct independent validation for research purposes. The
insurance agency does conduct routine audits to prevent fraudulent claims.

1.6 Governance and Ethical Issues

The Taiwan government owns all data described in this chapter and has invested
public funding to develop the data infrastructure. Access to the data can be granted
through the Department of Statistics, Ministry of Health and Welfare.

1.6.1 Department of Statistics, Ministry of Health and Welfare

A repository of health data has been established at the Health and Welfare Data
Science Center, Department of Statistics. In addition to the NHI, cancer registry,
vaccinations and mortality data, data from population-based surveys are available
and linkable. Access to the full datasets is available at the 'clean rooms' at 11 sites
across Taiwan, where investigators and analysts work with dedicated computers that
are not connected to the internet. The computing area is closely monitored and no

cell phones or other electronic equipment are allowed. Analytic results are reviewed by Center staff before their release to the investigators. Analytic results must be consistent with objectives specified in the protocol, and cell counts of two or smaller in a table are not allowed. Investigators need to prepare a study protocol, obtain research ethics approval at their home institution, and have a budget for the data and processing fees. The principle investigator must be Taiwan-based and affiliated with an academic or research institution in Taiwan.

1.6.2 National Health Research Institute (NHRI)

The NHRI is a non-profit research organization established by the Taiwan government. Historically de-identified datasets derived from the NHI were made available through the NHRI for research, but there was no linkage capability with other health data at the NHRI. Three datasets labeled as LHID2000, LHID2005, and LHID2010, each comprising health insurance claims data for a representative sample of one million NHI enrollees in 2000, 2005, and 2010, respectively, were developed. These datasets were provided on electronic media at nominal costs and could be analyzed on investigators' computers within Taiwan. Per government policy, the NHRI has stopped providing the one million subject datasets on November 30, 2015.

1.7 Documents and Publications

Detailed descriptions of data elements and data files are available in Chinese at the website of the Health and Welfare Data Science Center (Ministry of Health and Welfare 2020). Some university-based research centers have prepared documents in English in order to promote collaboration with international colleagues. For example, additional information is available at the website of the National Taiwan University Health Data Research Center (2020). Since the late 1990s, NHI data has been used extensively for clinical and public health research. Selected peer-reviewed articles of original investigations in recent years are those of Chang et al. (2012), Wu et al. (2012), Yang et al. (2015), and Lee et al. (2019).

An editorial of Hsing and Ioannidis in a major medical journal reviewed the strengths and limitations of this data environment (2015). A review by Hsieh et al. described the NHI (2019).

1.8 Administrative Information

The Department of Statistics, Ministry of Health and Welfare is responsible for maintaining the electronic health data environment for public health and clinical research. International investigators interested in collaboration may contact one of the university-based research centers. The data environment is open for all qualified investigators in Taiwan, and no center has exclusive access.

Contact Details

Organization: National Taiwan University Health Data Research Center*
　　33 Linsen South Road, Room 526
　　Taipei, Taiwan

Administrative contact
　　Email: ntuhdrc@ntu.edu.tw
　　Telephone 886 2 3366 8688

Scientific contact: K. Arnold Chan, MD, ScD, FISPE
　　Email: kachan@ntu.edu.tw
　　Telephone: 886 2 3366 8688
　　Website http://hdrc.ntu.edu.tw
　　*One of several research centers with experience in international collaboration

References

Chang CH, Lin JW, Wu LC et al (2012) Association of thiazolidinediones with liver cancer and colorectal cancer in type 2 diabetes mellitus. Hepatology 55(5):1462–1472. https://doi.org/10.1002/hep.25509

Hsieh CY, Su CC, Shao SC et al (2019) Taiwan's National Health Insurance Research Database: past and future. Clin Epidemiol 11:349–358. https://doi.org/10.2147/clep.s196293

Hsing AW, Ioannidis JP (2015) Nationwide population science: lessons from the Taiwan National Health Insurance research database. JAMA Intern Med 175(9):1527–1529. https://doi.org/10.1001/jamainternmed.2015.3540

Lee TY, Hsu YC, Tseng HC et al (2019) Association of daily aspirin therapy with risk of hepatocellular carcinoma in patients with chronic hepatitis B. JAMA Intern Med 179(5):633–640. https://doi.org/10.1001/jamainternmed.2018.8342

Ministry of Health and Welfare (2020) https://dep.mohw.gov.tw/DOS/np-2497-113.html. Accessed 20 Jan 2020

National Taiwan University Health Data Research Center (2020) Real World Evidence. https://hdrc.ntu.edu.tw/. Accessed 20 Jan 2020

Wu CY, Chen YJ, Ho HJ et al (2012) Association between nucleoside analogues and risk of hepatitis B virus-related hepatocellular carcinoma recurrence following liver resection. JAMA 308(18):1906–1914. https://doi.org/10.1001/2012.jama.11975

Yang CY, Chen CH, Deng ST et al (2015) Allopurinol use and risk of fatal hypersensitivity reactions: a nationwide population-based study in Taiwan. JAMA Intern Med 175(9):1550–1557. https://doi.org/10.1001/jamainternmed.2015.3536

Printed in the United States
by Baker & Taylor Publisher Services

Printed in the United States
by Baker & Taylor Publisher Services